WHAT'S NORMAL?

§

Literature and Medicine
MARTIN KOHN AND CAROL DONLEY, EDITORS

What's Normal?

❧

Narratives of
Mental & Emotional
Disorders

❧

Edited by

Carol Donley &

Sheryl Buckley

❧

The Kent State

University Press

KENT, OHIO, &

LONDON

❧

© 2000 by The Kent State University Press, Kent, Ohio 44242
ALL RIGHTS RESERVED
Library of Congress Catalog Card Number 99-048190
ISBN 0-87338-653-1
Manufactured in the United States of America

06 05 04 03 02 01 00   5 4 3 2 1

Due to the length of the permissions acknowledgments,
a continuation of the copyright page appears following the text.

Library of Congress Cataloging-in-Publication Data
What's Normal? narratives of mental and emotional disorders / edited by
Carol Donley and Sheryl Buckley.
    p.   cm. — (Literature and medicine ; 3)
Includes index.
ISBN 0-87338-653-1 (paper : alk. paper) ∞
1. Mental illness—Literary collections. 2. Emotional problems—Literary collections.
3. Mentally ill—Literary collections. 4. Emotional problems. 5. Mental illness. 6. Mentally
ill. I. Donley, Carol C. II. Buckley, Sheryl, 1946–   III. Literature and medicine (Kent,
Ohio) ; 3.
PN6071.M4 W49 2000
808.8'0353—dc21   99-048190

British Library Cataloging-in-Publication data are available.

Contents

§

Section Six: *Alzheimer's and Dementia*

Preface

§

"WHAT'S NORMAL?" is the title of a course in literature and medicine that we have team-taught annually in the weekend college at Hiram College for more than ten years. Growing out of our experiences with that course and with the stimulating contributions of our students have come two anthologies: *The Tyranny of the Normal* (Kent State University Press, 1996), in which we focused on physical abnormalities, and this volume, *What's Normal?* with its focus on mental and behavioral deviations from the norm.

People with marked physical abnormalities provoke at least three reactions from society: one is an assumption that these "Others" should get fixed so they look more like us (the obese should lose weight; the disfigured should have plastic surgery); another is a long tradition of using them for entertainments, exhibiting them in freak shows or, as in the case of the Elephant Man, in hospitals; a third is the common tendency to shut them out because they make us normal people feel so uncomfortable. Until very recently, physically challenged people had little access to public buildings, effectively keeping them out of sight. Some cities even had "ugly laws" to keep the disfigured off the streets so they could not disturb the rest of us.

Leslie Fiedler, whose powerful essay gave the title to *The Tyranny of the Normal*, shows how cultural norms pressure people to conform, to fit in with acceptable ranges for appearance. In America, the idealized norms of thinness and youth, for example, drive many people to try diets, exercise programs, cosmetics, plastic surgery, hormone treatments—all in an effort to bring one's appearance in line with the images on magazine covers and TV advertisements. The many who cannot make their physical appearance conform to cultural norms are often degraded and alienated, enduring what Jonathan Carey calls the Quasimodo Complex. These "abnormals"—whether they be obese or disfigured from disease or injury—understand the severity of their alienation, not by looking in the mirror, but by reading the reactions of fear and disgust in people who meet them. Like Quasimodo, they learn how deeply alienated they are by watching how their appearance repulses even kind and thoughtful people.

As *What's Normal?* demonstrates, a similar tyranny of the normal dominates those who do not fit within the culture's norms for mental ability, mental health and acceptable behavior. Like their physically abnormal fellows, those deviating from mental and/or behavioral norms suffer basic social reactions: we expect them to be normalized through drugs and/or other therapies; we use them for entertainments, as the objects of jokes about the retarded or demented or crazy; or we expect them to be removed from sight by being put in jails or mental hospitals. We are often afraid of them, fearing that somehow we might be like them. We protest if someone suggests opening a halfway house in our neighborhood. Those who slip through the cracks make up a large percentage of the homeless, barely visible outcasts off on the margins of our consciousness unless we have to step over them on our way to the subway. The tyranny of the normal effectively demeans and ostracizes the mentally ill and disabled, adding social cruelties to the anguish they already suffer.

In order to examine these issues, this anthology is divided into two parts: one, an opening collection of articles and essays which address clinical, ethical, and social issues related to mental illness and disorders; and two, a section of fiction, poetry and drama portraying mental and behavioral abnormalities, sometimes from inside the perspective of the deviant and sometimes from the experience of family, friends, and other engaged observers. The clinical and bioethical essays address issues and principles (such as autonomy, beneficence, and justice) as they apply to cases of the mentally ill or disabled. Some essays argue against the concept of mental illness itself, suggesting that our culture has medicalized deviant behavior and has socially constructed many of our diseases and disorders.

The second part of the anthology gets inside the experiences of particular people in the often messy contexts of their lives. Thus the two sections complement each other. In the first, authors are speaking more from a detached and objective standpoint (though still with biases) while in the second, narrators are immersed in the experience and know how it feels. The first section is usually expressed in the discourse of scientific/philosophical argument and exposition while the second gives the engaged personal narratives of people suffering mental and emotional disorders.

This collection owes much to our students in the Hiram Weekend College who over several years of our teaching "What's Normal?" have given us thoughtful insights in class discussions and critical evaluations of the readings. These selections have, in other words, been tested in the crucible of the classroom.

Additional help came from the faculty in the Bioethics program at Case Western Reserve University, particularly Thomas Murray, Stephen Post, Eric

Juengst, Stuart Youngner, Rebecca Dresser, Peter Whitehouse, Anita Weiss, Beth O'Toole, and two especially challenging and stimulating visiting scholars: Kathryn Hunter and Grant Gillett. We also appreciate the support of Martin Kohn, our colleague and codirector of the Center for Literature, Medicine and the Health Care Professions at Hiram College.

Special thanks go to the Foote Committee on Programs in Ethics and Values at Hiram which generously helped cover some of the copyright expenses.

This project would never have been completed without the careful, thorough and committed effort of Hiram alumna Amy Daniel, who worked on everything from copyright permissions to editing text. Other Hiram students who helped with the manuscript include Paul Cockeram, Dawn Santabarbara, Karen Stocz, and Joaquin Uy, each of whom provided thoughtful and diligent editing.

Finally we want to thank Marge Buckley and Alan Donley, whose loving support, patience, and humor made our work much easier.

Editors' Commentary on Narrative

§

THE WRITER Scott Sanders describes storytelling as "the most human art," which serves us in many ways, from creating and sustaining community to helping us see through the eyes of people different from us. Through narrative, women can try on the experiences of men and vice versa; young people can vicariously experience what it means to be old; people of different races, classes, cultures can get a chance to walk in each other's shoes, however briefly. The sane can get into the narrative of the manic-depressive or the paranoid schizophrenic or the clinically depressed, and can get a taste of their experiences.

All of us have our own life stories which give us our identities, placing us in our families, our religious and social communities, our jobs, our own histories. Illness and disability change our stories; mental problems may seriously disconnect us from who we are (were) or may certainly redefine that identity, telling a different story. Families dealing with Alzheimer's disease in a loved one recognize how radically that story may change.

Good stories, Sanders says, teach us how we ought to live. They "educate our desires." They can "lead our desires in new directions—away from greed, toward generosity; away from suspicion, toward sympathy" (Utne 55). Because most narratives move in cause and effect patterns, they show us how our present actions and words produce effects, some of which we might not have anticipated. Whether we are reading the children's story of the "Fisherman and His Wife," or the parable of the Good Samaritan, or the play *Oedipus Rex*, they teach us to choose wisely and carefully what we do and say. And stories help us cope with despair, with suffering and death; they can comfort and console and offer hope; they give us models of how others have coped.

For all these reasons, narratives "teach us how to be human" (Utne 56) and thus are essential for our understanding of each other. Especially in the health care professions, where the patient may be referred to by symptom or diagnosis (i.e., the schizophrenic, the neurotic, the manic-depressive), narratives remind us there is a whole complex person with a life story in which this particular illness may be just a small anecdote. Labeling closes down our thinking.

Once we put a label on someone, we often act as if that is all there is. Rosenhan points out that once a person is designated as "abnormal," everything he does or says in interpreted in that light. Even normal behavior is likely to be misinterpreted by those who think the person is mentally ill.

Susan Sontag, James Childress, and many others have shown that the metaphor of war dominates much medical treatment. The foreign invader (cancer, virus, bacteria) attacks the body's defense systems, often overwhelming resistance; so the physician warriors battle the enemy with weapons of surgery and medicines, or target the enemy cancer cells and bombard them with radiation. The patient himself often becomes a battleground on which the physicians fight the disease, sometimes long after the patient has recognized that it's a losing battle and that to continue struggling is fruitless and painful. The patient may admit defeat and seek peace long before the physicians give up. That metaphor makes it very hard for some people to seek hospice or other palliative care for the terminally ill, because the metaphor makes us think we are cowards or losers or incompetent fighters. We need to adopt a different metaphor if we are to understand the dying process differently.

Similarly, metaphors and their embedded assumptions affect how we see and think about the mentally ill and mentally retarded (or disadvantaged or handicapped or disabled). They, too, battle against insanity or depression; they, too, often seem to be invaded and defeated. We want them to fight their depressions, to "snap out of it," to get control of themselves. Since we will always have metaphors embedded in our language and in the ways we see the world, at the very least we have an obligation to be aware of them and be sensitive to how they direct and limit our thinking.

Narratives also teach us to pay attention to the narrator who always has a particular point of view, a context which allows certain ways of describing and interpreting what is going on. No narrator has a God's eye view. Each of our descriptions and analyses of events, no matter how objective, is told from a particular perspective, colored by the education, experience and ability of the narrator. Ways of seeing and interpreting may vary greatly, even over a short time. Note, for example, in Hacking's essay, how the diagnosis and treatment of multipersonality disorder occurs almost exclusively in the last two decades of the twentieth century in America. Whether we are listening to a psychiatrist, a child, or a depressed suicidal patient, we have to pay attention to the perspective of the storyteller as well as to the content of the story.

Realizing the limited perspectives of narrators does not mean we read a scientific essay the same way we read a story. Wayne Booth, in *The Company We Keep: An Ethics of Fiction*, points out that "we read differently when we think a story is true rather than 'made up.' Whether or not we are critically innocent, we never read a story without making a decision, mistaken or justified, about the implied author's answer to a simple question: Is this 'once-upon-a-time' or is it a claim about events in real time? . . . The answers we hear them giving create solid differences in the company we *think* we keep—and at any one moment, that is the company we *do* keep" (16–17). As readers we bring a whole set of expectations and assumptions to a writing which we believe to be true, and a different set to a writing we think is fiction. In this anthology, we keep several different kinds of company, from the scientific/philosophical exposition and argument of Part 1 to the autobiography, story, and poetry of Part 2. Each work can be a valuable companion in itself and can serve as a measure and balance for the others, revising our expectations, challenging our assumptions, and, we hope, increasing our understanding and compassion.

PART ONE

Clinical & Bioethical Perspectives

Introduction to Part One

§

THE OPENING ESSAY in this section addresses the obvious but often over-looked question about what we mean when we say something is normal. Davis and Bradley, in "The Meaning of Normal," show how the term "normal" has widely different meanings in different contexts and how our failure to realize these differences can have serious consequences. Normal can mean "healthy" (as in normal body temperature), "typical" (as in a normal routine at work), "average" (as in normal winter snowfall). It has a specific definition in statistics. In medicine, normal can be taken to be a defined standard, such as normal blood pressure. As they point out, "When the ideal is taken as the norm, variation becomes defined as disease." Too often we convert normal and healthy variabilities into diseases or disorders because they differ from the ideal norm. This reluctance to accept normal variations makes people who are only slightly different from the norm feel unacceptable.

Several of the selections in this section of the anthology raise questions about how we diagnose and label mental illnesses and disorders. In *The Myth of Mental Illness,* his famous critique of psychiatry, Thomas Szasz said that problems in human conduct, misbehaviors or deviant behaviors, became medicalized—they became diseases caused by physiological problems that could be treated with drugs, shock therapies, and other interventions. For Szasz, mental illness is a myth. Psychiatrists have taken a metaphor—that mental problems are *like* illnesses—and have converted it to "fact": now they *are* illnesses. By converting antisocial behavior into symptoms of illness, we undermine personal responsibility for our actions. How many bad behaviors have been blamed on PMS or ADD or any number of other three-and-four-letter disorders described in the Diagnostic and Statistical Manual of Mental Disorders (DSM-III and IV), thereby relieving the patient of responsibility?

Seth Farber opens his essay with the comment that he has seen "the best minds of his generation destroyed by the mental health system." He worries that patients are reduced to labels and their so-called disorders are treated with drugs, but the psychiatrists do not really listen to the patient's story. The doctors "see" the expert diagnosis and treatment and construct a standard case study of a damaged individual, but they do not see the whole person whose life story might be read and interpreted very differently. Kristin's story is an effective example of what Farber means by this contrast.

In another well-known critique of psychiatry, R. D. Laing argues that there is no generally agreed-upon objective clinical criteria for the diagnosis of schizophrenia; there are no pathological anatomical findings post mortem, no general acceptance of any treatment as proven. Psychiatrists act as if schizophrenia is a fact, and they often label and pigeonhole patients. But there have been many cases of misdiagnosis and inappropriate interventions. D. L. Rosenhan's article from *Science* in this section documents several instances of healthy people being labeled as schizophrenics and admitted to mental hospitals even though nothing was wrong with them.

Rosenhan's famous experiment, "On Being Sane in Insane Places," demonstrates that we cannot always tell the normal from the abnormal. We cannot always distinguish the sane from the insane, even in psychiatric hospitals. Rosenhan had eight normal people pretend they were hearing voices. All eight were admitted to mental hospitals, whereupon they stopped having any symptoms. Although they acted normally, they were kept in the mental hospitals an average of nineteen days, and each was discharged with a diagnosis of schizophrenia in remission (although none was actually ill). Rosenhan showed that the diagnosis stuck to the pseudopatients. None of the professionals realized these were not mentally ill patients, though often other patients in the hospital did.

Ian Hacking, in the first chapter of his *Rewriting the Soul*, raises questions about why, in the last fifteen years, North America has experienced an epidemic of multiple personality disorders (MPD), while at the same time most psychiatrists contend there is no such thing. The European International Classification of Diseases (ICD-10 of 1992) does not even have a category of MPD, while the American Diagnostic and Statistical Manual of Mental Disorders describes the disorder in detail. Hacking asks if this is real, or is it a culturally permissible way to express unhappiness? A dominant theory of causation is that MPD is a coping mechanism some women show in response to physical and sexual abuse in their childhood. Many therapists of multiples are also feminists who find that "the roots of a patient's troubles come from the home, from neglect, from cruelty," from oppressive men. Considerable evidence exists that these multiple personalities may be generated in the counseling environment and that hunting for them to support the evidence of child abuse actually encourages the patient to dissociate herself into various components. Linked with this problem are instances of false memory syndrome, where patients recall abuse that never happened. Hacking is very concerned about our use of value-loaded language, even the term "disorder," which becomes a stigmatizing label that may stick to someone for a lifetime.

One way society has marginalized and manipulated "abnormal" people is in the eugenics movements. As Stephen Jay Gould points out, eugenics movements to eliminate "undesirables," or at least prevent them from reproducing, were powerfully active in the first half of this century in both America and Europe. "Sterilization could be imposed upon those judged insane, idiotic, imbecilic, or moronic, and upon convicted rapists or criminals when recommended by a board of experts." By 1935, more than "20,000 forced 'eugenic' sterilizations had been performed in the U.S." Nazi Germany sterilized almost 400,000 people who were supposedly feebleminded. In the famous U.S. Supreme Court case *Buck v Bell* (1927), Oliver Wendell Holmes wrote: "It is better for the world, if instead of waiting to execute degenerate offspring for crime, or to let them starve for their imbecility, society can prevent those who are manifestly unfit from continuing their kind . . . . Three generations of imbeciles are enough." That decision led to the forced sterilization of Carrie Buck, who was supposed to be the feebleminded daughter of a feebleminded mother. Carrie's infant daughter was also labeled an imbecile. It turned out much later, in 1972, that Carrie Buck was a woman of normal intelligence, reading newspapers daily, working crossword puzzles. Gould points out that Carrie Buck grew up with foster parents and was raped by one of their relatives and "then blamed for the resulting pregnancy. Almost surely she was (as they used to say) committed to hide her shame (and her rapist's identity). . . . In short, she was sent away to have her baby. Her case never was about mental deficiency." The claim that her baby girl was not normal came from a social worker who saw the child at six months. The child was adopted by the same family who sent her mother away (perhaps because they were related to her father). She was a perfectly normal student in school, even making the honor roll in 1931, not what one would expect of a third-generation imbecile. But Carrie Buck was sterilized so that she (as one supposed imbecile) could not produce anymore "idiotic" children.

The wrong labeling of all three generations as imbeciles should give us sobering pause about who has the authority and wisdom to do this labeling, how much labeling is caught up in current fads and assumptions such as a eugenics movement, and what actions the state can take on the basis of those labels.

Another essay in this section serves as a "counter" story in that it demonstrates a successful and encouraging relationship between a psychiatrist and his patient. Irving Yalom's descriptions of his psychotherapy sessions with his patient Elva give us a much more positive picture of how experts really can help those with mental distress. Yalom shows the doctor growing and learning as well as healing the patient. He has a refreshing humility and sense of humor.

To close this section, three cases brought up in a Hastings Center discussion serve as good models for these complex questions of making decisions for the mentally incompetent. From one debate about the right of a mentally compromised man to refuse treatment ("Ain't Nobody Gonna Cut on My Head!") to another argument about the right of a parent to sterilize a mentally challenged daughter, these cases and their commentaries reveal the complexities of the issues.

The Meaning of Normal

Phillip V. Davis & John G. Bradley

Everyone knows what "normal" is. Imbedded in nearly every judgment that we make, every comparison, and every weighing of possibilities is a firmly developed concept of what's "normal." And, while the definition varies with the referent, it generally describes some commonly held understanding, a culturally accepted belief about what is typical, usual, and natural. The "normal price of goods," for example, describes the typical cost of items when discounts and sales are ignored. "Normal body temperature" refers to the usual temperature measured in a healthy person. "Normal behavior" describes natural, expected actions. We depend, in fact, on having a common understanding of "normal" in order to make a number of judgments. In medicine, particularly, beliefs about what is normal are central in making judgments about disease.

In a classic article entitled "The Normal, and the Perils of the Sylleptic Argument," Edmund Murphy posits a number of different uses of the word *normal* that illustrate just how complicated this common understanding can be.[1] *Normal*, Murphy suggests, means "typical" when appealing to a commonly accepted practice. It means "average" when describing what is most representative of a class or group. When used to give assurance in a clinical setting, *normal* means "innocuous" or "harmless." In genetics, it defines what is "most suited" for survival. When used in statistics, Murphy suggests that the meaning is technically specific. Finally, Murphy notes that when we make judgments about absolute goals, when we talk about what is desirable, we sometimes use the word *normal* as a synonym for "perfection."

Murphy's observations suggest two potential dangers in the belief that we genuinely understand what *normal* means. The first is the hazard of assuming that we understand the *intended* use of the word *normal* in any given context (as in what the word *normal* means in the phrase "normal sexual relations"). The second is that the contextual meaning of the word may be revised and thereby change our understanding of the phenomenon it describes. "Normal highway speed," for instance, is often more dependent on the speed of surrounding traffic than on the posted speed limits. In the same way, the concept of "normal social behavior" changes. For example, Daniel Moynihan suggests in an article entitled "Defining Deviancy Down" that societies can criminalize actions only to the extent that their justice systems can handle the results.[2] When more deviant behavior exists than the structure can deal with—e.g., than prisons can hold—the range of acceptable behaviors is broadened. What had been "criminal" becomes "normal."

In medicine, there is particular danger in shifting the contextual meanings of the word *normal*, in part because of the large range of meanings that the discipline allows the word, and in part because the result of allowing one definition to take the place of another changes the way in which physicians define disease itself. Medicine uses the word *normal* to express all of the various meanings that Murphy describes, and it appears to extend the use of the word to include a number of other meanings. In medicine, *normal* can refer to a "defined standard," such as normal blood pressure; a "naturally occurring state," such as normal immunity; or simply mean "free from disease," as in a normal Pap smear. It can mean "balanced" as in a normal diet, "acceptable" as in normal behavior, or it can be used to describe a "stable physical state." In all of these meanings, the word *normal* is used to describe an "ordinary finding" or an "expected state." But medicine allows another meaning for the word *normal* that differs significantly from the ordinary. In many ways, medicine has come to understand *normal* as a "description of the ideal."

Medicine's identification of the normal with the ideal may stem from a related concept: the definition of the clinical term *norm. Dorland's Medical Dictionary* defines *norm* as a "fixed or ideal standard"—that is, an ideal standard against which some measurement is compared.[3] The definition of normal blood cholesterol levels, for example, represents an "ideal standard" rather than the average blood cholesterol value found in the adult population. Medicine has defined clinical norms for many laboratory findings by deriving mathematical values from the results of clinical tests and then deciding which of these values are included within a normal range. While normal values are determined in various ways—by averaging, by empirical decisions about what is healthy, by guessing what the optimal state should be—many have increasingly come to define what we consider to be "perfect" or "desirable" or "healthiest." The "norm" represents not what is common, typical, or customary, but instead what we believe normal "ought to be."

Defining the norm as an ideal leads to significant problems. All of us understand that it is an illusion to believe that perfection is even theoretically possible and that it is certainly a practical impossibility. Perfect health, across the lifeline, is unattainable. Disease and ill health are a normal part of the human condition. The constant pursuit of health (and the concomitant inability to constantly achieve it) leads easily to blaming those who bear the burden of ill-

ness for being irresponsible enough to contract it. The need to see within illness an organism's manifest destiny is critical. As Freud notes in *Analysis Terminable and Interminable,* "Every normal person, in fact, is only normal on the
average."[4]

More important for medicine, however, are the problems that result from
defining variation from the ideal as "abnormal." When the ideal is taken as
the norm, variation becomes defined as disease—an especially peculiar cir-
cumstance insofar as much variation has no particular clinical significance or
biological consequence. Accepting the ideal as the norm begs the question
of how uncommon something must be to be considered abnormal. The use
of growth-stimulating hormones in children who are small for their chrono-
logical age, for example, posits a range of assumptions about normality that
appear, at a minimum, to suggest that small physical stature is a condition that
should be corrected—a suggestion underscored by our willingness to tolerate
considerable variation at the other extreme.

The notion of variation as pathology has been powerfully apparent for several decades. A 1964 *Lancet* article by Marc Steinbach, for example, presents
the following point of view:

> A man of 60 should be considered normal only if he has the same blood-
> pressure and blood–cholesterol as a healthy man of 25. The fact that in his popu-
> lation group most "healthy" men of 60 have an increased blood-pressure may
> reassure him but should not mislead the physician. If it is true that people have
> the age of their arteries, it is likewise true that they have the arteries of their
> age. . . . There should be only one set of normals—namely, the values character-
> istic of young adults between 20 and 30 years.[5]

Implicit in the idea of a clinical norm is not only the notion of perfection but also the notion of measurement. Measurement, in turn, suggests that
the definition of normal results from a set of comparative judgments that
are made either against a dichotomous scale (normal vs. abnormal) or within
a prescribed range of possibilities (the statistical norm). When the judgment is
dichotomous, as is often the case with behavior, for example, the measurement
can also be relatively ambiguous. A mother who wonders whether her baby's
behavior is "normal" has already made a judgment about a number of behaviors that are acceptable; she is concerned about whether some other behaviors (or lack of behaviors) should also be accepted. The ambiguity results from
varying levels of comfort or discomfort with the observed behaviors. When
the measurement depends on statistical manipulation, however, it has the appearance of being more precise. Normal intelligence, for example, falls within

two standard deviations of the mean on accepted intelligence tests. Along with this appearance of precision comes a curious phenomenon. The measurement does more than contribute to the definition of what is normal quantitatively; rather, by defining the norm, it actually becomes the norm in a more absolute sense.

As we have become increasingly more dependent on measurement to define what is or what can be taken to support a judgment of the normal, we have also tended to ignore problems inherent in the process. Two central issues result: first, our ability to make very sensitive measurements has resulted in a tendency to refine the definition of normal to ever smaller and smaller ranges; second, the range of abnormality has proportionately increased.

Cancer of the prostate provides a clear example. We now have a laboratory test that is simple and inexpensive to perform, the Prostate Specific Antigen (PSA) test. Elevated PSA levels are associated with the presence of cancer of the prostate. Fully 80 percent of clinically verifiable cases of prostate cancer show elevated PSA levels.[6] While this has allowed us the ability to more easily screen for the pathology, the importance of the measurement remains unclear. In a recent review of the usefulness of PSA as a screening tool, Steven Woolf identifies two significant problems.[7] First, the number of false positive results may be as high as two–thirds of all men screened. In such cases, the measurement has suggested the presence of a disease that is not pathologically verifiable. Second, the existence of prostate cancer may not be clinically relevant. At autopsy, 30 percent of men over the age of 50 have histological evidence of prostate cancer. Extrapolated to the population at large, nearly 9 million American men may have latent prostate cancers. Some 40,000 deaths result from the disease each year, but there is little evidence that screening affects either mortality or morbidity. We can take a measurement which suggests the presence of the disease, and we have accepted the absence of the measurement as normal, despite the fact that virtually all men may get cancer of the prostate if they live long enough, and the overwhelming preponderance of them suffer no clinically significant ill effects from the disease. We have taken the presence of an abnormal laboratory value and concluded that it signifies a disease process which should be treated. We are so convinced of the significance of the measurement that it supersedes clinical relevance. We have allowed a measurement to guide our pursuit of perfection.

Similarly, we are so enamored of our ability to intervene that we frequently ignore whether intervention is actually necessary. Lynn Payer, writing in *Medicine and Culture*, a fascinating book on cultural differences in health care, suggests the following: American medicine is aggressive. From birth—which is more likely to be by caesarean than anywhere in Europe—to death in the hospital, from invasive examination to prophylactic surgery, American doctors want to *do* something, preferably as much as possible.[8]

The process by which medicine has moved from a concept of normal as representing the "ordinary state" to normal as a "description of the ideal" is noteworthy. It is a history, first of all, of medical progress. Man has long developed compensatory strategies for dealing with the undesirable aspects of the human condition. Before the scientific revolution, most of those strategies were religious responses to life's vicissitudes. The great strides made in epidemiological understanding of disease transmission around the turn of the last century and the introduction of effective anti-bacterial agents following World War II have resulted in medicine's striking successes at controlling the morbidity and mortality of infectious disease. More recently, our faith in technology has led us to believe that we can escape much of life's unpleasantness. Medicine, in particular, has been charged with identifying ways to "fix" these undesirables and hold off mortality.

Faithful conduct of the charge, however, asks us to ignore certain fundamental truths. Disease and death are natural phenomena. Despite increases in longevity, the actual mortality rate for humans is 100 percent. Despite advances in the treatment of disease, illnesses plague mankind. Despite our most effective interventions, perfection remains elusive. And, perhaps even more importantly, despite our sureness of aim in the pursuit of physical perfection, the target keeps shifting. Cultural beliefs about what constitutes perfection change with time. Personal beliefs about what constitutes perfection change with age. No matter how well intentioned, the pursuit of the perfect is fraught with dilemmas.

Several such dilemmas come readily to mind. First, because of its cultural variability, its contextual meaning, and its necessarily temporal nature, the definition of perfection is completely arbitrary. The image of a perfect physique, for example, differs today from that of a century ago; it differs between bodybuilders and advertising executives; and it conjures up different pictures in a 16–year–old's mind than it does in a septuagenarian's. Second, the pursuit of perfection is dis-economic. The consumption of resources expended in pursuit of health in the United States, for example, is widely recognized as excessive, although the actual health status of the population is far from ideal. Our cultural obsession with being healthy has led to ever-increasing expenditures with at best only marginal health gains. Third, perfection is biologically maladaptive. Variation is an important biological advantage for the survival of a species, and any movement toward uniformity decreases the overall adaptability. Fourth, there is an inbred arrogance in the assumptions that we know what constitutes perfection, that we are able to manipulate the human organism to achieve it, and that we are able to control any unanticipated effects.

Nathaniel Hawthorne explores the theme of man's perfectibility in several short stories, but perhaps most powerfully in a piece entitled "The Birthmark."[9] Here, Hawthorne recounts a tale of a man of science who marries a lady of exquisite beauty, a beauty he finds marred by a small birthmark on her face. The scientist is obsessed with removing the birthmark and uses all his considerable intellect to concoct a therapy that will efface it forever. And, while his therapy is successful in removing the offending stain, it also kills his wife. Her dying words to him make the point: "[y]ou have aimed loftily; you have done nobly. Do not repent that with so high and pure a feeling, you have rejected the best the earth could offer." Fifth, since the time of Copernicus, one of the most powerful and persistent metaphors for human life has been an understanding of the body as a machine. While the metaphor has been an extremely useful one, it also suggested that the body can be seen as simply a collection of replaceable parts—a point made powerfully by Renee Fox and Judith Swazey in their profoundly moving book about organ transplantation, *Spare Parts*.[10] As they note in the book, the Jarvick artificial heart represents perhaps the most striking proof of our belief in the body-as-machine metaphor. The metaphor has also driven a great deal of medical research around the mechanical stabilization of failing physical systems—renal dialysis, ventilator support, and the entire armamentarium of intensive care units provide ready examples. It has led our society, in particular, to a belief that physical perfection can be achieved by rearranging pieces according to a "correct" template or replacing defective parts.

There is another set of problems inherent in the pursuit of perfect health as well, problems that stem from the effects of the pursuit. The most obvious in contemporary American life is that the achievement of perfect health is symbolized by cosmetic changes rather than meaningful changes in health status or lifestyle. To be sure, the way a person looks is an obvious and "easy" measurement of health. The first clinical signs a physician looks for are gross abnormalities in physical appearance. The confusion between appearance and health, however, is insidious precisely because appearance too easily substitutes for reality. In the words of the comic Billy Crystal, "It is more important to look marvelous than to be marvelous." The confusion of appearance and health is especially prevalent in advertising—shampoos that promise healthy-looking hair, dairy products that promise healthy bodies, and an entire plethora of products ranging from alcoholic beverages to zinc supplements whose use by attractive models implicitly promises consumers who use their products the look of health. Madison Avenue has promulgated its own version of the norm, a standard which in turn helps inform how science interprets normality.

A second significant problem inherent in the pursuit of perfect health is found in the psychological costs involved in punishing ourselves for failure to live up to these ideals. The health care establishment, spurred perhaps by Madison Avenue, is busy engendering a national neurosis of inadequacy as our cultural expectations make it clear that one should be taller, more beautiful, stronger, or healthier. Implicit in the message is that failure to achieve perfection is the fault of the individual. If only we would have tried harder, eaten better, exercised more regularly, used the right products, and even relaxed more effectively, the message goes, perfect health certainly would have followed. Conversations with medical students (who are experiencing the peak of their own physical health) make it frighteningly clear that many believe that the illnesses which beset their patients are self-imposed. In a recent classroom session, for instance, students discussing a patient with lung cancer noted their belief that after "thirty years of smoking" patients deserve what happens. The fact that most smokers don't die from lung cancer and a significant number of patients who do have never smoked fails to mitigate against these kinds of attitudes. Belief in personal responsibility for ill health is seductively misleading. In a recent letter to medical school deans, for example, Cloe Milne recounts the way in which her husband's life was shortened by physicians who, after diagnosing the early stages of lung cancer in a 74-year-old, looked no further for the eminently treatable conditions which rapidly killed him.[11] It is a kind of medical Puritanism that bespeaks a need for a more liberal understanding of human frailty. In fact, popular notions about what constitutes healthy lifestyles may have more to do with cultural bias than scientific evidence, but physicians are as influenced by cultural values as the rest of the population. Faith Fitzgerald, in a recent issue of the *New England Journal of Medicine*, makes the point powerfully:

> We excoriate the smoker but congratulate the skier. Yet both skiing and smoking may lead to injury, may be costly, and are clearly risky. We have created a new medical specialty to take care of sports injuries, an acknowledgment of the hazardous sequelae. And though there are no doubt benefits to exercise and sports, the literature on the complications of some activities is such that were they drugs, they would probably have been banned by the Food and Drug Administration years ago.[12]

Yet a third problem arises in the way in which the pursuit of perfection systematically disenfranchises those identified as imperfect. A person who is crippled or lame, a person with limited mental ability, a person with diabetes or hypertension, are all unhealthy (abnormal) by definition. Their personal feelings of good health aside, they are weighed in society's balance and found lacking. Marjorie Kagawa-Singer, reporting on the feelings of cancer patients, noted that of 50 people interviewed, all defined themselves as "healthy":

> These participants understood the gravity of their disease, but they were able
> to continue to be self-sufficient within the limitations imposed by their condition, and they maintained their functional social roles. They saw themselves as
> healthy with cancer.[13]

A fourth, more subtle set of problems arises from the pursuit of perfection within the structure of our health care system. As advances in nutrition, sanitation, and the control of infectious diseases have occurred, medical practice is slowly changing its emphasis from treating disease to preventing disease. Inherent in prevention is the concept of early detection.

Two distinct problems are central to early detection. The first is related to measurement. In our haste to identify subclinical presentations of disease, we have developed the ability to measure disease states (or the precursors of disease states) without any assurance that the actual illness event will happen. As previously noted, the identification of a biologic marker for prostate cancer, for example, has given us the ability to test for prostate cancer in entire populations. Unfortunately, a positive test result doesn't necessarily mean that the cancer will develop into a clinically significant illness that can or should be treated.

A related phenomenon is described by Black and Welch, reporting on research conducted by Harach, et al., about the incidence of thyroid cancer among Finnish adults at autopsy.[14] Black and Welch note that "for diseases defined microscopically, such as cancer, the reservoir of detectable subclinical disease is huge." They report, for example, that based on Harach's work it appears that if one can look at thin enough slices of the thyroid gland, the prevalence of histologically verifiable papillary carcinoma could equal 100 percent. The irony, of course, lies in the fact that the incidence of clinically significant thyroid cancer is very small.

The second problem with early detection is economic. Under fee-for-service medicine, it is in physicians' economic interest to aggressively seek out and treat disease. Health care economists criticize the inflationary pressures of such a system. The process, however, claims a certain justification through its implicit promise of perfect health.

Economically based paradigms for prevention, on the other hand, suggest that we should "incentivise" providers to keep people healthy (a basic tenet of many Health Maintenance Organizations). With the exception of immunizations, however, virtually all preventive strategies are behavioral, and, in the final analysis, naively suggest that if people are simply kept healthy they will never get sick. This is analogous to an idea popularized in the geriatric medical literature of "squaring the curve"—that is, living in perfect health to a certain age and then suddenly, painlessly, and at no cost to the system, dropping dead. It simply doesn't happen.

It is another kind of mistake, however, to write off the pursuit of perfection as an ill-conceived endeavor or vainglorious folly. There is a long-standing belief in our culture, and in virtually all others, that people should strive to be "better" than we are. In the Judeo-Christian heritage, for example, striving toward redemption is man's central task. In the Hindu tradition, the point of reincarnation is perfection. In Buddhist sects, nirvana is achieved by a process of freeing yourself of undesirable traits. Each of these religious traditions, and many others as well, celebrate the pursuit of perfection without promising its actual fulfillment in earthly life. What these traditions suggest is both a universal need for the quest and a clear understanding of man's limitations.

Our pursuit of perfect health must likewise take the genuine limitations of what is normal into account. The World Health Organization's definition of health as "a state of complete physical, mental, and social well-being and not merely the absence of disease and infirmity" is too ideological to be of much relevance to medical practice.[15] We need a more functional approach to understanding what constitutes good health, one which accepts variability as normal rather than as a deviation from perfection. The definition must take human limitations into account. It must enfranchise the lame and the chronically ill and allow them their claims to health by applauding the way they cope with their diseases. It should allow for the inevitable changing physical and mental status of people over time. In short, it should concentrate on the process rather than the product as the important part of health.

Health will always be defined in relation to a number of critically important societal assumptions. Our belief in the validity of scientific measurement is one such assumption. A genuine respect for the inherent advantages of variability should be equally important. The medical concept of what is normal must be expansive enough to recognize the variability and even the frailty of the human condition. We must be humble enough to realize that our notion of perfection is necessarily subjective, elusive, and transient. We must recognize that disease is a normal part of human existence.

NOTES

1. Murphy, E. A. The normal, and the perils of the sylleptic argument. *Persp. Biol. Med.* 15:566–582, 1972.

2. Moynihan, D. Defining deviancy down. *Amer. Schol.* 62:17–30, 1993.

3. *Dorland's Illustrated Medical Dictionary,* 25th ed. Philadelphia: W. B. Saunders, 1974. 1057.

4. Freud, S. *Analysis Terminable and Indeterminable,* as quoted in *On Freud's "Analysis Terminable and Indeterminable,"* edited by J. Sandler. New Haven: Yale Univ. Press, 1987. 22.

5. Steinbeck, M. The normal in cardiovascular diseases. *Lancet* 7369:1117, 1964.

6. Catalona, W. J., et al. Comparison of digital-rectal examination and serum-prostate specific antigen in the early detection of prostate cancer: Results of a multi-center clinical trial of 6,630 men. *J. Urol.* 151:1283–1290, 1994.

7. Woolf, S. H. Screening for prostate cancer with prostate specific antigen: An examination of the evidence. *N. Eng. J. Med.* 33(21):1401–1405, 1995.

8. Payer, L. *Medicine and Culture.* New York: Henry Holt, 1988. 124.

9. Hawthorne, N. The Birthmark, in *The Complete Short Stories of Nathaniel Hawthorne.* Garden City, NY: Doubleday, 1959. 227–238.

10. Fox, R., and Swazey, J. *Spare Parts.* New York: Oxford Univ. Press, 1992.

11. Milne, C. Open letter to the deans of U.S. medical schools, 1994.

12. Fitzgerald, F. T. The tyranny of health. *N. Eng. J. Med.* 330:440–441, 1994.

13. Kagawa-Singer, M. Redefining health: Living with cancer. *Soc. Sci. Med.* 37 (3):295–304, 1993.

14. Black, W. C., and Welch, H. G. Advances in diagnostic imaging and overestimations of disease prevalence and the benefits of therapy. *N. Eng. J. Med.* 328:1237–1243, 1993.

15. World Health Organization. Principles of world health. *WHO Chron.* 27:300, 1973.

From Madness, Heresy, and the Rumor of Angels: The Revolt against the Mental Health System

SETH FARBER

INTRODUCTION

"I SAW THE BEST MINDS of my generation destroyed by madness," wrote Allen Ginsberg in *Howl*. I believe this statement is inaccurate: I contend that he saw the best minds of his generation destroyed by the 'mental health' system. Contrary to popular opinion (encouraged by a formidable public-relations campaign) the mental health system has not changed significantly since Ginsberg wrote *Howl* in the 1950s. But there has been one rather significant change since Ginsberg saw his friends destroyed: at least *some* of the best minds of *my* generation have survived this system. They triumphed. This book tells how and why.

As to madness, most of the psychiatric survivors I interviewed (and others with militant viewpoints I've spoken to) agree with the late psychiatrist R. D. Laing: 'madness,' however painful it may be, can provide the opportunity to re-create one's self and expand one's possibilities. In their time of madness the subjects interviewed here became aware of the 'spiritual' dimension of human existence; they experienced their oneness with all beings.

I have interviewed and told here the story of seven individuals. If we could look at their 'case records' we would be able to verify that they were classified by the numerous professionals who 'treated' them as 'chronically mentally ill.' Each person was typically given various diagnoses by different professionals: 'schizophrenic,' 'manic-depressive' ('bipolar disorder'), 'borderline personality disorder,' and so forth. From the point of view of the mental health expert, they were clearly severely mentally ill. The 'expert' would say they are still ill or that their illness is 'in remission.' They exhibited the 'symptoms' that typically warrant the diagnosis of schizophrenia or manic-depression. Yet they do not conform to the mental health experts' expectations: they are not taking psychiatric drugs, collecting disability funds from the government, or manifesting an inability to work and form intimate relationships. To the contrary, those individuals are leaders: keenly aware of the inequities in society, highly socially responsible and strongly determined to change the world, to save the Earth, and to redress injustice.

A sequence of events and experiences can be *storied* in a variety of different fashions. The *meaning* of these events is determined by the particular narrative ploys and metaphors that we utilize in order to shape and organize these events, by the way in which the raw material of life is configured. In order to demonstrate this to the reader I decided to construct two competing narrative lines for each subject I interviewed.

The dominant narrative line was the product of the fusion of my psyche with that of the subject. Each person interviewed felt that the narrative line which emerged did justice to the complexity of their experience and to the mystery of their soul's quest for meaning and fulfillment. The narrative line I counterpoised to this is one standardly constructed by mental health experts. On the one hand is the experts' case study of a damaged individual afflicted with the symptoms of mental illness. On the other hand is the story that seemed evident to me, the story of quest, of descent into madness, of spiritual vision, of existential crisis, of triumph, of self-discovery and spiritual transformation.

This format enables the reader to see how 'mental illness' stories are constructed and how they come to acquire their plausibility. It allows the reader to compare and judge for himself or herself: Is this officially sanctioned story the Truth? Or is it a banal and demeaning way of *storying* the events and experiences in a person's life? Many readers will be led to ponder the next logical question: Why do we continue to place our trust in a community of experts who have become skilled in construing and interpreting events in such a way that they fail to do justice to the dignity of the individual and to the value of the human quest for meaning and happiness?

This format forces readers to experience *themselves* the desecration of the human spirit involved in the 'mental health' enterprise. At times this will be an aggravating or painful process for the reader. Those experiences that are most *intimate* to the individual cannot be communicated to mental health professionals who work in mental hospitals without risking the violation of the self. On the one hand the most precious and inspiring experiences the individual has and on the other hand those experiences that reveal most starkly the individual's human vulnerability are typically not understood or appreciated by mental health experts. On the contrary it is these experiences that are most likely to be seized upon and interpreted as proof of the individual's 'psychopathology.'

My purpose is not primarily to entertain. It is to jar and disturb the reader as well as to awaken his or her reverence for the indomitability of the human spirit. Hopefully, the perspective presented here will inspire the reader and give to him or her an enhanced sense of human possibility.

CHAPTER TWO

Kristin's Story

Kristin is a 34-year-old woman. She is a survivor of several psychiatric incarcerations. She has been a psychotherapist for several years. She completed her master's degree in counseling in 1988. She has not been in a mental hospital in seven years. She does not take psychiatric drugs. Throughout her hospitalizations she has consistently refused to take neuroleptic drugs. She took antidepressants for two years in her early twenties. She has been diagnosed as a 'depressive neurotic,' a 'pseudo-neurotic schizophrenic,' and a 'manic-depressive.'

Kristin's first encounter with the mental health system occurred when she was seven. Her mother thought Kristin was too active and took her to a psychiatrist who diagnosed her as hyperactive. Kristin's sister, who was one year older than her, was physically handicapped and consequently did not move around much. Kristin believed that her mother would have felt more comfortable with a child who "just lay around." "I was just real active, a normal child." The psychiatrist gave her phenobarbital. It had an adverse affect on her. "I remember taking the stuff and running into walls." The administration of the drug was discontinued.

When Kristin was in third grade she had another encounter with the mental health system. Kristin got A's in all her classes except math, where she consistently got D's and F's. An IQ test was administered to her. She did very well on the verbal sub-test and poorly on the performance sub-test. The school psychologist said she had a 'minimal brain dysfunction' that caused a 'learning disability.' No 'remedial' measures were taken at that time.

Home Life

Kristin's childhood and adolescence were not happy. Kristin's mother and father did not have a happy marriage. Her mother drank heavily and her father was in the Air Force so that he was usually out of town. When he was in town he seemed to have a closer bonding with Kristin than he did with his wife. Kristin was his favorite daughter. She thought that her mother was very critical of her. "No matter what I did, my mother didn't like it." But the mother was not critical of Kristin's two sisters. Kristin says that she believes her sisters would corroborate her perception that her mother was more critical of her.

When Kristin was a young adolescent her mother would frequently get drunk and accuse her of having sex with her father.

Kristin recounts one incident that typifies the pattern that persisted in her family. "When I was 15 Dad got me a horse. I loved horseback riding. Shortly afterwards he got himself a horse and the two of us would go on trips together. I enjoyed this because I loved my dad and I wasn't getting any attention from my mother. This made my mother furious, of course, since my dad was neglecting her."

Throughout Kristin's adolescence a similar sequence of events would recur continually. Her mother would get drunk and accuse her of "doing things" with her father. Both she and her mother would go into their own bedrooms crying. Later her father would come to her bedroom and say to Kristin, "I know you were right. It was wrong of your mother to criticize you like that, but I couldn't say anything. I had to stick by her because she is my wife."

The situation at school was hardly more felicitous. Kristin's older sister had skipped three grades, and was in college by age 16. "To keep up with this woman was impossible." The teachers would constantly say to Kristin, "You're sure not as smart as your sister." Her little sister, who was two years younger, got straight A's. "I decided to be bad. I started smoking cigarettes, running around with kids who drank." She never did anything serious enough to get involved with the police. But she and her friends would play pranks, such as stuffing the school toilets up with buns that they had gotten from the cafeteria. Whereas previously her grades had been satisfactory, now she started getting D's and F's.

Her mother and her father took her to a psychologist to find out what was wrong with her. He was an unusual psychologist who had studied family therapy. After hearing Kristin's story about her family life he told her that the problem was not in her but in the way that the family related to each other. He explained to Kristin that she was 'triangulated': that her parents fought out their problems through her. He said that he needed to get the family to change. She responded, "Good luck!" He made an appointment for all the family members to come in. When she left his office, she thought to herself, "God, there is actually someone who put into words what I've been feeling for 15 years."

Kristin remembers well the family session. The psychologist was blunt with her parents. "What would you talk about if you didn't have problems with Kristin?" he asked directly. "You need to communicate with each other and to stop putting her in the middle." Kristin's sisters started crying and yelling, "Stop it! Stop it!"

The therapist tried to get Kristin's mother and father to talk to each other about their problems and their conflicts. Her mother got angry and insisted that Kristin had deep emotional problems. Her father was silent but he gave Kristin a look as if to say, "I know he's right but your mother can't take it." Of course she realized that this act was a repetition of the same pattern that the therapist was attempting to change. Her mother led the family members out of the office and said that she was not coming back. Kristin remained. The therapist looked at her and said, "You must convince them to come back."

From a family-therapy perspective—from a systems perspective—this therapist had clearly identified the problem. But he had failed to respond in a competent manner. The therapist's task is not just to correctly identify a problem, but to motivate people to change their behavior. This therapist had attempted to prematurely force a reorganization of the family. As a consequence he alienated them and they walked out. The prominent family therapist Salvador Minuchin would have said that he had challenged the dysfunctional patterns of interaction and assumptions of the family before he had succeeded in 'joining' with them, that is, before he had gained their trust. A family therapist must first gain the trust of all the family members—must be accepted as part of the family—before he can motivate them to change.

Kristin was about 17 at this time. She decided to run away to Florida. "I couldn't stand it any more." She would call her parents from time to time to tell them that she was safe. Her mother threatened to kill Kristin's cat if she did not return. She found some friends in Florida and she survived by panhandling, stealing from grocery stores, and eating turtle eggs, which they would dig up from the sand on the beaches. She explained that this was a good source of protein. She had been reported as a runaway child and the police were looking for her.

Six months after she had left home she was caught by the police and sent home. It was the middle of the year, too late to return to school, so she got a job working in a restaurant. Her two sisters had left home. She was alone with her parents. She was miserable. That summer she stopped working and got her G. E. D.

She considered going to college but at this point her confidence in her intellectual abilities had been shaken. One can easily infer some of the sources of this lack of confidence. Earlier she had been 'diagnosed' as having 'minimal brain dysfunction' and a 'learning disability.' Her triangulation in her parents' marriage was a source of great distress that had a deleterious effect on her performance in school. Her siblings' relative freedom from the marital conflict helped them to excel in school. Her teachers had continually made negative comparisons between her and her sister, further undermining her confidence.

The Expert: The patient's low sense of self-esteem is a result of impairment of the ego, suggesting that the classical Oedipal neurosis is complicated by a narcissistic disorder stemming from early childhood. This diagnosis is further corroborated by the persistent pattern of rebellion and the patient's denial of any pathology.

Marriage and Divorce

She stayed at her parents and went back to work as a waitress. Then a new development occurred. "This guy came along who raced horses and I liked horses, so we ended up getting married." It must have seemed to her as if a golden opportunity had fallen before her: finally an escape from the insufferable conditions at home with her family.

The honeymoon was short-lived. They lived together in a one-room trailer and spent all day working together raising the horses. The constant association caused a lot of tension between them. This was made worse by the fact that he felt threatened when she did a better job training a horse than he did.

One day, approximately six months after the marriage, one of Kristin's girlfriends came down to visit her from a neighboring town. It had been decided before that Kristin and her husband Jack and the girlfriend Sue and a friend of Jack's would go out dancing together. But Jack had been drinking quite heavily that day, something that he infrequently did, and he had passed out on the bed. Kristin said to her girlfriend, "Well, we'll just go out without him." Apparently Jack had awoken and overheard her statement. Almost immediately after she made the suggestion he got up from the bed and walked into the room where they were sitting. He said, "You're going to do what?" Before she had a chance to reply he smacked her a couple of times in the face. He was 6'6" and muscular, she was 5'4" and delicate. At that point she kicked him "in the balls." "He started beating the hell out of me. There was blood everywhere." Kristin's girlfriend was not able to stem the tide of his fury. Finally she ran out of the house crying.

She was taken to the hospital. She had a broken nose. Plastic surgery was performed six months later. She immediately filed for divorce and at his urging dropped the criminal charges against him.

She moved back into her parents' home. "I was emotionally mortified. I love someone enough to marry him and he half kills me. I was paralyzed. I was so stressed out I didn't know what to do. I started hallucinating. Things looked different, as if they were breathing. I went into Mom's bed and was crying. I was seeing colored dots on the wall and I told her about it. I wanted her to hold me and talk to me. I'd always wanted that to happen but I never got it." She tried halfheartedly but it felt awkward. "It didn't feel real."

In the Psychiatric Ward

Her mother begged her to go to the psychiatric ward of the general hospital. She agreed. The psychiatrist in the ward told her that she was suffering from a depressive neurosis. She would meet with him regularly when she was in the hospital. He was a Freudian and he had some unusual ideas. He told her that she was having sex with her father, that she had repressed the memory of it.

He called her father and asked him to come for a session. Dr. Cox said to him, "I know about your incestuous relationship with your daughter."

Kristin's father responded, "I think you have the wrong idea."

Dr. Cox said, "I do not. I will now leave you two alone to talk."

She said neither of them knew what to say. Her father said, "I'm sorry if I haven't been as good a parent as I could have."

He got up to leave the psychiatric ward. Kristin reached up to hug him goodbye. He recoiled. He said, "I'll call you."

Kristin thought, "Dr. Cox, you asshole. Maybe my dad did triangulate me. But at least he was a parent close to me that I did get some kind of affection from. It's been funny since then. My dad is not that kind of person. He never touched me physically at all." Dr. Cox had the idea that he would "re-parent"Kristin.

While she was in the hospital she was forced to take antidepressant drugs, which made her nervous. One of her main fears was that she would be 'electro-shocked.' Dr. Cox had told her, "If you do what you're told you will not have to have it." She remembers that Tuesday and Thursday were electro-shock days and Dr. Cox would line everybody up.

One woman, Frankie, was bummed out because she had walked home one day and found her husband in bed with her best friend. She made a suicide attempt. I don't think it's that abnormal—a reaction to losing the two most important people in your life at once. And Dr. Cox gave her ECT the next day, before the drugs were even out of her system. Then she came back delirious. ECT causes brain damage, which makes you temporarily euphoric. Frankie was giddy and euphoric for a couple of days. She acted silly. But two days later she was sitting right back in the corner, moaning and crying. I would go into the room and try to talk to her. I would say to her, "Do you want to talk?" But the nurses would always come in and say, "Leave her alone. She needs to be alone." Then two or three days later Dr. Cox would come to give her another ECT treatment and she would say, "Oh, no! Not again!"

I was scared to death they'd give it to me. I thought to myself, 'Don't look depressed, whatever the hell you do. And eat all your supper, for God's sake, and try to think what this 70-year-old man wants you to act like and look like so he doesn't think you are depressed.'

Kristin didn't see anyone who was helped by the ECT. Another woman who had it seemed indifferent when she came back. Kristin noticed that she would just sleep a lot more.

After a month in the hospital Dr. Cox released her. She went home and resumed working as a waitress in a restaurant. She continued to see Dr. Cox once a month for antidepressants and psychotherapy. I asked her why she continued to see him. She said, "The first year and a half I thought he was really going to help. I didn't know what else to do. I thought, 'Maybe he knows something I don't know.' I knew later on, of course, that he didn't. But I thought maybe there was some pill that would make things stop hurting. I know better now."

The sessions did nothing to stimulate her or to boost her self-confidence or to motivate her. "Dr. Cox would ask me questions about my childhood first, and then he would just get bored. Several times he even fell asleep when I was talking. And then he'd just give me another prescription."

The drugs did nothing to make her pain go away. "Why should they?" she asked. "My living situation hadn't changed at all." Her sisters had both escaped from the home and were in college getting all A's. The same pattern persisted in her relationship with her parents. Her mother would get drunk and hit her father, who would sit there passively. She would criticize Kristin viciously. "She told me that she and Dad had a wonderful relationship until I came along." Later in the evening Kristin's father would go to her bedroom and apologize for not sticking up for her. She would ask, "Why didn't you protect me?"

He would start crying and saying, "I just can't."

Sometimes he would go to sleep at the foot of her bed. "He seemed like a lost kid to me. He'd always talk to me about their problems. I felt stuck right in the middle and terrified my mother was going to walk in and hear my father confiding in me."

New Diagnosis, New Drugs

This went on for a year and a half after she got out of the hospital. It was around this time that Dr. Cox decided that she was not a depressive-neurotic after all, but a 'pseudo-neurotic schizophrenic.' He decided to put her on Stelazine and Prolixin. He gave her these new drugs and told her to take them. She agreed.

She went home. "I took the drug and I thought I was going to die. I couldn't walk. I felt a strong disinclination to live. I could not get out of bed. My arms were like metal and the bed was like a magnet. My tongue was all rolled up in my mouth. My toes were in spasms. I couldn't move. I peed in my bed."

The next day she called Dr. Cox and told him that the drugs were making her sick. He said, "I gave you the smallest dosage. It's not possible that you feel that way."

Kristin was shocked. She responded, "But I do! And when I don't take them I don't feel that bad. When I do take them I do."

Dr. Cox responded, "Well, that's just part of your illness. It's a deeper psychosis coming on. I could have predicted this."

"I said to him, 'My eyes were rolling back in my head, my tongue was hanging out of my mouth jerking around and once I could move again I found myself constantly pacing up and down the floor.'"

Dr. Cox was adamant. "This is part of your illness."

"I said to him, 'Before I went into the hospital all I felt was sad.'"

At this point, her confidence in Dr. Cox was thoroughly undermined. She began to think about things differently. "I felt that I was sad because I had a terrible relationship with my mom and dad, and I went to another relationship that I really depended on and he about half-killed me. I was just very grieved. I was never given the opportunity to grieve. And that's what turned into what they called a 'depression.'"

The next visit that she was scheduled to see him, she got to the office early and snuck into the room where her chart was. It was on the desk. She looked at it. She saw that the diagnosis had been changed from "depressive neurosis" to "pseudo-neurotic schizophrenia." This explained why he had decided to put her on different drugs.

"Were you doing anything differently?" I asked.

She responded that she had started working in a new restaurant and she was dating the grill cook. She thought that Dr. Cox did not approve of her going out with someone with such a lowly occupation, particularly as she herself came from an upper middle-class professional family. Her relationship with the grill cook ended after several months.

By this time she was 24 years old. She'd made friends with Jeff, a man about ten years older than she was and she moved into his three-bedroom house. After living there for several months they became lovers. She felt more confident in herself and she started college.

Her relationship with Jeff was complicated by her parents' opposition. Despite the fact that she was living away from them and had a boyfriend, her parents attempted to include her once again in their relationship. The family would not reorganize to accept Kristin's independence. "I'd call my mom and she said, 'Don't call me, we're not your family any more. Jeff and Timmy are your family now. You have a retarded stepson now to take care of.' " (Jeff's eight-year-old son was slightly retarded.)

Kristin was having a hard time separating from her parents because she had such a strong yearning for their approval. "Jeff was a working-class guy and my parents never approved. I loved him but I was torn. I thought if I got rid of this guy, if I get my college degree, then I'll get approval from my parents. I finally realized that no matter what I did they wouldn't approve."

She remembers vividly one incident that occurred shortly before she and Jeff broke up. Her parents were coming over to visit her and Jeff. Her father called to say that her mother was drunk and had jumped out of the car on the way over. "Please help me find your mother," he pleaded.

Jeff and Kristin got in a car and began to look for her. They found her in a field and brought her back to their home. She started hitting Jeff. "I pulled her off Jeff. She started punching me. She kept hitting me repeatedly, over and over again. Jeff finally succeeded in pulling her off me."

Jeff thought formalizing their relationship might make it stronger. He asked Kristin to marry him. She agreed. He gave her a ring. She was talking to her mother one day on the phone and her mother was criticizing her, saying, "Why do you want to marry him? He's just a factory worker."

She said, "I'm not really engaged to him, I'm going to give him back the ring. I just don't know how to tell him yet."

Jeff heard her. He was very hurt. Two days later he said to her, "When are you going to give back the ring?"

At that point she did not know what to do. She felt torn in different directions. She went out, started getting drunk and sleeping around. On the one hand she felt she loved him; on the other hand she felt that she was "supposed to end up with somebody more educated and more intellectual. I relied on my parents to give him the stamp of approval."

One day she came home from a bar late at night to find that Jeff had taken all her stuff out of the house and loaded it up in her station wagon. She called her mother and went over to her parents' house. She was sleeping on the couch and her mother came out and was "peering" at Kristin. "I started seeing malicious expressions on her face. I thought to myself, 'She's going to kill me.' It's not as crazy as it seems, considering that just several weeks ago she had almost beaten me to death and that she had undermined my relationship with my fiance. I cried out to my father, 'Daddy, she's going to kill me!' "

New Diagnosis, More New Drugs

She agreed to go with her parents to the psychiatric ward at the hospital. When she got there her mother told the psychiatrist that she had delusions. She was diagnosed as a manic-depressive. She refused to take the Lithium. They then changed her diagnosis to 'undifferentiated schizophrenia.' They tried to persuade her to take Triliphon. She took one pill and she had to go to bed for two days, she was so sick. She continued to refuse to take any drugs. The doctors threatened to give her ECT but no action was taken.

While she was there a woman that she had become friendly with committed suicide. This was right after the woman had been given ECT. She'd jumped through a plate-glass window 15 minutes after the treatment and fell three stories to her death. Kristin wanted to know what drug this woman had been on. She asked the nurse if she could see the Physician's Desk Reference. The nurse threatened to put her in seclusion.

They told her that if she did not take the Lithium she would not be released from the hospital. So she took it.

"It made everything monotonous. I didn't care about anything. If someone had told me that my mother or father had died I would have just said, 'Hmm-mmm.' I couldn't get excited about anything. When I got out of the hospital they sent me to a mental health center. They said I'd have to take Lithium for the rest of my life. They said I was a manic-depressive."

I said to them, "I've never been manic."

They said, "Well, you're depressed, then."

I said, "No, I'm not depressed, I'm sad."

They can't understand that. It didn't mean that I was mentally ill or defective. It was natural for me to be sad. My marriage had failed, my parents sucked rocks, I had nowhere to go except back to the fiance that I was fighting with because of my parents. What was I supposed to be so thrilled about?

The Expert: The denial of pathology demonstrates the fragility of the patient's ego. She must accept that she must stay on Lithium for the rest of her life in order to prevent a more serious decompensation. She will never be able to lead a normal life or to have intimate heterosexual relationships. The damage is too severe and the ego is not strong enough to withstand the re-activation of the initial transference. She should avoid over-stimulation and be given supportive therapy to help her cope and to form friendships that are not too demanding.

She moved in with one of her closest girlfriends. The woman was divorced, with two kids. Kristin helped to take care of the kids. "She made me feel it was nice to have me around. That was the closest thing I'd had to having a family. I had never felt that before. That was one of the happiest times of my life."

Kristin finished college and eventually moved several hours away from her mother's home to go to graduate school. She decided to get a master's degree in counseling. She thought that she could work within the system to help people to change. She finished her master's degree in two years and has been working as a counselor for several years now. She has not taken any psychiatric drugs since her last hospitalization, over eight years ago.

She is not pleased with her job.

"The mental health system has ripped me off twice, first as a patient then as a counselor. I thought I could work within the system. I was wrong. You can't show any human emotion because they're mental-health trained. They look for symptoms in everything and everybody, especially at work. They look down on me because I was a mental patient. They even told me not to tell any of the clients that I had ever been in a mental hospital because the clients wouldn't respect me. Sometimes I think I'm in a room filled with psychoanalysts and they're analyzing me all day long. For example, they seem to have no respect for the clients. All the things I feared that the mental health professionals thought about us are worse than what I thought it was from the other side. They think less of us and more degrading of us than I would have ever imagined in my most horrible dreams in the hospital. They've confirmed everything I've ever dreaded."

One of the clients had gotten mad at one of the mental health workers because they were treating him in a condescending manner, as if he were a child. This "patient," Conrad, said, "Just because I am a mental patient doesn't mean I don't know how to brush my teeth or shower, or that I can't take care of myself." So of course they said he had a paranoid delusion. The patient is paranoid if he or she thinks therapists talk about them. But we do. You do talk about them when they're gone. You all get together and talk about how paranoid they are that they think you're talking about them. It's crazy.

A psychiatrist said about this one patient who showed some independence, "He's a good paranoid schiz." I thought to myself, "Did you hear *anything* he said?" They didn't hear anything he said. And he quit today and I don't blame him. They engage continually in client-bashing in the treatment team. I brought in some writings that one of my clients had composed, and they just passed them around and they laughed and they laughed.

They listen to them in their sessions and they feel sorry for them but they basically don't care what they do with their lives. They don't help them to get their lives together.

Kristin feels that she has for the most part extricated herself from the marital triangle that her parents attempted to involve her in. She now lives three hours away from her parents and sees them less frequently. Sometimes she finds herself yearning once again for her parents' approval of what she's doing, but she is learning to break that habit and rely more on her own instincts. "If I tell my mother what I really feel about the mental health establishment she starts screaming, 'Wait a minute, wait a minute! You're supposed to be in the mental health establishment. You're just setting yourself up for a failure and you're going to end up back in the hospital and all this shit.' I can't talk to them at all."

She regrets that her parents do not have a more happy life together, but she knows that this is outside her power to change. Kristin is at a turning point in her life. From her own independent perspective, she sees all the flaws in the mental health system. She has developed the confidence to trust her own judgment and common sense.

She had escaped being inducted into the role of a chronic mental patient. But she is now stuck within a new role, a role with which she does not identify but which remains her source of livelihood. She is a social control agent whose job it is to attempt to induce individuals to accept the role of chronic mental patients. Her position in the agency is precarious and she refuses to perform this function and encourages 'patients' to become more independent. But she is keenly aware of the narrow limits of her power within a system that is organized in such a manner as to undermine individuals' confidence in their ability to function competently. Once again she is trapped and once again she is looking forward to the day when she will finally make her escape. She remains a rebel with a cause.

Six months after the above was written, Kristen left her job. "There was too much pressure on me to manipulate and intimidate the clients into taking drugs. When I helped people to get off drugs, the staff threatened to have me fired. I quit first."

Kristen has now been living with a new boyfriend for two years, and is happy in that relationship. She is about to commence a new career.

From The Flamingo's Smile: Reflections in Natural History

STEPHEN JAY GOULD

CARRIE BUCK'S DAUGHTER

THE LORD really put it on the line in his preface to that prototype of all prescription, the Ten Commandments:

> ... for I, the Lord thy God, am a jealous God, visiting the iniquity of the fathers upon the children unto the third and fourth generation of them that hate me (Exod. 20:5).

The terror of this statement lies in its patent unfairness—its promise to punish guiltless offspring for the misdeeds of their distant forebears.

A different form of guilt by genealogical association attempts to remove this stigma of injustice by denying a cherished premise of Western thought—human free will. If offspring are tainted not simply by the deeds of their parents but by a material form of evil transferred directly by biological inheritance, then "the iniquity of the fathers" becomes a signal or warning for probable misbehavior of their sons. Thus Plato, while denying that children should suffer directly for the crimes of their parents, nonetheless defended the banishment of a personally guiltless man whose father, grandfather, and great-grandfather had all been condemned to death.

It is, perhaps, merely coincidental that both Jehovah and Plato chose three generations as their criterion for establishing different forms of guilt by association. Yet we maintain a strong folk, or vernacular, tradition for viewing triple occurrences as minimal evidence of regularity. Bad things, we are told, come in threes. Two may represent an accidental association; three is a pattern. Perhaps, then, we should not wonder that our own century's most famous pronouncement of blood guilt employed the same criterion—Oliver Wendell Holmes's defense of compulsory sterilization in Virginia (Supreme Court decision of 1927 in *Buck v. Bell*): "three generations of imbeciles are enough."

Restrictions upon immigration, with national quotas set to discriminate against those deemed mentally unfit by early versions of IQ testing, marked the greatest triumph of the American eugenics movement—the flawed hereditarian doctrine, so popular earlier in our century and by no means extinct today, that attempted to "improve" our human stock by preventing the propagation of those deemed biologically unfit and encouraging procreation among the supposedly worthy. But the movement to enact and enforce laws for compulsory "eugenic" sterilization had an impact and success scarcely less pronounced. If we could debar the shiftless and the stupid from our shores, we might also prevent the propagation of those similarly afflicted but already here.

The movement for compulsory sterilization began in earnest during the 1890s, abetted by two major factors—the rise of eugenics as an influential political movement and the perfection of safe and simple operations (vasectomy for men and salpingectomy, the cutting and tying of Fallopian tubes, for women) to replace castration and other socially unacceptable forms of mutilation. Indiana passed the first sterilization act based on eugenic principles in 1907 (a few states had previously mandated castration as a punitive measure for certain sexual crimes, although such laws were rarely enforced and usually overturned by judicial review). Like so many others to follow, it provided for sterilization of afflicted people residing in the state's "care," either as inmates of mental hospitals and homes for the feebleminded or as inhabitants of prisons. Sterilization could be imposed upon those judged insane, idiotic, imbecilic, or moronic, and upon convicted rapists or criminals when recommended by a board of experts.

By the 1930s, more than thirty states had passed similar laws, often with an expanded list of so-called hereditary defects, including alcoholism and drug addiction in some states, and even blindness and deafness in others. These laws were continually challenged and rarely enforced in most states; only California and Virginia applied them zealously. By January 1935, some 20,000 forced "eugenic" sterilizations had been performed in the United States, nearly half in California.

No organization crusaded more vociferously and successfully for these laws than the Eugenics Record Office, the semiofficial arm and repository of data for the eugenics movement in America. Harry Laughlin, superintendent of the Eugenics Record Office, dedicated most of his career to a tireless campaign of writing and lobbying for eugenic sterilization. He hoped, thereby, to eliminate in two generations the genes of what he called the "submerged tenth"—"the most worthless one-tenth of our present population." He proposed a "model sterilization law" in 1922, designed to prevent the procreation of persons socially inadequate from defective inheritance, by authorizing and providing for eugenical sterilization of certain potential parents carrying degenerate hereditary qualities.

This model bill became the prototype for most laws passed in America, although few states cast their net as widely as Laughlin advised. (Laughlin's categories encompassed "blind, including those with seriously impaired vision; deaf, including those with seriously impaired hearing; and dependent, including orphans, ne'er-do-wells, the homeless, tramps, and paupers.") Laughlin's suggestions were better heeded in Nazi Germany, where his model act inspired the infamous and stringently enforced *Erbgesundheitsrecht*, leading by the eve of World War II to the sterilization of some 375,000 people, most for "congenital feeblemindedness," but including nearly 4,000 for blindness and deafness.

The campaign for forced eugenic sterilization in America reached its climax and height of respectability in 1927, when the Supreme Court, by an 8-1 vote, upheld the Virginia sterilization bill in *Buck v. Bell*. Oliver Wendell Holmes, then in his mid-eighties and the most celebrated jurist in America, wrote the majority opinion with his customary verve and power of style. It included the notorious paragraph, with its chilling tag line, cited ever since as the quintessential statement of eugenic principles. Remembering with pride his own distant experiences as an infantryman in the Civil War, Holmes wrote:

> We have seen more than once that the public welfare may call upon the best citizens for their lives. It would be strange if it could not call upon those who already sap the strength of the state for these lesser sacrifices. . . . It is better for all the world, if instead of waiting to execute degenerate offspring for crime, or to let them starve for their imbecility, society can prevent those who are manifestly unfit from continuing their kind. The principle that sustains compulsory vaccination is broad enough to cover cutting the Fallopian tubes. Three generations of imbeciles are enough.

Who, then, were the famous "three generations of imbeciles," and why should they still compel our interest?

When the state of Virginia passed its compulsory sterilization law in 1924, Carrie Buck, an eighteen-year-old white woman, lived as an involuntary resident at the State Colony for Epileptics and Feeble-Minded. As the first person selected for sterilization under the new act, Carrie Buck became the focus for a constitutional challenge launched, in part, by conservative Virginia Christians who held, according to eugenical "modernists," antiquated views about individual preferences and "benevolent" state power. (Simplistic political labels do not apply in this case, and rarely in general for that matter. We usually regard eugenics as a conservative movement and its most vocal critics as members of the left. This alignment has generally held in our own decade. But eugenics, touted in its day as the latest in scientific modernism, attracted many liberals and numbered among its most vociferous critics groups often labeled as reactionary and antiscientific. If any political lesson emerges from these shifting allegiances, we might consider the true inalienability of certain human rights.)

But why was Carrie Buck in the State Colony and why was she selected? Oliver Wendell Holmes upheld her choice as judicious in the opening lines of his 1927 opinion:

> Carrie Buck is a feeble-minded white woman who was committed to the State Colony. . . . She is the daughter of a feeble-minded mother in the same institution, and the mother of an illegitimate feeble-minded child.

In short, inheritance stood as the crucial issue (indeed as the driving force behind all eugenics). For if measured mental deficiency arose from malnourishment, either of body or mind, and not from tainted genes, then how could sterilization be justified? If decent food, upbringing, medical care, and education might make a worthy citizen of Carrie Buck's daughter, how could the State of Virginia justify the severing of Carrie's Fallopian tubes against her will? (Some forms of mental deficiency are passed by inheritance in family lines, but most are not—a scarcely surprising conclusion when we consider the thousand shocks that beset us all during our lives, from abnormalities in embryonic growth to traumas of birth, malnourishment, rejection, and poverty. In any case, no fair-minded person today would credit Laughlin's social criteria for the identification of hereditary deficiency—ne'er-do-wells, the homeless, tramps, and paupers—although we shall soon see that Carrie Buck was committed on these grounds.)

When Carrie Buck's case emerged as the crucial test of Virginia's law, the chief honchos of eugenics understood that the time had come to put up or shut up on the crucial issue of inheritance. Thus, the Eugenics Record Office sent Arthur H. Estabrook, their crack fieldworker, to Virginia for a "scientific" study of the case. Harry Laughlin himself provided a deposition, and his brief for inheritance was presented at the local trial that affirmed Virginia's law and later worked its way to the Supreme Court as *Buck v. Bell*.

Laughlin made two major points to the court. First, that Carrie Buck and her mother, Emma Buck, were feebleminded by the Stanford-Binet test of IQ, then in its own infancy. Carrie scored a mental age of nine years, Emma of seven years and eleven months. (These figures ranked them technically as "imbeciles" by definitions of the day, hence Holmes's later choice of words—though his infamous line is often misquoted as "three generations of idiots." Imbeciles displayed a mental age of six to nine years; idiots performed worse, morons better, to round out the old nomenclature of mental deficiency.) Second, that most feeblemindedness resides ineluctably in the genes, and that Carrie Buck surely belonged with this majority. Laughlin reported:

> Generally feeble-mindedness is caused by the inheritance of degenerate qualities; but sometimes it might be caused by environmental factors which are not hereditary. In the case given, the evidence points strongly toward the feeblemindedness and moral delinquency of Carrie Buck being due, primarily, to inheritance and not to environment.

Carrie Buck's daughter was then, and has always been, the pivotal figure of this painful case. I noted in beginning this essay that we tend (often at our peril) to regard two as potential accident and three as an established pattern. The supposed imbecility of Emma and Carrie might have been an unfortunate coincidence, but the diagnosis of similar deficiency for Vivian Buck (made by a social worker, as we shall see, when Vivian was but six months old) tipped the balance in Laughlin's favor and led Holmes to declare the Buck lineage inherently corrupt by deficient heredity. Vivian sealed the pattern—*three* generations of imbeciles are enough. Besides, had Carrie not given illegitimate birth to Vivian, the issue (in both senses) would never have emerged.

Oliver Wendell Holmes viewed his work with pride. The man so renowned for his principle of judicial restraint, who had proclaimed that freedom must not be curtailed without "clear and present danger"—without the equivalent of falsely yelling "fire" in a crowded theater—wrote of his judgment in *Buck v. Bell:* "I felt that I was getting near the first principle of real reform."

And so *Buck v. Bell* remained for fifty years, a footnote to a moment of American history perhaps best forgotten. Then, in 1980, it reemerged to prick our collective conscience, when Dr. K. Ray Nelson, then director of the Lynchburg Hospital where Carrie Buck had been sterilized, researched the records of his institution and discovered that more than 4,000 sterilizations had been performed, the last as late as 1972. He also found Carrie Buck, alive and well near Charlottesville, and her sister Doris, covertly sterilized under the same law (she was told that her operation was for appendicitis), and now, with fierce dignity, dejected and bitter because she had wanted a child more than anything else in her life and had finally, in her old age, learned why she had never conceived.

As scholars and reporters visited Carrie Buck and her sister, what a few experts had known all along became abundantly clear to everyone. Carrie Buck was a woman of obviously normal intelligence. For example, Paul A. Lombardo of the School of Law at the University of Virginia, and a leading scholar of *Buck v. Bell*, wrote in a letter to me:

> As for Carrie, when I met her she was reading newspapers daily and joining a more literate friend to assist at regular bouts with the crossword puzzles. She was not a sophisticated woman, and lacked social graces, but mental health professionals who examined her in later life confirmed my impressions that she was neither mentally ill nor retarded.

On what evidence, then, was Carrie Buck consigned to the State Colony for Epileptics and Feeble-Minded on January 23, 1924? I have seen the text of her commitment hearing; it is, to say the least, cursory and contradictory. Beyond the bald and undocumented say-so of her foster parents, and her own brief appearance before a commission of two doctors and a justice of the peace, no evidence was presented. Even the crude and early Stanford-Binet test, so fatally flawed as a measure of innate worth (see my book *The Mismeasure of Man*, although the evidence of Carrie's own case suffices) but at least clothed with the aura of quantitative respectability, had not yet been applied.

When we understand why Carrie Buck was committed in January 1924, we can finally comprehend the hidden meaning of her case and its message for us today. The silent key, again as from the first, is her daughter Vivian, born on March 28, 1924, and then but an evident bump on her belly. Carrie Buck was one of several illegitimate children borne by her mother, Emma. She grew up with foster parents, J. T. and Alice Dobbs, and continued to live with them as an adult, helping out with chores around the house. She was raped by a relative of her foster parents, then blamed for the resulting pregnancy. Almost surely, she was (as they used to say) committed to hide her shame (and her rapist's identity), not because enlightened science had just discovered her true mental status. In short, she was sent away to have her baby. Her case never was about mental deficiency; Carrie Buck was persecuted for supposed sexual immorality and social deviance. The annals of her trial and hearing reek with the contempt of the well-off and well-bred for poor people of "loose morals." Who really cared whether Vivian was a baby of normal intelligence; she was the illegitimate child of an illegitimate woman. Two generations of bastards are enough. Harry Laughlin began his "family history" of the Bucks by writing: "These people belong to the shiftless, ignorant and worthless class of antisocial whites of the South."

We know little of Emma Buck and her life, but we have no more reason to suspect her than her daughter Carrie of true mental deficiency. Their supposed deviance was social and sexual; the charge of imbecility was a cover-up, Mr. Justice Holmes notwithstanding.

We come then to the crux of the case, Carrie's daughter, Vivian. What evidence was ever adduced for her mental deficiency? This and only this: At the original trial in late 1924, when Vivian Buck was seven months old, a Miss Wilhelm, social worker for the Red Cross, appeared before the court. She began by stating honestly the true reason for Carrie Buck's commitment:

> Mr. Dobbs, who had charge of the girl, had taken her when a small child, had reported to Miss Duke [the temporary secretary of Public Welfare for Albemarle County] that the girl was pregnant and that he wanted to have her committed somewhere—to have her sent to some institution.

Miss Wilhelm then rendered her judgment of Vivian Buck by comparing her with the normal granddaughter of Mrs. Dobbs, born just three days earlier:

> It is difficult to judge probabilities of a child as young as that, but it seems to me not quite a normal baby. In its appearance—I should say that perhaps my knowledge of the mother may prejudice me in that regard, but I saw the child at the same time as Mrs. Dobbs' daughter's baby, which is only three days older than this one, and there is a very decided difference in the development of the babies. That was about two weeks ago. There is a look about it that is not quite normal, but just what it is, I can't tell.

This short testimony, and nothing else, formed all the evidence for the crucial third generation of imbeciles. Cross-examination revealed that neither Vivian nor the Dobbs grandchild could walk or talk, and that "Mrs. Dobbs' daughter's baby is a very responsive baby. When you play with it or try to attract its attention—it is a baby that you can play with. The other baby is not. It seems very apathetic and not responsive." Miss Wilhelm then urged Carrie Buck's sterilization: "I think," she said, "it would at least prevent the propagation of her kind." Several years later, Miss Wilhelm denied that she had ever examined Vivian or deemed the child feebleminded.

Unfortunately, Vivian died at age eight of "enteric colitis" (as recorded on her death certificate), an ambiguous diagnosis that could mean many things but may well indicate that she fell victim to one of the preventable childhood diseases of poverty (a grim reminder of the real subject in *Buck v. Bell*). She is therefore mute as a witness in our reassessment of her famous case.

STEPHEN JAY GOULD 37

When *Buck v. Bell* resurfaced in 1980, it immediately struck me that Vivian's case was crucial and that evidence for the mental status of a child who died at age eight might best be found in report cards. I have therefore been trying to track down Vivian Buck's school records for the past four years and have finally succeeded. (They were supplied to me by Dr. Paul A. Lombardo, who also sent other documents, including Miss Wilhelm's testimony, and spent several hours answering my questions by mail and Lord knows how much time playing successful detective in researching Vivian's school records. I have never met Dr. Lombardo; he did all this work for kindness, collegiality, and love of the game of knowledge, not for expected reward or even requested acknowledgment. In a profession—academics—so often marred by pettiness and silly squabbling over meaningless priorities, this generosity must be recorded and celebrated as a sign of how things can and should be.)

Vivian Buck was adopted by the Dobbs family, who had raised (but later sent away) her mother, Carrie. As Vivian Alice Elaine Dobbs, she attended the Venable Public Elementary School of Charlottesville for four terms, from September 1930 until May 1932, a month before her death. She was a perfectly normal, quite average student, neither particularly outstanding nor much troubled. In those days before grade inflation, when C meant "good, 81–87" (as defined on her report card) rather than barely scraping by, Vivian Dobbs received A's and B's for deportment and C's for all academic subjects but mathematics (which was always difficult for her, and where she scored D) during her first term in Grade 1A, from September 1930 to January 1931. She improved during her second term in 1B, meriting an A in deportment, C in mathematics, and B in all other academic subjects; she was placed on the honor roll in April 1931. Promoted to 2A, she had trouble during the fall term of 1931, failing mathematics and spelling but receiving A in deportment, B in reading, and C in writing and English. She was "retained in 2A" for the next term—or "left back" as we used to say, and scarcely a sign of imbecility as I remember all my buddies who suffered a similar fate. In any case, she again did well in her final term, with B in deportment, reading, and spelling, and C in writing, English, and mathematics during her last month in school. This daughter of "lewd and immoral" women excelled in deportment and performed adequately, although not brilliantly, in her academic subjects.

In short, we can only agree with the conclusion that Dr. Lombardo has reached in his research on *Buck v. Bell*—there were no imbeciles, not a one, among the three generations of Bucks. I don't know that such correction of cruel but forgotten errors of history counts for much, but I find it both symbolic and satisfying to learn that forced eugenic sterilization, a procedure of such dubious morality, earned its official justification (and won its most quoted line of rhetoric) on a patent falsehood.

Carrie Buck died last year. By a quirk of fate, and not by memory or design, she was buried just a few steps from her only daughter's grave. In the umpteenth and ultimate verse of a favorite old ballad, a rose and a brier—the sweet and the bitter—emerge from the tombs of Barbara Allen and her lover, twining about each other in the union of death. May Carrie and Vivian, victims in different ways and in the flower of youth, rest together in peace.

From Rewriting the Soul

IAN HACKING

CHAPTER 1: IS IT REAL?

AS LONG AGO as 1982 psychiatrists were talking about "the multiple personality epidemic."[1] Yet those were early days. Multiple personality—whose "essential feature is the existence within the individual of two or more distinct personalities, each of which is dominant at a particular time"—became an official diagnosis of the American Psychiatric Association only in 1980.[2] Clinicians were still reporting occasional cases as they appeared in treatment. Soon the number of patients would become so overwhelming that only statistics could give an impression of the field.

Ten years earlier, in 1972, multiple personality had seemed to be a mere curiosity. "Less than a dozen cases have been reported in the last fifty years."[3] You could list every multiple personality recorded in the history of Western medicine, even if experts disagreed on how many of these cases were genuine. None? Eighty-four? More than one hundred, with the first clear description given by a German physician in 1791?[4] Whatever number you favored, the word for the disorder was *rare.*

Ten years later, in 1992, there were hundreds of multiples in treatment in every sizable town in North America. Even by 1986 it was thought that six thousand patients had been diagnosed.[5] After that, one stopped counting and spoke about an exponential increase in the rate of diagnosis since 1980. Clinics, wards, units, and entire private hospitals dedicated to the illness were being established all over the continent. Maybe one person in twenty suffered from a dissociative disorder.[6]

What has happened? Is a new form of madness, hitherto almost unknown, stalking the continent? Or have multiples always been around, unrecognized? Were they classified, when they needed help, as suffering from something else? Perhaps clinicians have only recently learned to make correct diagnoses. It is far easier, they say, now that we know the most common cause of dissociated personalities—early and repeated sexual abuse in childhood. Only a society prepared to acknowledge that family violence is everywhere could find multiple personalities everywhere.

Or, as a majority of psychiatrists still contend, is there simply no such thing as multiple personality disorder? Is the epidemic the work of a small but committed band of therapists, unwittingly aided and abetted by sensational stories in the tabloids and afternoon TV talk shows?

We at once arrive at what sounds like the big question: *Is it real?* That is the first question people ask me when they hear I am interested in multiple personality. It is not only amateurs who ask. The American Psychiatric Association staged a debate at its annual meeting of 1988: "Resolved That Multiple Personality Is a True Disease Entity." For: Richard Kluft and David Spiegel. Against: Fred Frankel and Martin Orne. The debaters, all leading professionals, remain in bitter disagreement today. The rest of us, once we see how vehemently the two camps of experts oppose each other, are bewildered. Multiple personality has become the most contested type of diagnosis in psychiatry. So we bystanders repeat, rather helplessly: Is it real?

What is "it," this controversial multiple personality? Not schizophrenia. Schizophrenia is often called split personality, so we reason that multiple personality = split personality = schizophrenia. Not so. The name *schizophrenia* was introduced at the beginning of the twentieth century. It is Greek for "split brain." The metaphor of splitting has been used in many different ways—Freud, for example, used it in three distinct ways at different stages in his career.[7] The idea behind the name schizophrenia was that a person's thoughts, emotions, and physical reactions are split off from each other, so that the emotional reaction to a thought, or the physical response to an emotion, is completely inappropriate or bizarre. There are delusions, thought disorders, and a terrible range of suffering. It is unclear whether schizophrenia is one disease or several. One form of it develops in the late teens or early twenties, so that this disease was once called *dementia praecox,* or premature senility. Schizophrenia probably has neurochemical causes; some forms of it might be genetic. Since the 1960s there has been an increasing battery of drugs that radically improve the quality of life for many schizophrenics.

None of the things I have just said about schizophrenia is true of multiple personality. No medication has specific effects on multiple personality as such, although switches in personality, like any other exceptional behavior, can be damped down by mood-altering drugs. Multiple personality has most commonly been first diagnosed in patients over thirty years of age, not in adolescence. It is not characterized by a splitting of thought, emotion, and bodily response. Multiple personality may mimic schizophrenia, in that there may be short periods of "schizophreniform" behavior, but these episodes do not endure. I shall return to schizophrenia, but for the present we must put it to one side.

So what is multiple personality? I will begin by being quite formal, using official guidelines. There are two widely used standard classifications of mental illness. One is part of the International Classification of Diseases, published by the World Health Organization in Geneva. The tenth edition of 1992, called *ICD-10,* does not have a separate category for multiple personality, although it does have an extended classification of types of dissociation.[8] *ICD-10* is used primarily in Europe, where most psychiatric establishments are disdainful of the multiple personality diagnosis. Another classification is the *Diagnostic and Statistical Manual of Mental Disorders,* authorized by the American Psychiatric Association. It sets the standard in North America and, despite *ICD-10,* is widely used overseas. In its third edition of 1980, called *DSM-III,* the diagnostic criteria for multiple personality disorder were:

A. The existence within the individual of two or more distinct personalities, each of which is dominant at a particular time.
B. The personality that is dominant at any particular time determines the individual's behavior.
C. Each individual personality is complex and integrated with its own unique behavior pattern and social relationships.[9]

These criteria, abstract as they are, matter to both research and practice. The great American psychiatric journals require that results be written up according to the classification of the current *Diagnostic and Statistical Manual.* Insurance companies and publicly funded health plans reimburse doctors, hospitals, and clinics according to a schedule coded by the current *DSM.*

The criteria were made less restrictive in the revised *Manual* of 1987, *DSM-III-R,* where condition C was deleted. The personalities no longer had to be complex and integrated, or to manifest distinct social relationships.[10] Hence more individuals could be diagnosed with multiple personality. But in research at the National Institute of Mental Health, Frank Putnam insisted on criteria more stringent than *DSM-III,* not less. "The diagnosing clinician must: (1) witness a switch between two alter personality states; (2) must meet a given alter personality on at least three separate occasions to assess the degree of uniqueness and stability of the alter personality state; and (3) must establish that the patient has amnesias, either by witnessing amnesic behavior or by the patient's report."[11] The amnesia condition, as we shall see, was built in to the criteria of *DSM-IV* in 1994.

The changes do not seem to matter to the pressing question: whether there is such a thing as multiple personality. The straightforward answer is plainly yes. There were patients who satisfied the criteria of 1980. More satisfied the criteria of 1987. Some satisfy Putnam's more stringent protocol. No matter what criteria are used, the rate of diagnosis has been growing apace. There are plenty of questions about what multiple personality is, and how to define it, but the simple conclusion is that there is such a disorder.

So that's the answer? There really is such a thing as multiple personality, because this or that book of rules lists some symptoms, and some patients have those symptoms? We should be more fastidious than that. To begin with, the question "Is it real?" is not of itself a clear one. The classic examination of the word "real" is due to the doyen of ordinary language philosophers, J. L. Austin. As he insisted, you have to ask, "A real *what?*" Moreover, "a definite sense attaches to the assertion that something is real, a real such-and-such, only in the light of a specific way in which it might be, or might have been *not* real."[12] Something may fail to be real cream because the butterfat content is too low, or because it is synthetic creamer. A man may not be a real constable because he is impersonating a police officer, or because he has not yet been sworn in, or because he is a military policeman, not a civil one. A painting may fail to be a real Constable because it is a forgery, or because it is a copy, or because it is an honest work by one of John Constable's students, or simply because it is an inferior work of the master. The moral is, if you ask, "Is it real?" you must supply a noun. You have to ask, "Is it a real *N?*" (or, "Is it real *N?*"). Then you have to indicate how it might fail to be a real *N*, "a real *N* as opposed to what?" Even that is no guarantee that a question about what's real will make sense. Even with a noun and an alternative, we may not have a real anything: there is no such thing as the "real" color of a deep-sea fish.

The American Psychiatric Association debate asked whether multiple personality "is a true disease entity." Colin Ross, a leading advocate of multiple personality, says that "the APA debate was incorrectly titled because MPD is not a true *disease* entity in the biomedical sense. It is a true psychiatric entity and a true disorder, but not a biomedical disease."[13] The APA provided a noun phrase ("disease entity"), and Ross offered two more terms ("psychiatric entity" and "disorder"). Do they help? We need to know what a true or real psychiatric entity *is*. A true or real disorder *as opposed to what?*

One question would be: Is multiple personality a real disorder as opposed to a kind of behavior worked up by doctor and patient? If we have to answer yes-or-no, the answer is yes, it is real—that is, multiple personality is not usually "iatrogenic."[14] That answer of course allows for some skepticism, for it might still be that many of the more florid bits of multiple behavior are iatrogenic.

A second question would be: Is multiple personality a real disorder as opposed to a product of social circumstances, a culturally permissible way to express distress or unhappiness? That question makes a presupposition that we should reject. It implies that there is an important contrast between being a real disorder and being a product of social circumstances. The fact that a certain type of mental illness appears only in specific historical or geographical contexts does not imply that it is manufactured, artificial, or in any other way not real. This entire book is about the relationships between multiplicity, memory, discourse, knowledge, and history. It must allow a place for historically constituted illness.

Throughout the history of psychiatry, that is, since 1800, there have been two competing ways to classify mental illness. One model organizes the field according to symptom clusters; disorders are sorted according to how they look. Another organizes according to underlying causes; disorders are sorted according to theories about them. Because of the enormous variety of doctrine among American psychiatrists, it seemed expedient to create a merely symptomatic classification. The idea was that people of different schools could agree on the symptoms, even if disagreeing on causes or treatment. From the very beginning, American *DSMs* have tried to be purely symptomatic. That is one reason for their limited relevance to the question of whether multiple personality is real. A mere collection of symptoms may leave us with the sense that the symptoms may have different causes.

We need to go beyond symptoms, and hence beyond the *DSM*, to settle a reality debate. In all the natural sciences, we feel more confident that something is real when we think we understand its causes. Likewise we feel more confident when we are able to intervene and change it. The questions about multiple personality seem to come down to two issues, familiar in all the sciences: intervention and causation.

Intervention is serious indeed. Does it help a sizable number of clients, who satisfy suitable criteria, to treat them as if they suffer from multiple personality disorder? At present such therapy often involves coming to know numerous personality states, and working with each in order to achieve some sort of integration. Or is that strategy virtually always a bad one—even when someone walks in off the street and claims to be controlled, successively, by three different personalities? The skeptics say that fragmenting should be discouraged from the start. Instead of eliciting more alter personalities and thus causing the patient to disintegrate further, we should focus on the whole individual and help one person deal responsibly with immediate crises, dysfunction, confusion, and despair. Advocates call that "benign neglect" and say it is ineffective in the long run. But more cautious multiple clinicians do discourage fragmenting, even when they are willing to diagnose multiple personality in the long haul.[15]

The argument is not only about how to interact with some troubled people. The working clinician is seldom a total empiric; disease and disorder are identified according to an underlying vision of health and of humanity, of what kinds of beings we are, and what can go wrong with us. That is why, as we shall see, the multiple personality field is so full of models of dissociation. We want to understand as well as to heal: practice demands theory. One kind of theory is causal, and so we pass from intervention to causation. The multiple personality field has been solidified by the causal idea that multiplicity is a coping mechanism, a response to early and repeated trauma, often sexual in nature.

When seen to be connected with child abuse, multiple personality prompts strong opinions about the family, about patriarchy, about violence. Many therapists of multiples are also feminists who are convinced that the roots of a patient's trouble came from the home, from neglect, from cruelty, from overt sexual assault, from male indifference, from oppression by a social system that favors men. It is no accident, they say, that most multiples are women, for women have had to bear the brunt of family violence from the time they were infants. Dissociation begins when babies and children are abused. A commitment to multiple personality becomes a social commitment. What kind of healer do you want to be? That is not only a question about how you conduct your practice: it is a question about how you want to live your life.

We hear moral conviction on all sides. Psychiatrists who reject multiple personality are accused of complacently dismissing the victims, the abused, the women and children. Is that true? Do the majority of doctors need to have their consciousness raised? There are less inflammatory explanations for their opposition. One has to do with institutions, training, and power. There has been a populist, grassroots air to the multiple personality movement. Many of the clinicians are not M.D.s or Ph.D. psychologists but hold another credential—a master of social work degree, a nursing qualification, right down (in the pecking order) to people who have taken a couple of weekend courses in memory regression and are in no strict sense qualified at all. There is a motley of believers drawn from the rich mixture of eclectic therapies that run rampant in America. Hence the more skeptical psychiatrists distrust the feminism, the populism, the New-Age babble that they hear. These doctors, most of whom are men, not only are at the top of their profession's power structure but also see themselves as scientists, dedicated to objective fact, not social movements. They resent the media hype that surrounds multiple personality. They are dubious about the sheer scope of the epidemic. How can a mental disorder be so at the whim of place and time? How can it disappear and reappear? How can it be everywhere in North America and nonexistent in the rest of the world until it is carried there by missionaries, by clinicians who seem determined to establish beachheads of multiple personality in Europe and Australasia? The only place that multiples flourish overseas is in the Netherlands, and that florescence, say skeptics, was nourished by intensive visiting by the leading American members of the movement.[16]

There are further grounds for professional caution. In the course of some types of therapy, multiples have been encouraged to recover ghastly scenes of long ago, painfully reliving them. Each alter, it is argued, was created to cope with some appalling incident, usually in childhood, and often involving sexual assault by father, stepfather, uncle, brother, baby-sitter. Any supportive therapist committed to multiple personality would, at least during therapy, accept such memories as they surface. But increasingly bizarre events are recalled: cults, rituals, Satan, cannibalism, innocents programmed to do terrible things later in life, adolescent girls used as breeders of babies intended for human sacrifice. These memories include allegations about real people, relatives or neighbors. The resulting accusations seldom stand up to police inquiry, or charges collapse when brought to trial. The credibility of the memory structure of multiples in therapy has thus become suspect, and hence the alters themselves come to look more like a way to act out fantasies.

Such doubts are now institutionalized in a False Memory Syndrome Foundation, established in 1992. This action group is dedicated to supporting accused parents, to litigation, and to publicizing the dangers of irresponsible psychotherapy. It accuses gullible clinicians, including those who work with multiple personality, of generating memories of child abuse that never happened. In return, activists on the other side say that the foundation is a support group for child abusers.

These events are unfolding day by day, but we should not ignore an older complaint about multiple personality. Multiples have always been associated with hypnosis and hypnotic therapy. Some people are more readily hypnotized than others. Multiples are at the top of the scale. They are terribly suggestible. Isn't the elaborate personality structure of multiples unwittingly (or worse, wittingly) encouraged by all-too-willing therapists who use hypnosis or related techniques? Hypnosis is, and has always been, a notorious problem area for psychiatry and the allied arts. Doctors who have favored the use of hypnosis in therapy have tended to be marginalized. It does no good for advocates of multiple personality therapy to protest that multiples seem to develop in therapy in much the same way whether or not the clinician uses hypnosis, for multiple personality is irrevocably tainted with hypnosis. Advocates protest: the suggestibility of the patients is an important clue to their disorder. Multiple personality is only one extreme in a continuum of what are called *dissociative* disorders. Opposition scientists who study hypnosis reply that hypnosis is too complex to be arranged on a linear scale of hypnotizability, and there is no one continuum of dissociation to range alongside of it.[17]

The debate rages. We are not on purely medical terrain. We are deeply involved in morality. Susan Sontag has movingly described how tuberculosis, and then cancer, and then AIDS have been relentlessly inscribed with judgements about the characters of the diseased. Childhood trauma gives a whole new dimension to the morality of the disorder. The most sensational trauma of recent times is child abuse. Abuse, as trauma, enters the equations of morality and medicine. It exculpates, or passes the guilt up to the abuser. Not only is a person with multiple personality genuinely ill: someone else is responsible for the illness. Lest you think that I exaggerate the emphasis on morality and metaphor, consider the opening words at the 1993 annual conference on multiple personality: "AIDS is a plague which attacks individuals. *Child abuse* damages individuals and is the cancer of our society: all too often it flourishes unrecognized and metastasizes across families and generations."[18] AIDS, plague, cancer, metastasizes: we do not need Susan Sontag to help us notice the hyperbolic moral metaphors of multiple personality.

Now let us complete the circle back from morality to causation. It is common, in some psychiatric practice, to diagnose a patient as suffering from several different *DSM* disorders. If we had a system of classification based on causes, that would mean that a person had problems arising from two or more distinct and logically unrelated causes. But *DSM* is symptomatic, so it is not surprising that the life and behavior of a patient should exhibit several different symptom clusters, such as depression, substance abuse, and panic disorder, say. Now the clinician may suspect that one of these clusters gets at the heart of the problem. For example, a classical psychiatrist may give a primary diagnosis of schizophrenia and hold that other behavior—including, perhaps, multiple personality behavior—is subordinate to that underlying cause. Hence he will treat the patient with some cocktail of neuroleptic drugs. The real disorder, he may say, is schizophrenia. The disorder to which all the other disorders are subordinate is sometimes called the superordinate. Primary treatment is for the superordinate disorder, and other symptoms are expected to remit, to some extent, as the superordinate disorder is relieved. Is multiple personality disorder a superordinate diagnosis? Is it the problem to be treated, in the expectation that other problems such as depression, or bulimia, or panic disorder are subordinate to it? Advocates are affirmative.[19] Skeptics completely disagree. In the skeptical opinion, patients who evince multiple personality have problems, but the mutually amnesic personality fragments are mere symptoms of some underlying disorder. "The diagnosis of MPD represents a misdi-

rection of effort which hinders the resolution of serious psychological problems in the lives of the patients."[20]

You may be beginning to think I'm of two minds, just a little bit split myself, when it comes to multiple personality. One moment I am sketching part of
the general theory proposed by experts who take for granted that multiple personality is a real disorder. The next moment I am repeating grounds for skepticism about the very idea of multiple personality. What do *I* think? Is it real, or
is it not?

I am not going to answer that question. I hope that no one who reads this
book will end up wanting to ask exactly that question. This is not because I
have some hang-up about reality or the idea of reality. There is a current fashion, among intellectuals who identify themselves as postmodern, to surround
the word *reality* with a shower of ironical quotation marks. That is not my
fashion. I do not use scare-quotes, and I am not ironical about reality. I expect
that both advocates and opponents of multiple personality will find some of
my discussion distasteful. I have no inclination to take sides. My concern is
not, directly, with uncovering a fundamental timeless truth about personality
or the relationship of fragmentation to psychic pain. I want to know how this
configuration of ideas came into being, and how it has made and molded our
life, our customs, our science.

My very neutrality makes me cautious about even the name of our topic.
Names organize our thoughts. Between 1980 and 1994 the official diagnosis was
"Multiple Personality Disorder." Most people involved in the field said or wrote
simply "MPD." I never do that, except when quoting—because there is nothing
like an acronym to make something permanent, unquestioned. (I use only two
acronyms systematically throughout this book, both for very real entities. One
is *DSM,* abbreviating the name of the manual. The other is ISSMP&D, which
stands for the original name of the multiple movement's professional society,
the International Society for the Study of Multiple Personality and Dissociation.) I shall talk about multiple personality, but very seldom do I even say
"multiple personality disorder." That is partly because I am wary of the word
"disorder." It is the standard all-purpose word used in the *DSM.* It is a good
choice but it cannot help being loaded with values. The word is code for a
vision of the world that ought to be orderly. Order is desirable, it is healthy, it
is a goal. Truth, the true person, is disrupted by disorder. I am cautious about
that picture of pathology. Others actively protest the very word "disorder" for
multiple personality. These radicals suggest that perhaps we are all multiples
really. A few established clinicians have gone almost that far, and one hears the
same thing in some patient support groups.[21]

Another word has attracted more criticism than "disorder"—"personality." In fact Multiple Personality Disorder has just gone out of existence. The official heading in the *DSM-IV* of 1994 is "Dissociative Identity Disorder (*formerly* Multiple Personality Disorder)." Personality has been bracketed. What is happening?

As early as 1984 Philip Coons warned, in one of the most scrupulous essays on the topic during that decade, that "it is a mistake to consider each personality totally separate, whole or autonomous. The other personalities might best be described as personality states, other selves, or personality fragments."[22] That was not at first agreed. In 1986 B. G. Braun suggested a nomenclature distinguishing alter personalities from "fragments."[23] The meaning was that, yes, there are fragments, but there are also personalities.[24]

There is one textbook of our subject, *Diagnosis and Treatment of Multiple Personality Disorder*, by Frank Putnam. It is humane and clear; at its appearance in 1989 it was up-to-the-minute. I shall occasionally take issue with Putnam's work, but that is a sign of real respect, for he is the clearest and most careful authority in the field. In his textbook he emphasized a treatment that involves intensive interaction with all the alters in a personality system. These alters, in his account, have very distinct characters and behaviors. One does get the picture of rather rounded "personalities." He nevertheless issued a salutary warning:

> Overemphasis on multiplicity per se is a common mistake made by therapists new to the disorder. MPD is a fascinating phenomenon that makes one question most of what one has learned about the human mind. A reading of the case report literature from the earliest cases to the present shows that one of the common impulses on the part of therapists is an attempt to document the differences among the alter personalities of their patients. This fascination with the differences of the alters sends a clear message to patients that these are what makes them interesting to therapists and to others.[25]

In a 1992 talk Putnam candidly stated that "very little is known about the alter personalities and what they represent."[26] His increasing reservations about alter personalities are shared by an influential group of psychiatrists within the multiple movement who have long held that the emphasis on personalities is wrongheaded. In 1993 David Spiegel, chair of the dissociative disorders committee for the 1994 *DSM-IV*, wrote that "there is a widespread misunderstanding of the essential psychopathology in this dissociative disorder, which is failure of integration of various aspects of identity, memory, and consciousness. The problem is not having more than one personality; it is having less than one personality."[27] Spiegel asked who originated this aphorism on being less than one personality. One is reminded of Alice (in Wonderland), "for this curious child was very fond of pretending to be two people. 'But it's no use now,' thought poor Alice, 'to pretend to be two people! Why, there is hardly enough of me left to make *one* respectable person!'"[28]

The emphasis on treating alter personalities almost as persons has not, however, gone away. In 1993, the same year that Spiegel made the comment I have just quoted, a clinician and a clergyman were describing the problems of treating a patient who was a devout Christian. Her alters were not. "Because some alter personalities have experienced so little religious involvement, their questions often require very basic religious education."[29] Although there is no inconsistency, it is hard to think in terms of giving religious instruction to a mere fragment.

An emphasis on fragments as opposed to whole personalities is having its effects. The replacement name "Dissociative Identity Disorder" is intended to dispel simplistic ideas that go along with "multiple personality." As Spiegel put it,

> I want to in a sense mainstream this disorder—I don't want it to be seen as some kind of circus sideshow. I want it to be considered as seriously as any other mental disorder. And we took great pains to make the language consistent with that of other disorders. But I felt that the important thing was to emphasize that the main problem is the difficulty in integrating disparate elements of memory, identity and consciousness, rather than the proliferation of personalities.[30]

Spiegel has been strongly criticized for railroading the name change. "The primary constituency of the Dissociative Disorders field is abused men, women and children, and the professionals who treat them."[31] And that constituency was not consulted! Will not the American Psychiatric Association be accused of "acting in a sexist and/or political manner"? The leaders in the movement quickly acknowledged the lay of the land. There was no longer such a thing as multiple personality to study, so the International Society for the Study of Multiple Personality and Dissociation had to change its name. This was done by overwhelming vote at the spring meeting in May 1994; we now have the International Society for the Study of Dissociation.

According to Spiegel, "the name change does not correspond to any change in diagnostic criteria."[32] Yet that is not strictly true. In 1994 the criteria became:

A. The presence of two or more distinct identities or personalities or personality states (each with its own relatively enduring pattern of perceiving, relating to and thinking about the environment and self).

B. At least two of these identities or personality states recurrently take control of the person's behavior.

C. Inability to recall important personal information that is too extensive to be explained by ordinary forgetfulness.

D. The disturbance is not due to the direct physiological effects of a substance (e.g., blackouts or chaotic behavior during Alcohol Intoxication) or a general medical condition (e.g., complex partial seizures). *Note:* In children the symptoms are not attributable to imaginary playmates or other fantasy play.[33]

The final "note" has a subtext. Many advocates wanted a new diagnostic category of childhood multiple personality disorder. They did not succeed but got their foot in the door. They hope to open the door wider in *DSM-V.*

Subtle differences in definition can be a surprisingly useful way to begin to understand how the disorder itself is changing.[34] *DSM-III* required the *existence* of more than one personality or personality state. In 1994 we require only the *presence*. What's the difference between existence and presence? Spiegel explained, "We felt that *existence* conveys some belief that there really are twelve people, when really what we want to underscore is that they experience themselves that way."[35] This tiny change in wording moves us away from actual multiple personalities to an experience that the patient has. Second, "presence" is the word used for the delusions characteristic of the schizophrenias. The parallelism was deliberate. Thus the alters of a multiple personality are, through the change of a mere word, made more analogous to delusions. Spiegel is, in effect, saying that multiple personality is not the main disturbance. The problem is disintegration of the sense of identity. We shall find over and over again that multiple personality is a moving target. Perhaps it has just moved out of sight.

Yet two things are constantly in view, memory and psychic pain. Whether the illness involves more than one personality or less than one, whether we have dissociation or disintegration, the disorder is supposed to be a response to childhood trauma. Memories of the early cruelties are hidden and must be recalled to effect a true integration and cure. Multiple personality and its treatment are grounded upon the supposition that the troubled mind can be understood through increased knowledge about the very nature of memory. I do not intend to question beliefs in multiple personality. I intend instead to find out why it is so taken for granted, by both sides, that memory is the key to the soul.

NOTES

1. M. Boor 1982, The Multiple Personality Epidemic: Additional Cases and Inferences Regarding Diagnosis, Dynamics and Cure. *Journal of Nervous and Mental Disease* 170:302–304.

2. American Psychiatric Association 1980, *Diagnostic and Statistical Manual of Mental Disorders*, 3d ed., 257, Washington, D.C.: American Psychiatric Association, called *DSM-III*.

3. P. Horton and D. Miller 1972, The Etiology of Multiple Personality, *Comparative Psychology* 13:151. Such figures are always underestimates; more extensive literature surveys inevitably turn up more cases.

4. None: see H. Merskey 1992, The Manufacture of Personalities: The Production of Multiple Personality Disorder, *British Journal of Psychiatry* 160:327–340. Eighty-four: this is one count up to 1969; see G. B. Greaves 1980, Multiple Personality: 165 Years after Mary Reynolds, *Journal of Nervous and Mental Disease* 168:578. The 1791 case was noticed in H. Ellenberger 1970, *The Discovery of the Unconscious*, 127, New York: Basic Books.

5. P. M.. Coons 1986, The Prevalence of Multiple Personality Disorder, *Newsletter. International Society for the Study of Multiple Personality and Dissociation* 4(3):6–8.

6. Incidence rates are discussed in chapter 7. For the 5 percent figure, see C. A. Ross, R. Norton, and K. Wozney 1989, Multiple Personality Disorder: An Analysis of 236 Cases. *Canadian Journal of Psychiatry* 34:413–418. For "exponential increase" see Ross 1989, *Multiple Personality Disorder: Diagnosis, Clinical Features and Treatment*, 45, New York: Wiley.

7. J. A. Brook 1992, Freud and Splitting, *International Review of Psychoanalysis* 19:335. The first type of splitting involves dissociation. The second type is the splitting of objects and affects into those which are good and those which are bad, into objects of affection and objects of hostility. The third type is the splitting of the ego into an acting part and a self-observing part. Freud made comments about splitting throughout the whole of his forty-five years of writing about psychology and psychoanalysis.

8. World Health Organization 1992, *The ICD-10 classification of Mental and Behavioural Disorders: Clinical Descriptions and Diagnostic Guidelines*, 151–161, Geneva: World Health Organization. For critical comments on *ICD-10*, from members of the multiple movement, see the essays by F. O. Garcia, Philip Coons, David Spiegel, and W.C. Young in *Dissociation* 3 (1990): 204–221.

9. American Psychiatric Association 1980, 259. S. Kirk 1992 (*The Selling of DSM: The Rhetoric of Science in Psychiatry*, New York: de Gruyter) is a study of how *DSM* criteria have become established, and how the manual itself achieved its present status as definitive.

10. 1987 criteria of *DSM-III-R* (American Psychiatric Association 1987, *Diagnostic and Statistical Manual of Mental Disorders*, 3d ed, rev., 272, Washington, D.C.: American Psychiatric Association, called *DSM-III-R*,) were:

A. The existence within the person of two or more distinct personalities or personality states (each with its own relatively enduring pattern of perceiving, relating to, and thinking about the environment and self).
B. At least two of these identities or personality states recurrently take full control of the person's behavior.

11. This summary is from F. W. Putnam 1993 (Diagnosis and Clinical Phenomenology of Multiple Personality Disorder: A North American Perspective, *Dissociation* 6:80–86) but was in force for the first survey of patients with multiple personality, Putnam et al. 1986 (The Clinical Phenomenology of Multiple Personality Disorder: A Review of One Hundred Recent Cases. *Journal of Clinical Psychiatry* 47:285–293).

12. Austin 1962, *Sense and Sensibilia*, 72, Oxford: Clarendon Press.

13. Ross 1989, 52. "True" is not the same word as "real." Austin held that "real" is the most general adjective of a class of which "true" was an instance. I am not sure he was right, but here it seems immaterial whether the APA or Colin Ross used the adjective "real" or the adjective "true."

14. For one review, see C. B. Wilbur and R. P. Kluft 1989, Multiple Personality Disorder, in *Treatments of Psychiatric Disorders*, Washington, D.C.: American Psychiatric Association, 2197–2198. The most usually addressed question about iatrogenesis is whether multiple personality is induced by hypnosis. The skeptic has something more general in mind and may observe with some justice that the most reliable predictor of the occurrence of multiple personality is a clinician who diagnoses and treats multiples.

15. For the phrase "benign neglect," see, for example, ibid., 2198. For the cautious approach see J. A. Chu 1991, On the Misdiagnosis of Multiple Personality Disorder, *Dissociation* 4:200–204. Chu is not a skeptic; he is the director of the Dissociative Disorders unit at McLean Hospital, Belmont, Mass. He has written about how to help patients overcome their own resistance to the diagnosis of multiple personality; see Chu 1988 (Some Aspects of Resistance in the Treatment of Multiple Personality Disorder. *Dissociation* 1[2]:34–38).

16. For a proud statement of Dutch contributions, see O. van der Hart 1993a (Guest Editorial: Introduction to the Amsterdam Papers, *Dissociation* 6:77–78) and 1993b (Multiple Personality in Europe: Impressions, *Dissociation* 6:102–118). In 1984 and thereafter leading American advocates of multiple personality—Bennet Braun, Richard Kluft, Roberta Sachs—conducted workshops in Holland. For these and other events of the early days, see O. van der Hart and S. Boon 1990 (Contemporary Interest in Multiple Personality in the Netherlands *Dissociation* 3:34–37).

17. F. H. Frankel 1990, Hypnotizability and Dissociation. *American Journal of Psychiatry* 147:823–829. For the extraordinarily ambiguous relationships between hypnotism and psychiatry, especially in France, from 1785 to the present, see L. Chertok and I. Stengers 1992, *A Critique of Psychoanalytic Reason: Hypnosis as a Scientific Problem from Lavoisier to Lacan*, trans. by M. N. Evans, Stanford: Stanford University Press.

18. B. G. Braun 1993, Dissociative Disorders: The Next Ten Years. In *Proceedings of the Tenth International Conference on Multiple Personality/Dissociative States*, ed. B. G. Braun and J. Parks, 5, Chicago: Rush–Presbyterian–St. Luke's Medical Center. This was the opening talk of the conference, in the first plenary session; I have quoted the first paragraph of Braun's abstract.

19. Ross, Norton, and Wozney 1989, 416. For a balanced discussion of the idea of superordinate diagnosis in this context, see C. S. North et al. 1993, *Multiple Personalities, Multiple Disorders: Psychiatric Classification and Media Influence*. New York: Oxford University Press.

20. Merskey 1992, 327. Merskey's denunciation of multiple personality produced an outpouring of angry letters in subsequent issues of the journal in which he published. So did Freeland et al. 1993 (Four Cases of Supposed Multiple Personality Disorder: Evidence of Unjustified Diagnoses, *Canadian Journal of Psychiatry* 38:245–247), an account of how Merskey and his colleagues treated four apparent cases of multiplicity.

21. One pioneering book which gives the impression that multiplicity is part of human nature is Crabtree 1985 (*Multiple Man: Explorations in Possession and Multiple Personality*, Toronto: Collins). Another work with a milder version of this idea is Beahrs 1982 (*Unity and Multiplicity*, New York: Brunner/Mazel). For one patient who also rejects the idea that multiple personality is a disorder, see note 28, chapter 2 below. Rowan 1990 (*Subpersonalities: The People Inside Us*, London and New York: Routledge) is a fascinating account of group therapies in which every member of the group creates a number of subpersonalities, expressing different aspects of character. Each individual's subpersonalities interact with other subpersonalities that emerge in group discussion. But although these subpersonalities acquire distinct names, there is no suggestion that they were "really there" as entities all along, waiting to be revealed by therapy.

22. P. M. Coons 1984, The Differential Diagnosis of Multiple Personality: A Comprehensive Review, *Psychiatric Clinics of North America* 7:53.

23. B. G. Braun 1986, Issues in the Psychotherapy of Multiple Personality Disorder. In *Treatment of Multiple Personality Disorder*, ed. by B. G. Braun, 1–28, Washington, D.C.: American Psychiatric Press.

24. To get a sense of evolving opinions, notice how in 1989 Colin Ross agreed to this way of speaking: "I personally use the terms alter, alter personality and personality as synonyms. I call more limited states fragments, fragment alters, or fragment personalities." But in 1994 he opined that "although MPD patients are, by definition, diagnosed as having more than one personality, in fact they don't." And: "Much of the scepticism about MPD is based on the erroneous assumption that such patients have more than one personality, which is, in fact, impossible." Ross 1989, 81; Ross 1994, *The Osiris Complex: Case Studies in Multiple Personality Disorder*, ix, Toronto: University of Toronto Press.

25. Putnam 1989, *Diagnosis and Treatment of Multiple Personality Disorder*, 161, New York: The Guildford Press.

26. Putnam 1993; cf. Putnam 1992, Are Alter Personalities Fragments or Fictions? *Psychoanalytic Inquiry* 12:95–111.

27. D. Spiegel 1993b, Letter, 20 May 1993, to the Executive Council, International Society for the Study of Multiple Personality and Dissociation, *News. International Society for the Study of Multiple Personality & Dissociation* 11(4):15.

28. Lewis Carroll, *Alice's Adventures in Wonderland* (1865), the third to last paragraph of chapter 1.

29. E. S. Bowman and W. E. Amos 1993, Utilizing Clergy in the Treatment of Multiple Personality Disorder. *Dissociation* 6:47–53.

30. Spiegel 1993a, Dissociation, Trauma and *DSM-IV*. Lecture to the Tenth International Conference on Multiple Personality/Dissociative States, Chicago, 15–17 October; Tape VII-860-93. Alexandria, VA.: Audio Transcripts.

31. M. S. Torem et al. (ISSMP&D Executive Council) 1993, Letter, 17 May 1993, to David Spiegel. *News. International Society for the Study of Multiple Personality & Dissociation* 11(4):14. I have spelled out the abbreviation DD as Dissociative Disorders.

32. Spiegel 1993b, 15.

33. American Psychiatric Association 1994, *Diagnostic and Statistical Manual of Mental Disorders*, 4th ed., 487, Washington, D.C. American Psychiatric Association. [Called *DSM-IV*.] The addition of the amnesia condition C was the culmination of a decade-long debate.

34. *DSM-IV*, clause B, deletes the word "full" from the corresponding clause of *DSM-III-R*, note 10 above. An alter need no longer take full control—just control. This is because in the current phenomenology of multiple personality, an alter in control may still be forced to listen to the jabbering of another alter who is sitting just inside the left ear. The one in control is not in full control.

35. Spiegel 1993a.

From "On Being Sane in Insane Places"

D. L. ROSENHAN

IF SANITY and insanity exist, how shall we know them?

The question is neither capricious nor itself insane. However much we may be personally convinced that we can tell the normal from the abnormal, the evidence is simply not compelling. It is commonplace, for example, to read about murder trials wherein eminent psychiatrists for the defense are contradicted by equally eminent psychiatrists for the prosecution on the matter of the defendant's sanity. More generally, there are a great deal of conflicting data on the reliability, utility, and meaning of such terms as "sanity," "insanity," "mental illness," and "schizophrenia." Finally, as early as 1934, Benedict suggested that normality and abnormality are not universal. What is viewed as normal in one culture may be seen as quite aberrant in another. Thus, notions of normality and abnormality may not be quite as accurate as people believe they are.

To raise questions regarding normality and abnormality is in no way to question the fact that some behaviors are deviant or odd. Murder is deviant. So, too, are hallucinations. Nor does raising such questions deny the existence of the personal anguish often associated with "mental illness." Anxiety and depression exist. Psychological suffering exists. But normality and abnormality, sanity and insanity, and the diagnoses that flow from them may be less substantive that many believe them to be.

At its heart the question of whether the sane can be distinguished from the insane (and whether degrees of insanity can be distinguished from each other) is a simple matter: do the salient characteristics that lead to diagnoses reside in the patients themselves or in the environments and contexts in which observers find them? . . . The belief has been strong that patients present symptoms, that those symptoms can be categorized, and, implicitly, that the sane are distinguishable from the insane. More recently, however, this belief has been questioned. Based in part on theoretical and anthropological considerations, but also on philosophical, legal, and therapeutic ones, the view has grown that psychological categorization of mental illness is useless at best and downright harmful, misleading, and pejorative at worst. Psychiatric diagnoses, in this view, are in the minds of the observers and are not valid summaries of characteristics displayed by the observed.

Gains can be made in deciding which of these is more nearly accurate by getting normal people (that is, people who do not have, and have never suffered, symptoms of serious psychiatric disorders) admitted to psychiatric hospitals and then determining whether they were discovered to be sane and, if so, how. If the sanity of such pseudopatients were always detected, there would be prima facie evidence that a sane individual can be distinguished from the insane context in which he is found. Normality (and presumably abnormality) is distinct enough that it can be recognized wherever it occurs, for it is carried within the person. If, on the other hand, the sanity of the pseudopatients were never discovered, serious difficulties would arise for those who support traditional modes of psychiatric diagnosis. . . .

This article describes such an experiment. Eight sane people gained secret admission to 12 different hospitals. . . . Immediately upon admission to the psychiatric ward, the pseudopatient ceased simulating *any* symptoms of abnormality. In some cases, there was a brief period of mild nervousness and anxiety, since none of the pseudopatients really believed they would be admitted so easily. Indeed, their shared fear was that they would be immediately exposed as frauds and greatly embarrassed. Moreover, many of them had never visited a psychiatric ward; even those who had, nevertheless had some genuine fears about what might happen to them. Their nervousness, then, was quite appropriate to the novelty of the hospital setting, and it abated rapidly.

Apart from that short-lived nervousness, the pseudopatient behaved on the ward as he "normally" behaved. The pseudopatient spoke to patients and staff as he might ordinarily. Because there is uncommonly little to do on a psychiatric ward, he attempted to engage others in conversation. When asked by the staff how he was feeling, he indicated that he was fine, that he no longer experienced symptoms. He responded to instructions from attendants, to calls for medication (which was not swallowed), and to dining-hall instructions. Beyond such activities as were available to him on the admissions ward, he spent his time writing down his observations about the ward, its patients, and the staff. Initially, these notes were written "secretly," but as it soon became clear that no one much cared, they were subsequently written on standard tablets of paper in such public places as the dayroom.

The pseudopatient, very much as a true psychiatric patient, entered a hospital with no foreknowledge of when he would be discharged. Each was told that he would have to get out by his own devices, essentially by convincing the staff that he was sane. The psychological stresses associated with hospitalization were considerable, and all but one of the pseudopatients desired to be discharged almost immediately after being admitted. They were, therefore, motivated not only to behave sanely, but to be paragons of cooperation. That their behavior was in no way disruptive is confirmed by nursing reports . . . [which]

uniformly indicated that the patients were "friendly," "cooperative," and "exhibited no abnormal indications."

THE NORMAL ARE NOT DETECTABLY SANE

Despite their public "show" of sanity, the pseudopatients were never detected. Admitted, except in one case, with a diagnosis of schizophrenia, each was discharged with a diagnosis of schizophrenia "in remission.". . . The evidence is strong that once labeled schizophrenic, the pseudopatient was stuck with that label. If the pseudopatient was to be discharged, he must naturally be "in remission," but he was not sane, nor in the institution's view, had he ever been sane.

The uniform failure to recognize sanity cannot be attributed to the quality of the hospitals, for although there were considerable variations among them, several are considered excellent. Nor can it be alleged that there was simply not enough time to observe the pseudopatients. Length of hospitalization ranged from 7 to 52 days, with an average of 19 days. The pseudopatients were not, in fact, carefully observed, but this failure clearly speaks more to traditions within psychiatric hospitals than to lack of opportunity. . . .

It was quite common for the patients to "detect" the pseudopatients' sanity. During the first three hospitalizations, when accurate counts were kept, 35 of a total of 118 patients on the admissions ward voiced their suspicions, some vigorously. "You're not crazy. You're a journalist, or a professor. You're checking up on the hospital." . . . The fact that the patients often recognized normality when staff did not raises important questions.

Failure to detect sanity during the course of hospitalization may be due to the fact that physicians operate with a strong bias towards what statisticians call the type 2 error. This is to say that physicians are more inclined to call a healthy person sick (a false positive, type 2) than a sick person healthy (a false negative, type 1). The reasons for this are not hard to find: it is clearly more dangerous to misdiagnose illness than health. Better to err on the side of caution, to suspect illness even among the healthy.

But what holds for medicine does not hold equally well for psychiatry. Medical illnesses, while unfortunate, are not commonly pejorative. Psychiatric diagnoses, on the contrary, carry with them personal, legal, and social stigmas (12). It was therefore important to see whether the tendency toward diagnosing the sane insane could be reversed. The following experiment was arranged at a research and teaching hospital whose staff had heard these findings but doubted that such an error could occur in their hospital. The staff was informed that at some time during the following 3 months, one or more pseudopatients would attempt to be admitted into the psychiatric hospital. Each staff member was asked to rate each patient who presented himself at admissions or on the ward according to the likelihood that the patient was a pseudopatient. A 10-point scale was used, with a 1 and 2 reflecting high confidence that the patient was a pseudopatient.

Judgments were obtained on 193 patients who were admitted for psychiatric treatment. All staff who had had sustained contact with or primary responsibility for the patient—attendants, nurses, psychiatrists, physicians, and psychologists—were asked to make judgments. Forty-one patients were alleged, with high confidence, to be pseudopatients by at least one member of the staff. Twenty-three were considered suspect by at least one psychiatrist. Nineteen were suspected by one psychiatrist *and* one other staff member. Actually, no genuine pseudopatient (at least from my group) presented himself during this period.

The experiment is instructive. It indicates that the tendency to designate sane people as insane can be reversed when the stakes (in this case, prestige and diagnostic acumen) are high. But what can be said of the 19 people who were suspected of being "sane" by one psychiatrist and another staff member? Were these people truly "sane," or was it rather the case that in the course of avoiding the type 2 error the staff tended to make more errors of the first sort— calling the crazy "sane"? There is no way of knowing. But one thing is certain: any diagnostic process that lends itself so readily to massive errors of this sort cannot be a very reliable one.

The Stickiness of Psychodiagnostic Labels

. . . . The data speak to the massive role of labeling in psychiatric assessment. Having once been labeled schizophrenic, there is nothing the pseudopatient can do to overcome the tag. The tag profoundly colors others' perceptions of him and his behavior. . . . Once a person is designated abnormal, all of his other behaviors and characteristics are colored by that label. Indeed, that label is so powerful that many of the pseudopatients' normal behaviors were overlooked entirely or profoundly misinterpreted. . . .

As far as I can determine, diagnoses were in no way affected by the relative health of the circumstances of a pseudopatient's life. Rather, the reverse occurred: the perception of his circumstances was shaped entirely by the diagnosis. A clear example of such translation is found in the case of a pseudopatient who had had a close relationship with his mother but was rather remote from his father during his early childhood. During adolescence and beyond, however, his father became a close friend, while his relationship with his mother cooled. His present relationship with his wife was characteristically close and warm. Apart from occasional angry exchanges, friction was minimal. The children had rarely been spanked. Surely there is nothing pathological about such a history. Indeed, many readers may see a similar pattern in their own experiences, with no markedly deleterious consequences. Observe, however, how such a history was translated in the psychopathological context, this from the case summary prepared after the patient was discharged.

> This white 39-year-old male . . . manifests a long history of considerable ambivalence in close relationships, which begins in early childhood. A warm relationship with his mother cools during adolescence. A distant relationship with his father is described as becoming very intense. Affective stability is absent. His attempts to control emotionality with his wife and children are punctuated by angry outbursts and, in the case of the children, spankings. . . .

The facts of the case were unintentionally distorted by the staff to achieve consistency with a popular theory of the dynamics of a schizophrenic reaction . . . . Clearly the meaning ascribed to his verbalizations (that is, ambivalence, affective instability) was determined by the diagnosis: schizophrenia. An entirely different meaning would have been ascribed if it were known that the man was "normal."

All pseudopatients took extensive notes publicly. Under ordinary circumstances, such behavior would have raised questions in the minds of observers, as, in fact, it did among patients. . . . If no questions were asked of the pseudopatients, how was their writing interpreted? Nursing records for three patients indicate that the writing was seen as an aspect of their pathological behavior. "Patient engages in writing behavior" was the daily nursing comment on one of the pseudopatients who was never questioned about his writing. Given that the patient was in the hospital, he must be psychologically disturbed. And given that he is disturbed, continuous writing must be a behavioral manifestation of that disturbance, perhaps a subset of the compulsive behaviors that are sometimes correlated with schizophrenia. . . .

A psychiatric label has a life and an influence of its own. Once the impression has been formed that the patient is schizophrenic, the expectation is that he will continue to be schizophrenic. When a sufficient amount of time has passed, during which the patient has done nothing bizarre, he is considered to be in remission and available for discharge. But the label endures beyond discharge, with the unconfirmed expectation that he will behave as a schizophrenic again. Such labels, conferred by mental health professionals, are as influential on the patient as they are on his relatives and friends, and it should not surprise anyone that the diagnosis acts on all of them as a self-fulfilling prophecy. Eventually the patient himself accepts the diagnosis, with all of its surplus meanings and expectations and behaves accordingly. . . .

A broken leg is something one recovers from, but mental illness allegedly endures forever. A broken leg does not threaten the observer, but a crazy schizophrenic? There is by now a host of evidence that attitudes towards the mentally ill are characterized by fear, hostility, aloofness, suspicion and dread. The mentally ill are society's lepers.

That such attitudes infect the general population is perhaps not surprising, only upsetting. But when they affect the professionals—attendants, nurses, physicians, psychologists, and social workers—who treat and deal with the mentally ill is more disconcerting, both because such altitudes are self-evidently pernicious and because they are unwitting. . . . Such attitudes should not surprise us. They are the natural offspring of the labels patients wear and the places in which they are found. . . .

Powerlessness and Depersonalization

Eye contact and verbal contact reflect concern and indivduation; their absence, avoidance and depersonalization. . . . Neither anecdotal nor "hard" data can convey the overwhelming sense of powerlessness which invades the individual as he is continuously exposed to the depersonalization of the psychiatric hospital. It hardly matters *which* psychiatric hospital—the excellent public ones and the very plush private hospital were better than the rural and shabby ones in this regard, but, again, the features that psychiatric hospitals had in common overwhelmed by far their apparent differences.

Powerlessness was evident everywhere. The patient is deprived of many of his legal rights by dint of his psychiatric commitment. He is shorn of credibility by virtue of his psychiatric label. His freedom of movement is restricted. He cannot initiate contact with the staff, but only respond to such overtures as they make. Personal privacy is minimal. . . . At times, depersonalization reaches such proportions that pseudopatients had the sense that they were invisible, or at least unworthy of account. . . .

Summary and Conclusions

It is clear that we cannot distinguish the sane from the insane in psychiatric hospitals. The hospital itself imposes a special environment in which the meanings of behavior can easily be misunderstood. The consequences to patients hospitalized in such an environment—the powerlessness, depersonalization, segregation, mortification, and self-labeling—seem undoubtedly counter-therapeutic.

NOTE

The full article, "Being Sane in Insane Places," appeared in the journal *Science*, Vol. 179 (19 January 1973), 250–258.

From Love's Executioner and Other Tales
of Psychotherapy

IRVIN D. YALOM

CHAPTER 5: "I NEVER THOUGHT IT WOULD HAPPEN TO ME"

I GREETED Elva in my waiting room, and together we walked the short distance to my office. Something had happened. She was different today, her gait labored, discouraged, dispirited. For the last few weeks there had been a bounce in her steps, but today she once again resembled the forlorn, plodding woman I had first met eight months ago. I remember her first words then: "I think I need help. Life doesn't seem worth living. My husband's been dead for a year now, but things aren't getting any better. Maybe I'm a slow learner."

But she hadn't proved to be a slow learner. In fact, therapy had progressed remarkably well—maybe it had been going too easily. What could have set her back like this?

Sitting down, Elva sighed and said, "I never thought it would happen to me."

She had been robbed. From her description it seemed an ordinary purse snatching. The thief, no doubt, spotted her in a Monterey seaside restaurant and saw her pay the check in cash for three friends—elderly widows all. He must have followed her into the parking lot and, his footsteps muffled by the roaring of the waves, sprinted up and, without breaking stride, ripped her purse away and leaped into his nearby car.

Elva, despite her swollen legs, hustled back into the restaurant to call for help, but of course it was too late. A few hours later, the police found her empty purse dangling on a roadside bush.

Three hundred dollars meant a lot to her, and for a few days Elva was preoccupied by the money she had lost. That concern gradually evaporated and in its place was left a bitter residue—a residue expressed by the phrase "I never thought it would happen to me." Along with her purse and her three hundred dollars, an illusion was snatched away from Elva—the illusion of personal specialness. She had always lived in the privileged circle, outside the unpleasantness, the nasty inconveniences visited on ordinary people—those swarming masses of the tabloids and newscasts who are forever being robbed or maimed.

The robbery changed everything. Gone was the coziness, the softness in her life; gone was the safety. Her home had always beckoned her with its cushions, gardens, comforters, and deep carpets. Now she saw locks, doors, burglar alarms, and telephones. She had always walked her dog every morning at six. The morning stillness now seemed menacing. She and her dog stopped and listened for danger.

None of this is remarkable. Elva had been traumatized and now suffered from commonplace post-traumatic stress. After an accident or an assault, most people tend to feel unsafe, to have a reduced startle threshold, and to be hypervigilant. Eventually time erodes the memory of the event, and victims gradually return to their prior, trusting state.

But for Elva it was more than a simple assault. Her world view was fractured. She had often claimed, "As long as a person has eyes, ears, and a mouth, I can cultivate their friendship." But no longer. She had lost her belief in benevolence, in her personal invulnerability. She felt stripped, ordinary, unprotected. The true impact of that robbery was to shatter illusion and to confirm, in brutal fashion, her husband's death.

Of course, she knew that Albert was dead. Dead and in his grave for over a year and a half. She had taken the ritualized widow walk—through the cancer diagnosis; the awful, retching, temporizing chemotherapy; their last visit together to Carmel; their last drive down El Camino Real; the hospital bed at home; the funeral; the paperwork; the ever-dwindling dinner invitations; the widow and widower's clubs; the long, lonely nights. The whole necrotic catastrophe.

Yet, despite all this, Elva had retained her feeling of Albert's continued existence and thereby of her persisting safety and specialness. She had continued to live "as if," as if the world were safe, as if Albert were there, back in the workshop next to the garage.

Mind you, I do not speak of delusion. Rationally, Elva knew Albert was gone, but still she lived her routine, everyday life behind a veil of illusion which numbed the pain and softened the glare of the knowing. Over forty years ago, she had made a contract with life whose explicit genesis and terms had been eroded by time but whose basic nature was clear: Albert would take care of Elva forever. Upon this unconscious premise, Elva had built her entire assumptive world—a world featuring safety and benevolent paternalism.

Albert was a fixer. He had been a roofer, an auto mechanic, a general handyman, a contractor; he could fix anything. Attracted by a newspaper or magazine photograph of a piece of furniture or some gadget, he would proceed to replicate it in his workshop. I, who have always been hopelessly inept in a workshop, listened in fascination. Forty-one years of living with a fixer is powerfully comforting. It was not hard to understand why Elva clung to the feeling that Albert was still there, out back in the workshop looking out for her, fixing things. How could she give it up? Why should she? That memory, reinforced by forty-one years of experience, had spun a cocoon around Elva that shielded her from reality—that is, until her purse was snatched.

Upon first meeting Elva eight months before, I could find little to love in her. She was a stubby, unattractive woman, part gnome, part sprite, part toad, and each of those parts ill tempered. I was transfixed by her facial plasticity: she winked, grimaced, and popped her eyes either singly or in duet. Her brow seemed alive with great washboard furrows. Her tongue, always visible, changed radically in size as it darted in and out or circled her moist, rubbery, pulsating lips. I remember amusing myself, almost laughing aloud, by imagining introducing her to patients on long-term tranquilizer medication who had developed tardive dyskinesia (a drug-induced abnormality of facial musculature). The patients would, within seconds, become deeply offended because they would believe Elva to be mocking them.

But what I really disliked about Elva was her anger. She dripped with rage and, in our first few hours together, had something vicious to say about everyone she knew—save, of course, Albert. She hated the friends who no longer invited her. She hated those who did not put her at ease. Inclusion or exclusion, it was all the same to her: she found something to hate in everyone. She hated the doctors who had told her that Albert was doomed. She hated even more those who offered false hope.

Those hours were hard for me. I had spent too many hours in my youth silently hating my mother's vicious tongue. I remember the games of imagination I played as a child trying to invent the existence of someone she did not hate: A kindly aunt? A grandfather who told her stories? An older playmate who defended her? But I never found anyone. Save, of course, my father, and he was really part of her, her mouthpiece, her animus, her creation who (according to Asimov's first law of robotics) could not turn against his maker—despite my prayers that he would once—just once, please, Dad—pop her.

All I could do with Elva was to hold on, hear her out, somehow endure the hour, and use all my ingenuity to find something supportive to say—usually some vapid comment about how hard it must be for her to carry around that much anger. At times I, almost mischievously, inquired about others of her family circle. Surely there must be someone who warranted respect. But no one was spared. Her son? She said his elevator "didn't go to the top floor." He was "absent": even when he was there, he was "absent." And her daughter-in-law? In Elva's words, "a GAP"—gentile American princess. When driving home, her son would call his wife on his automobile telephone to say he wanted dinner right away. No problem. She could do it. Nine minutes, Elva reminded me, was all the time required for the GAP to cook dinner—to "nuke" a slim gourmet TV dinner in the microwave.

Everyone had a nickname. Her granddaughter, "Sleeping Beauty" (she whispered with an enormous wink and a nod), had two bathrooms—two, mind you. Her housekeeper, whom she had hired to attenuate her loneliness, was "Looney Tunes," and so dumb that she tried to hide her smoking by exhaling the smoke down the flushing toilet. Her pretentious bridge partner was "Dame May Whitey" (and Dame May Whitey was spry-minded compared with the rest, with all the Alzheimer zombies and burned-out drunks who, according to Elva, constituted the bridge-playing population of San Francisco).

But somehow, despite her rancor and my dislike of her and the evocation of my mother, we got through these sessions. I endured my irritation, got a little closer, resolved my countertransference by disentangling my mother from Elva, and slowly, very slowly, began to warm to her.

I think the turning point came one day when she plopped herself in my chair with a "Whew! I'm tired." In response to my raised eyebrows, she explained she had just played eighteen holes of golf with her twenty-year-old nephew. (Elva was sixty, four foot eleven, and at least one hundred sixty pounds.)

"How'd you do?" I inquired cheerily, keeping up my side of the conversation.

Elva bent forward, holding her hand to her mouth as though to exclude someone in the room, showed me a remarkable number of enormous teeth, and said, "I whomped the shit out of him!"

It struck me as wonderfully funny and I started to laugh, and laughed until my eyes filled with tears. Elva liked my laughing. She told me later it was the first spontaneous act from Herr Doctor Professor (so that was *my* nickname!), and she laughed with me. After that we got along famously. I began to appreciate Elva—her marvelous sense of humor, her intelligence, her drollness. She had led a rich, eventful life. We were similar in many ways. Like me, she had made the big generational jump. My parents arrived in the United States in their twenties, penniless immigrants from Russia. Her parents had been poor Irish immigrants, and she had straddled the gap between the Irish tenements of South Boston and the duplicate bridge tournaments of Nob Hill in San Francisco.

At the beginning of therapy, an hour with Elva meant hard work. I trudged when I went to fetch her from the waiting room. But after a couple of months, all that changed. I looked forward to our time together. None of our hours passed without a good laugh. My secretary said she always could tell by my smile that I had seen Elva that day.

We met weekly for several months, and therapy proceeded well, as it usually does when therapist and patient enjoy each other. We talked about her widowhood, her changed social role, her fear of being alone, her sadness at never being physically touched. But, above all, we talked about her anger—about how it had driven away her family and her friends. Gradually she let it go; she grew softer and more gentle. Her tales of Looney Tunes, Sleeping Beauty, Dame May Whitey, and the Alzheimer bridge brigade grew less bitter. Rapprochements occurred; as her anger receded, family and friends reappeared in her life. She had been doing so well that, just before the time of the purse snatching, I had been considering raising the question of termination.

But when she was robbed, she felt as though she were starting all over again. Most of all, the robbery illuminated her ordinariness, her "I never thought it would happen to me" reflecting the loss of belief in her personal specialness. Of course, she was still special in that she had special qualities and gifts, that she had a unique life history, that no one who had ever lived was just like her. That's the rational side of specialness. But we (some more than others) also have an irrational sense of specialness. It is one of our chief methods of denying death, and the part of our mind whose task it is to mollify death terror generates the irrational belief that we are invulnerable—that unpleasant things like aging and death may be the lot of others but not our lot, that we exist beyond law, beyond human and biological destiny.

Although Elva responded to the purse snatching in ways that *seemed* irrational (for example, proclaiming that she wasn't fit to live on earth, being afraid to leave her house), it was clear that she was *really* suffering from the stripping away of irrationality. That sense of specialness, of being charmed, of being the exception, of being eternally protected—all those self-deceptions that had served her so well suddenly lost their persuasiveness. She saw through her own illusions, and what illusion had shielded now lay before her, bare and terrible.

Her grief wound was now fully exposed. This was the time, I thought, to open it wide, to debride it, and to allow it to heal straight and true.

"When you say you never thought it would happen to you, I know just what you mean," I said. "It's so hard for me, too, to accept that all these afflictions—aging, loss, death—are going to happen to me, too."

Elva nodded, her tightened brow showing that she was surprised at my saying anything personal about myself.

"You must feel that if Albert were alive, this would never have happened to you." I ignored her flip response that if Albert were alive she wouldn't have been taking those three old hens to lunch. "So the robbery brings home the fact that he's really gone."

Her eyes filled with tears, but I felt I had the right, the mandate, to continue. "You knew that before, I know. But part of you didn't. Now you really know that he's dead. He's not in the yard. He's not out back in the workshop. He's not anywhere. Except in your memories."

Elva was really crying now, and her stubby frame heaved with sobs for several minutes. She had never done that before with me. I sat there and wondered, "*Now* what do I do?" But my instincts luckily led me to what proved to be an inspired gambit. My eyes lit upon her purse—that same ripped-off, much-abused purse; and I said, "Bad luck is one thing, but aren't you asking for it carrying around something that large?" Elva, plucky as ever, did not fail to call attention to my overstuffed pockets and the clutter on the table next to my chair. She pronounced the purse "medium-sized."

"Any larger," I responded, "and you'd need a luggage carrier to move it around."

"Besides," she said, ignoring my jibe, "I need everything in it."

"You've got to be joking! Let's see!"

Getting into the spirit of it, Elva hoisted her purse onto my table, opened its jaws wide, and began to empty it. The first items fetched forth were three empty doggie bags.

"Need two extra ones in case of an emergency?" I asked.

Elva chuckled and continued to disembowel the purse. Together we inspected and discussed each item. Elva conceded that three packets of Kleenex and twelve pens (plus three pencil stubs) were indeed superfluous, but held firm about two bottles of cologne and three hairbrushes, and dismissed, with an imperious flick of her hand, my challenge to her large flashlight, bulky notepads, and huge sheaf of photographs.

We quarreled over everything. The roll of fifty dimes. Three bags of candies (low-calorie, of course). She giggled at my question: "Do you believe, Elva, that the more of these you eat, the thinner you will become?" A plastic sack of old orange peels ("You never know, Elva, when these will come in handy"). A bunch of knitting needles ("Six needles in search of a sweater," I thought). A bag of sourdough starter. Half of a paperback Steven King novel (Elva threw away sections of pages as she read them: "They weren't worth keeping," she explained). A small stapler ("Elva, this is crazy!"). Three pairs of sunglasses. And, tucked away into the innermost corners, assorted coins, paper clips, nail clippers, pieces of emery board, and some substance that looked suspiciously like lint.

When the great bag had finally yielded all, Elva and I stared in wonderment at the contents set out in rows on my table. We were sorry the bag was empty and that the emptying was over. She turned and smiled, and we looked tenderly at each other. It was an extraordinarily intimate moment. In a way no patient had ever done before, she showed me everything. And I had accepted everything and asked for even more. I followed her into her every nook and crevice, awed that one old woman's purse could serve as a vehicle for both isolation and intimacy: the absolute isolation that is integral to existence and the intimacy that dispels the dread, if not the fact, of isolation.

That was a transforming hour. Our time of intimacy—call it love, call it love making—was redemptive. In that one hour, Elva moved from a position of forsakenness to one of trust. She came alive and was persuaded, once more, of her capacity for intimacy.

I think it was the best hour of therapy I ever gave.

Three Stories
from Cases in Bioethics

EDITED BY CAROL LEVINE

"AIN'T NOBODY GONNA CUT ON MY HEAD!"

A FIFTY-SIX-YEAR-OLD farmer, accompanied by his wife, consulted the Neurology Service of Veterans' Hospital because of memory difficulty. For two years the patient had been having increasing trouble with technical aspects of farming. More recently he had been talking about his brother George as if he were alive although he had died two years earlier. He gave his own age as 48 and the year as "1960, pause... er, no, 1970." Examination revealed that the patient walked with a wide-based gait (a standard sign of brain pathology) and decreased cerebral function but was otherwise normal. The patient had no difficulty with simple coin problems and could repeat six digits.

Pleading pressing business, the patient declined hospitalization to determine the cause of his decreasing cerebral function. His wife tried to persuade him to enter the hospital, but when the resident suggested that she might assume guardianship for her husband through court action she declined.

Six months later the patient's condition had worsened. Through the urging of the county agent the patient had leased most of his farmland to his neighbors and now did no work. His gait had become so wide-based that acquaintances mistakenly thought him inebriated. He urinated in his pants about once a week, and recently seemed not to care. He sat watching television all day, but never paid any attention to the program content.

Examination at this time showed an apparently alert man without speech difficulty but with considerable mental deterioration. The patient gave his age as thirty-eight, the year as 1949, the president as Eisenhower, and the location as a drug store in his home town. He failed to recognize the name Lyndon Johnson, but upon hearing the name John F. Kennedy he spontaneously volunteered knowledge of his assassination. The patient could not subtract 20 cents from a dollar but could name the number of nickels in a quarter. He could recite the months of the year and could upon request from his wife give fairly long quotations from the Bible.

The resident and the attending physician urged hospitalization. They told the patient they would evaluate him for treatable causes of mental deterioration and memory deficit. In view of his wide-based gait and urinary incontinence in association with dementia, it was likely he had occult hydrocephalus. It was explained that this disorder caused decreased mental abilities by interference with absorption of cerebrospinal fluid. The mental deterioration in these patients is partially (as in his case now) or completely (as in his case six months ago when first seen) reversible. The treatment is to place a plastic tube through the skull to drain the cerebrospinal fluid from the brain to the vascular system; this was explained to the patient with diagrams. The patient immediately rejected the surgery, summarizing his thoughts with these exact words: "Ain't nobody gonna cut on my head." The patient's wife again attempted to persuade the patient to accept hospitalization and, if tests confirmed the clinical impression, surgery. The attending physician argued to the wife that the patient did not have the mental competence to decide his own fate and the wife should become the patient's legal guardian through court action and force hospitalization. The wife politely but vigorously rejected this course of action, pointing out that in her family the husband made all important decisions.

The resident and the attending physician differed in opinions at this point. The resident thought the patient should be followed in the outpatient clinic until he perhaps changed his mind. The resident pointed out that though the patient had decreased mental abilities he still retained enough intelligence to decide his own fate. The attending physician wished for court action to make the patient the ward of one of his relatives or, if necessary, the temporary ward of the hospital, and to force hospitalization and therapy.

COMMENTARY

James M. Gustafson

The principal substantive moral issue in this case is the status of the right of the patient to determine his own bodily destiny. He refuses to consent to a procedure which is likely to relieve his disability, though apparently he understands in lay terms what is involved in the surgery. At his level of competence he is "informed," but he refuses to give "consent."

The principle of informed consent is based upon one moral assumption and upon one philosophical judgment. The moral assumption is that individuals have a right to refuse treatment even when in the judgment of others that treatment is in the patient's own best interests. A person has a right to determine his or her own destiny. The ground of this assumption is historically located in the libertarian tradition of Western culture; it stems from the same tradition that values civil liberties, that believes that the state exists properly only on the basis of the consent of the governed, and so forth. The philosophical justification for the individual's right to self-determination has been made in various ways: the right is "natural"; capacity for self-determination is what makes humans distinctive as a species and from this is derived both its value and the right; individual rights are conferred by God; excessive incursion on self-determination leads to repression and in turn to social unrest, and for this reason the right is to be protected.

The serious philosophical judgment on which the principle of informed consent is based is that persons actually have a capacity to determine their own destinies. Every case of this sort opens the historic debate about "free will" if the case is carried beyond the immediate clinical circumstances.

This case can be analyzed on the basis of two questions which follow from the two paragraphs. 1) Are there *moral* grounds for exerting persuasive, or legal and coercive, measures to override this man's presumed right of self-determination? Do his obligations to his family and to the community (or, to make the point in a weaker way, do the interests of his family and the community) provide a sufficient basis for intervention without his consent? How one would answer this question would depend upon the status of the right of self-determination in relation to the claims of communities (his family, the neighbors, etc.) to limit and even override that right. 2) Are this man's capacities to judge rationally and to act in accordance with a rational judgment impaired by his illness to the extent that he cannot properly exercise his moral right to self-determination? Is he, to use the common term, really "competent?" Does his impairment provide "excusing conditions" so that just as he is not held accountable for his wide gait, so he is not accountable for his rejection of the proposed therapy? Given the assumption of "free will" in the consent procedure, can his will be judged to be "less free" than is necessary and sufficient to make a sound judgment? The attending physician could justify his "wish" for court action on the basis of either or both of the matters raised by these questions.

In this case I would argue in favor of the attending physician's "wish." My principal argument would be on the basis of the patient's limited capacities to exercise his right of self-determination. Note that an empirical judgment about those limits is involved. A hypothesis (and that is all it is) would be required to support the argument, namely, if this man's capacities were not so impaired he would consent to the surgery. Procedurally, I would support the steps taken in the report of the case; that is, first seeking voluntary consent of the patient, then of his family, and only as a last resort seeking a court order. I am prepared also, however, to argue that this man has obligations to his family and to the community that he ought to take into account in making his own judgment. His failure to consent is, it appears, costly to others; others are dependent upon him and, thus, also have a claim on him to consent to a procedure that would permit him to fulfill his duties to them. Procedurally, if such a line of argument failed to persuade him, and then his family, there would be a moral justification for court action. At the base of my conviction here is a significant qualification of the individual libertarian tradition in the direction of a more "social" view of persons and of duties and obligations of persons to other individuals and to communities.

COMMENTARY

Francis C. Pizzalli

At first blush, the attending physician presents a fairly convincing case for initiating state intrusion into the patient's brain. As the title of the case implies, the proffered therapy is fairly characterized as "brain surgery" and thus avoids categorization as "psychosurgery," replete with its politically value-laden premise of experimental treatment for the purpose of controlling socially deviant behavior. If, indeed, the preliminary diagnosis of occult hydrocephalus is sound, the operation would be tailored to rectify an accepted organic brain pathology. Though this entails the concomitant effect of controlling aberrant behavior (e.g., urinary maintenance and dementia), the presence of excess cerebrospinal fluid calls into play a well-defined medical/disease model which makes less persuasive the need to inquire into the motives of the physician as a check against the potential transmogrification of psychiatrists into thought-controllers.

If one were to accept the physician's evaluation of the mental incompetency of the patient, coerced institutionalization and treatment could be defended on a number of grounds. The procedure is relatively non-intrusive; to wit, it is a safe, non-experimental operation which involves no destruction of brain tissue and is intended to control behavior that ranks rather low on the continuum of volitional and autonomous functions. Not only is this intrusion minimal, but an array of humanitarian and utilitarian impulses militate for intervention. Does not the state have a moral obligation to the patient's former self to restore it? Or an obligation to construct a new self for the person, at which point he would be released to exercise his autonomy to its fullest potential? And would not this restoration to optimal functionality redound to the benefit of his family and community?

Even if we were to assume the patient's competency, the cost of overriding his competent judgment would be measured in terms of a single interference with personal autonomy at a particular time, presumably to be outweighed by the personal and social interest in a long-term increase in autonomy achieved by effective treatment.

Is there a decisive rebuttal to the physician's benevolent despotism? From a traditional legal perspective the case for involuntary commitment (i.e., enforced hospitalization) in this instance is rather weak. There is no mention of antisocial activities by the patient, which would warrant a finding of "dangerousness to others." To say that occasional urinary incontinence and mindless fixation upon the boob tube—behavioral traits found in many "normal" persons—constitute dangerousness to oneself reflects a most extreme paternalistic bias.

Even if the criteria for involuntary commitment are met, the case against intervention by no means falls. We cannot conclude that because an individual may no longer be competent to care for himself generally (e.g., due to memory deterioration), he is thereby incompetent to pass informed judgment upon such an intrusion as the proposed organic therapy. The notion of limited competency, besides having legal recognition, is rooted in the empirical observation that certain mental illnesses do not completely obliterate a person's ability to make decisions. While the patient may no longer recall dates and ages, it is hard to envision how memory deficit can totally discredit the capacity to understand the consequences of an operation, and to immediately summarize the resident's explanation and conclude with a refusal, as the patient has done. Even if we were to adopt the simplistic view that there is no competency where the refusal only occurred because of the mental deterioration, there is no evidence to indicate that the patient is other than strongly individualistic, and would not have decided likewise prior to the onset of deterioration. Moreover, the competent spouse's concurrence in his decision might be construed as evidence of agreement with his lifelong views on brain surgery.

To respond to the invocation of a classic Benthamite calculus that would override limited, albeit informed, judgment to refuse therapy, we might profitably view the case from a rule-utilitarian perspective. While it may be true in this particular case that only a minimally intrusive operation is needed to arrest mental deterioration and partially restore memory function, we should ask what the consequences would be of a practice of substituting the state's judgment for individual informed consent in order to achieve the incremental gain in utility involved in curing those who suffer from marginal mental impairment. Is it too far-fetched to conclude that the result would be a society in which democratic values of personal autonomy, freedom, and privacy would be subjugated to the ideal of state control over various kinds of behavior?

There is one final barrier to coerced surgery, assuming for the sake of argument that there are grounds for civil commitment and that the patient does not have the limited competency to give informed refusal to treatment. Shall the next-of-kin be designated as the proxy, with the power to give or withhold consent? To argue in the negative, because it is suspected the spouse will only rubber-stamp the incompetent's decision, conflicts with the legal presumption of identity of interests among kin. Likewise, to propose a third-party guardian who will rubber-stamp the physician's decision, on the ground that it will enhance the well-being of the patient and his family, arrogates to the physician the right to define that well-being, instead of allowing it to be defined within the privacy of the family.

In sum, only a highly paternalistic society could tolerate the intrusions upon autonomy and privacy that would flow from a practice of coercion in cases such as that at hand.

THE WOMAN WHO DIED IN A BOX

One frigid January day Rebecca Smith, age sixty-one, was found dead of hypothermia in her makeshift home—a cardboard box covered by a rug—on a New York City street. The Red Cross had reported her unusual living arrangements to the police two weeks earlier. Social workers had visited her, offering food and help in moving to a city shelter. A mobile unit designed to help geriatric patients had approached her. A psychiatrist had visited her and declared her an "endangered adult," part of the procedure that would have allowed the authorities to hospitalize her under seventy-two-hour protective custody. But before the order could be carried out—the first time the city had attempted its implementation—Rebecca Smith died.

Before she joined the ranks of New York's homeless street people, Rebecca Smith had lived a rather different life. One of a family of thirteen children in Virginia, she had graduated from Hampton Institute as valedictorian. But she was hospitalized as a schizophrenic for ten years and underwent electroshock therapy. When she was released from the hospital, her daughter said, she was a changed woman.

In 1959 Mrs. Smith came to New York to live with her sister and then entered a mental hospital in Long Island. She was later released from the institution and decided to strike out on her own. That meant living on public assistance, taking Thorazine, and going to a medical clinic. In 1981 she failed to

appear for recertification interviews with social workers and from then on—
until her death—she lived on the streets.

Could Rebecca Smith's death have been prevented? How far do society's
obligations extend toward those who are in need but who refuse to conform?
Does society have different obligations to intervene in protecting those it con-
siders mentally ill?

COMMENTARY

Kim Hopper

On March 19 this year [1982], I joined a hundred others across from the White
House in a memorial service for the homeless poor who had died on the streets
of six American cities this winter. Forty crosses were driven into the ground of
Lafayette Park, joining over 500 already in place, the reported toll of the last
five years or so in eleven cities. As it happened, the name on the cross I carried,
the name I shouted out in the bright sunshine that day, was Rebecca Smith.

Rebecca Smith's death has drawn much more attention than her life ever
did; it has been the subject of two editorials in the *New York Times*, another
in the *Washington Post*, and of several commentaries on local TV news. But
listen for a moment to the words of Betty Higden in Dickens's *Our Mutual
Friend:* "You pray that your Granny may have the strength enough left her at
the last . . . to get up from the bed and run and hide herself, and sworn to death
in a hole, sooner than fall into the hands of those Cruel Jacks we read of, that
dodge and drive, and worry and weary, and scorn and shame, the decent poor"
(cited by Steven Marcus, "Their Brothers' Keepers," 1978).

What little we know of Rebecca Smith's life suggests that she may well have
read about, and directly encountered, "Cruel Jacks" in the course of her institutionalized life. Mental hospitals were forbidding places in the 1950s and
1960s, and patients often fared as badly there as the "decent poor" had a century earlier in England.

There is a danger in discussing Rebecca Smith's death—that it will be
taken more than it should be, as emblematic of a general refusal of assistance on the part of the homeless. From there, it is a small step to reviving the
stale myth that the legions of the homeless poor on our streets are there because they choose to be. The recent history of New York's sheltering efforts
suggests otherwise.

Since the *Callahan v. Carey* suit[1] was filed in October 1979, more than 1700
new emergency shelter beds have been provided by New York City. All were
filled this winter. An additional 175 homeless men and women avail themselves

each night of the twenty-four-hour drop-in facilities at the Moravian Church and Olivieri Center. Dozens more found respite this past winter, courtesy of the churches and synagogues that opened their doors to the wandering poor. Did these people materialize out of thin air? Or, as appears to be the case, were most of them making their way wretchedly until a more decent option presented itself?

It is difficult to attribute the recent surge in the sheltered population to more rational behavior by the homeless. If anything, observers agree that recent recipients of shelter have more tenuous mental health than traditional clients of the public shelters. The decisive difference appears to be the range of options offered the homeless poor: as that range has increased, so has their demonstrated willingness to come in out of the cold. It takes some flexibility, a modicum of decency, and respect for the heightened sense of self-protection that life on the streets can breed. It takes patience—but that is all.

But exceptions do occur. We don't know exactly what Rebecca Smith was offered, or what she understood the offer to be. A lot of people tried, but there was neither world enough nor time. City attorneys waited until a Friday afternoon to file papers in court, assuring inattention for another two days. Does that imply misgivings about their own resolve? This was, after all, the maiden application of the Protective Services Law. The process has since been streamlined to minimize gratuitous delays. Thus, several people may subsequently have been spared death by exposure. Clearly, once the protection of due process is secured, it is a civil obligation to take emergency action to save from imminent death one who is unaware of the peril.

But in the unforgiving light of hindsight, more than "what should have been done" is illuminated. Private shelters are filled with wary, once-desperate men and women who formerly saw no alternative to the degradation and danger of the public shelters than to live apart from them and to die decently when that failed. Betty Higden would have been one:

> Comprehending that her strength was quitting her, and that the struggle of her life was almost ended, she could neither reason out the means of getting back to her protectors, nor even form the idea. The overmastering dread, and the proud stubborn resolution it engendered in her to die undegraded, were the two distinct impressions left in her failing mind.

Betty Higden's prayer—"to die undegraded"—was heard. She died, alone and unseen, by the roadside one night, the money to pay for her burial sewn into her gown. There is a defiant dignity in such a death, one that refuses to exonerate a society inured to her suffering. It was as if she had demanded, not justice at last, but injustice consistently applied. There were to be no eleventh hour "heroics," no final capitulation to the indignity of a pauper's death. This recognition, that even the desperately poor may prize self-respect above a forced and servile dependency, should arrest easy ruminations about "what should have been done."

Rebecca Smith's is not a "right to die" case, anymore than Betty Higden's was. It is rather an object lesson in how comfortably we tolerate routine misery and how quickly we will pounce to sequester evidence of that fact.

Of course, there is an out. One could argue that others have found their way to refuge before death, that it needn't be shameful, and that were more decent shelter available, Rebecca Smith might not have had to die to force the issue. But to raise the question of intervention only at the hour of her death is seriously to cheapen the worth of her life.

COMMENTARY

Nicholas N. Kittrie

Despite my continuing concern for the excesses of the "therapeutic state"—which has permitted involuntary sterilization, lobotomies, electroshock, and indeterminate incarceration for those suffering from mental illness, while forbidding these procedures to be applied to convicted criminals—I believe that New York has failed in its duty toward Rebecca Smith. This conclusion follows from general principles of enlightened jurisprudence, which are applicable community-wide, regardless of the psychiatric status of Rebecca Smith or the mental illness laws of New York.

The balance between personal autonomy and communal responsibility is difficult to strike. Excessive stress on autonomy is likely to reinforce individualism, but also to introduce alienation and community disintegration. Emphasis on communal responsibility, on the other hand, while strengthening collective bonds, could result in paternalism and possibly even in authoritarian suppression. Different societies strike the balance differently. While American jurisprudence, in its commitment to liberty, has not usually articulated "Good Samaritan" laws for the community or individual citizens, both the Italian and French Penal Codes specify penalties for "any person who neglects to afford the necessary assistance" to a "person wounded or otherwise in danger."

One may doubt the desirability or effectiveness of decreeing that an individual citizen become a Good Samaritan under the penalty of criminal law or of interfering with an individual's voluntary exposure to danger—including motorcycle riding, smoking, or sky diving. Yet one can readily concede the importance of communal efforts on behalf of those who appear to be *involuntarily* stranded or in danger.

Rebecca Smith was exposed to evident, continuing, and increasing danger on the public streets of New York. Suppose she had stepped into the middle of oncoming traffic. Would the state agencies have felt the need for a complex and time-consuming procedure to remove her to safety? Would it have mattered whether or not she suffered from one mental illness or another, or from none? In a reasonably humanitarian, welfare-oriented society, at the moment of risk the state must step in, at least temporarily, to rescue those disabled from their own pursuit of "life, liberty and property." This rescue the state owes to its citizens regardless of color, creed, sex, fortune, or mental ability.

What if the citizen for a second time marches into the middle of the traffic, climbs onto the rooftop, or threatens to jump from the bridge? Even for a person who is sane, the state is expected to make a second rescue effort. Moreover, under common law such willful citizens could be charged with disturbing the peace, attempting suicide, or some other obscure legal violation, thus affording the state the justification for temporary restraint.

If minor sanctions are to be attached to deliberate, repeated risk takers, they should apply whether the risk takers are competent or incompetent. But I am strongly opposed to attaching a psychiatric label to people in order to permit greater intervention and control over their lives than over the community at large.

Rebecca Smith died before New York City authorities could implement her hospitalization under its new protective custody law. Yet for at least three decades, under special laws, the mentally ill, alcoholics, and drug addicts have been confined on the basis of psychiatric labels, without complying to the standards of "due process" and "probable cause" required under the criminal law. At the height of the therapeutic state, in the 1950s and 1960s, efforts were made to greatly and unduly broaden the insanity defense, as well as to altogether prohibit criminal sanctions against public drunkenness. But the late 1970s brought an antitherapeutic movement of similar extremity. While therapists of two decades ago called for voluntary and involuntary "treatment" of all deviants, today's therapeutic nihilists wish to totally abolish the insanity defense and to condemn to benign neglect those who require assistance.

Neither extreme supplies even and civilized justice for America. Rebecca Smith's life should have been saved, even at the cost of a temporary loss of freedom. But the same conclusion should apply to all citizens similarly situated, regardless of their psychiatric diagnosis. The New York seventy-two-hour temporary custody law, designed exclusively for those allegedly mentally disabled, proved not only unjust, but also ineffective.

Decisions on Behalf of the Incompetent

Sterilizing the Retarded Child

A retarded eleven-year-old girl from the city of Sheffield, England, had been booked to enter a hospital on May 4, 1975, for a sterilization operation. The girl, known as "D," suffers from Sotos Syndrome—also called cerebral giganticism—an unusual group of congenital abnormalities including epilepsy. Characteristics of the disease include large hands, feet, and skull; poor coordination; and endocrine problems of unknown etiology. Intelligence ranges from normal to severe retardation, with most mildly retarded. ("D" had a normal intelligence range, a fair academic standard, and the understanding of a nine- to nine-and-a-half-year-old.)

While authorities in the genetics of Sotos Syndrome are uncertain about its inheritability, they believe that it is not one disease but a heterogeneous group of disorders, and that it may be either a recessive trait or a new dominant mutation. Most cases of Sotos Syndrome have been sporadic, occurring equally in both sexes. Those afflicted do not seem to have a higher incidence of relatives affected than does the normal population, and the risk of genetic transmission is not known. There have been reports, however, of its occurrence among first cousins, identical twins, and between father and son.

"D's" father died in 1971, leaving the mother to raise the girl and two other daughters in very difficult circumstances. The mother, a part-time cleaner, is very hard-working, sincere, and devoted. The girl sleeps with her mother in one bed; their two-bedroom house has no toilet; and they live under conditions described as appalling.

In 1973 "D" was transferred to a school specializing in children's behavioral problems, a move reported to be a success. Her progress in education and behavior was evident. But by the time "D" reached puberty at the age of ten the mother had grown concerned, fearing her daughter might be seduced and have an abnormal baby, for which she would then have to care. She stated: "I don't think my daughter will ever be responsible enough to bring up a family. I don't think she will improve enough to look after children." However, "D" had not yet shown any interest in the opposite sex, and her opportunities for promiscuity were virtually nonexistent since her mother was always at her side.

Dr. Ronald Gordon, a consultant pediatrician at Sheffield Northern General Hospital who had taken an interest in the family, said that there was a risk that any child borne by "D" would be abnormal and that the girl's epilepsy might cause her to harm a child. He thought that she would always remain so substantially handicapped that she would be unable to care for herself or any children she might have. He maintained that his recommendation to operate was based on his clinical judgment; furthermore, he claimed that he and the gynecologist, Dr. Sheila Duncan, should be the sole judges of whether surgery should be performed, provided that there was parental consent. Dr. Gordon also asked the mother, who consented to the sterilization, to discuss the operation with her daughter.

Mrs. Margaret Dubberley, an educational psychologist at the school the girl attended, strongly opposed the operation and brought legal proceedings aimed at having the girl made a ward of the court. The headmaster at the girl's school believed it was unrealistic to be dogmatic about "D's" future, a view supported by some medical evidence. Mrs. Dubberley was further supported by the National Council for Civil Liberties and by a movement in the House of Commons opposing the operation.

COMMENTARY

LeRoy Walters

Before we examine the normative issues in "D's" case, it will be useful to analyze precisely what kind of sterilization is being proposed on her behalf. Since there is no evidence to indicate that the sterilization of "D" is medically required for the diagnosis or treatment of an existing illness or injury, the proposed sterilization can be categorized as *nontherapeutic.* A more complex question is the voluntariness of the proposed procedure. The surgery envisioned is clearly not compulsory, or involuntary, in the sense of being performed against the expressed wishes of the daughter. However, "D" is legally a minor and is probably not mentally competent to provide voluntary consent to the surgery on her own behalf. Perhaps a third category is required—nonvoluntary sterilization, or sterilization in the absence of the prospective sterilizee's consent or refusal. The proposed sterilization in "D's" case would seem to correspond most closely to this third category; that is, if performed, the sterilization would be nonvoluntary and would be authorized by the substituted judgment of the mother and the two physicians.

Under what conditions can nontherapeutic, nonvoluntary sterilization be morally justified? I would like to suggest three formal requirements which should be applied to this and similar cases. First, there should be *just cause,* or a sufficiently weighty reason, for the proposed sterilization. A just cause is required because sterilization in the absence of consent constitutes a significant invasion of the body and a rather massive intrusion into the sphere of reproductive privacy that has recently been recognized by Anglo-American law. The second requirement is that sterilization should be a *last resort,* since it is generally irreversible and since equally effective, reversible contraceptive techniques are available—for example, the pill. The third formal requirement is *due process,* or an adequate procedure for representing the interests and protecting the rights of all parties concerned.

The proposed sterilization of "D" satisfies none of these formal requirements. First, there is no just cause for the sterilization of "D." It is not clear whether sterilization was recommended by the mother and the pediatrician primarily for the benefit of "D" herself, for the benefit of her mother and sisters, or for the benefit of a child which might potentially be conceived and born to "D." (Another logical possibility, not mentioned in this case, would be sterilization for the benefit of society as a whole.) However, no convincing arguments are presented to support any of these possible justifications. The evidence concerning the probabilty of "D's" producing handicapped children is inconclusive at best. In addition, the prognosis for "D's" own intellectual development is uncertain. It is at least possible that with the aid of continued special education she will one day be able to make informed decisions concerning her reproductive capacities.

Second, the proposed sterilization of "D" is clearly not a last resort. In the case report there is no evidence to indicate that reversible contraceptive techniques were either considered or tried. Until such alternatives have been demonstrated to be infeasible, consideration of an irreversible surgical procedure is premature.

Third, the proposal to sterilize "D" also fails to satisfy the due process requirement. Quite possibly the physicians and the mother based their decision primarily on the best interest of the child, as they perceived that interest. However, the "clinical judgment" of the physicians extended far beyond the bounds of the medically indicated. Even the mother, whose response in very difficult circumstances is understandable, did not sufficiently consider the rights of her child. In cases where the performance of an irreversible, nontherapeutic procedure on a child is contemplated, due process seems to require either the appointment of a guardian for the child or formal approval by an independent review committee. This at least seems to be the view of the U. S. Department of Health, Education and Welfare (as expressed in the sterilization restrictions published in the *Federal Register,* February 6, 1974) and the British Department of Health and Social Security, as outlined in a discussion paper, "Sterilization of Children under 16 Years of Age" (cited in the *British Medical Journal,* November 8, 1975 p. 356).

It is easy to forget that the momentary act of nonvoluntary sterilization has lifetime consequences for the person undergoing the procedure. A sociological study by G. Sabagh and R. B. Edgerton in *Eugenics Quarterly* (December 1962) reported that, of forty retarded persons who had been sterilized prior to their release from the institution, many understood "the meaning and implications of sterilization" and 68 percent "disapproved of the sterilization procedure which they had undergone."

In sum, the proposed sterilization of "D" in this case fails to fulfill the requirements of just cause, last resort, and due process. The preferable alternative would be to employ nonpermanent contraceptive techniques as necesary, in the hope that one day "D" will attain sufficient intellectual maturity to make her own reproductive decisions.

COMMENTARY

Willard Gaylin

When analyzed in terms of the specific data presented in this case, a court decision to prevent irreversible surgery seems reasonable enough; and that is, in fact, what took place. The child is, after all, still young; the nature of the mental impairment is still unclear; the degree of retardation (and possible maturation that can be expected) has yet to be defined. There will be a time for a reevaluation when the facts of her destiny become clearer.

The actual response the court's decision elicited, however, was not what one would expect for a prudential compromise, but more like that which is accorded a victory of the forces of good over those of evil. The applause in Britain and elsewhere was as unanimous and hearty as though Tinkerbell's life depended on it. One suspects that it was not the eleven-year-old girl and her future that were being judged, but a cliché. For years sterilization of the mentally retarded has been an issue fraught with emotion. The ominous implications of genetic engineering, cast in the shadow of the recent Nazi past, make the problem too easy by evoking an instinctive and intuitive response to the connotation of the words employed rather than their explicit meaning. Here was an issue that managed to unite educational psychologists, the medical establishment, the civil libertarians, and the House of Commons on one side—with only the unfortunate girl's mother in opposition. Any moral issue in biomedicine these days that commands such unanimity warrants a reexamination.

What is needed is some understanding of the value of sterilization in the mentally retarded. An automatic negative response is not warranted; and the reason is precisely the one sometimes relied upon by opponents of sterilization—that we now recognize the mentally retarded as a broad spectrum of individuals who, while limited in their capacity for certain functions of the healthy mature adult, are not limited in all.

One of the great disadvantages of IQ as the measurement of retardation is that it forces us to see the retarded of all ages as children. We describe them as "having the mentality of a six-year-old." No mentally retarded individual has the mentality of a six-, eight-, twelve- or fourteen-year-old. A six year-year-old is a learner par excellence, with unbounded intellectual curiosity, and a potential for mastery of new material that a thirty-six-year-old would envy. He is, however, immature, childish, and incapable of making the decisions which his profound intelligence might imply. A thirty-six-year-old with severe retardation to a point where he can neither read, write, count, tell time, nor follow street directions, can still be a mature adult in a host of ways beyond the capacity of the six-year-old. The price we make the retarded pay for their incapacity in one area is the sacrifice of capacity in certain other areas which could be compensatory if allowed to develop.

Because we cast mentally retarded adults as children we are appalled, for example, at the thought of their having a sexual or even a social life. Deprived of the joy and privilege of parenthood, for which they may have no capacity, they are punished further by being denied the privilege and pleasure of affection, tenderness, romance, and sexual contact for which they may indeed have a capacity.

A mentally retarded individual ought not be given the responsibility of raising a child, and indeed a mentally retarded woman could be terrified of the changes in her body which pregnancy would produce. Sterilization could allow for the kind of innovation in social living lacking at most facilities for the mentally retarded. There is no reason why community living, even a family-type living, that involved affection, tenderness, and sexuality could not be a fundamental part of their lives and partly compensate for their lack of ordinary intellectual pleasures. Instead we punitively add one deprivation onto the other.

Sterilization is, after all, simply a word. There is nothing in the procedure itself that is innately evil. We allow sterilization when its benefits for the individual outweigh its costs. It is a legitimate procedure, offensive to some for religious reasons but not to others. In this matter society ought to respect the individual conscience and the individual value.

When, as with the retarded, the concepts necessary for intelligent decision making are beyond a person's intellectual grasp, we would be wise to leave the power of the delegated autonomy in the hands of the family. If that is abused all sorts of legal mechanisms exist for rectification. What state right warrants intrusion into the decision making? If it is established (first by the family, then if there is suspicion of abuse, by courts), that the mental retardation is of a degree that precludes the role of parent, the young woman will be deprived only of the "privilege" of conception and, presumably, abortion. She will gain, however, new freedoms, and her parents will gain peace of mind.

The incursion into the powers of the family by the state, here as in other places, is often cast in the noble language of rights. What is really at issue in many arguments about "fetal rights," "infant rights," and so on is in reality the relocation of delegated autonomy and power from one institution—the family—to another—the state. Too often the kind of government intervention we have been seeing in these difficult cases, where right and wrong are too finely balanced for comfort or coincidence in any decision, represents arrogance rather than compassion. It is unseemly and demeans the state, for more often than not the state is acting not *in loco parentis* but simply as Nosey Parker.

If "D's" incapacities to be a mother are still evidenced when she is fifteen years of age, she, through the agents of her care, that is, her family, ought to have the right to exercise the privilege of sterilization.

NOTE

1. This class action suit successfully argued that conditions in the public shelters for men were so dangerous, dirty, and degrading as to constitute a genuine deterrent to their use by homeless men. It was settled in August 1981 by means of a negotiated consent decree that not only recognized a legal right to shelter but also established certain qualitative standards that public shelters must henceforth meet.

PART TWO

Narrative Perspectives

Introduction to Part Two

§

WHILE PART 1 includes many challenges to our definitions of insanity and mental disorders, all the authors recognize that—however we define, diagnose, and treat—some people really do suffer from breaks with reality, from disabling fears, from depressions and behavior disorders. Great writers throughout history have given us literary portraits of these deviations from the norms, about the irrational and surprising things people do and say and about what might motivate or determine that behavior. Stories about the unusual and strange appeal to us more than stories about the normal—perhaps because we can try them on without risking too much.

This part of *What's Normal?* contains short stories, poems, and excerpts from plays, novels, and autobiographies—all portraying the experience of mental illnesses or disabilities. These works are grouped into six sections, each with its particular focus. The first section concentrates on children and adolescents suffering from mental disorders. Section two focuses on people with mental disabilities (retardation) and the problems experienced by their caregivers. Section three is devoted to portraits of women with mental disorders. Both four and five look at mental disturbances in men, but four focuses on men who suffer from "shell shock," or what is now termed Post Traumatic Stress Disorder. And, finally, section six explores the experience of senile dementia and Alzheimer's.

All these works offer insights and issues for us to consider when we are thinking about mental deviations from the norm. Sometimes they help us walk in the shoes of those who are suffering from mental distresses or of those who are trying to care for them. They help us to understand the pain of being treated as mentally abnormal, perhaps labeled that way forever. As Wayne Booth comments in *The Company We Keep,* narratives supplement and interpret life; they make and remake our primary experiences, and therefore ourselves. When we read any work, or listen to any story, we are keeping company for a while with that storyteller. We sometimes wonder if we should believe the storyteller and if we are willing to be the kind of person the storyteller is asking us to be. We absorb the values of what we read, at least as long as we are reading it. Sometimes, as is the case with most of the works in this collection, keeping that company opens us to "otherness," to people who experience the world in ways that may be radically different from ours. Such encounters with those "others" undermine our conventional attitudes about the mentally ill and disabled and help us learn new ways of seeing.

It is important, therefore, to pay careful attention to the narrators in each of these works. Some are "unreliable" because of their mental disorder or disability. Or at least a "normal" reader might consider them to be unreliable. As readers we need to listen carefully to them, because we are not used to their perspectives. Some narrators are stressed by their roles as caregivers of mentally disabled loved ones. Some may be intolerant and judgmental. Rarely can we accept a narrator as neutral and objective, as giving us the "straight" story without filters and biases.

Some of the works are first-person accounts, narrated by the person inside the experience of the illness or disorder (these accounts may be fiction as well as autobiography). A first-person narration produces several effects. It seems more real. As the narrator says, "I saw it happen," the "I" seems to be speaking from experience, as an "eyewitness," even if the work is fiction. The reader tends to trust and believe the narrator, at least as long as the story does not stray too far from the normal (though many of these stories do deviate rather far). First-person narration is often deeply personal and subjective, concentrating on the truths of feelings and emotions rather than on verifiable experiments. First-person narration lacks the "corrective" balance of a neutral outside observer, so the reader can be "taken in" by the intimate, interior perspective and not be at all sure whether the narrator is normal.

In the first section, on children and adolescents, Conrad Aiken's remarkable story is told by a disturbed autistic child as he withdraws deeper and deeper into his own world. Since he is the only narrator, we do not have access to what his parents or the doctor think except for occasions when he quotes them. Somehow we align with him and do not want to hear from the parents. Susanna Kaysen, in the excerpt from *Girl Interrupted,* has her teenaged narrator describe her own suicide attempt as well as her experiences in a mental hospital. Both the youth of the narrators and their mental disturbances cause us to be cautious about taking everything they say at face value, but we share their distrust of the adults. But the child narrator of Graham Greene's "The End of the Party" quite convincingly persuades us that his brother was literally scared to death at a children's party. Finally, the excerpt from the play *Equus* presents the narrative dramatically as the play evolves—the doctor gradually drawing out the teenager's story of why he blinded six horses with a hoof pick. While we cannot share this disturbed boy's beliefs, we can be convinced that he believed them and acted on them, and we can even sympathize some with the doctor's reluctance to make the boy normal.

Not surprisingly, none of the works in the second section—on mental disability—is narrated from "within" the experience, although the parents in *Joe Egg* do invent voices and personalities for their severely retarded daughter. (One of the few attempts in literature to articulate what the inarticulate might be thinking and feeling appears in the Benji chapter of William Faulkner's *The Sound and the Fury*—"a tale told by an idiot, signifying nothing.") Out of the works in this section, the somewhat handicapped Lennie in John Steinbeck's *Of Mice and Men* has the clearest voice, though he cannot remember much or control his impulses. Most of these stories are told from the outside, the narrator observing and reporting on what happens, and sometimes getting inside the thoughts of the "normal" characters. Seamus Heaney, in his poem "Two Stick Drawings," offers a bemused description of the inexplicable importance of walking sticks to the town's mentally handicapped "Simple" Jim. Often the author's tone colors how we interpret what the narrator tells us. Eudora Welty, for example, looks with amusement and gentle satire on the retarded Lilly and the busybody townswomen who try to get her committed to an institution before she gets pregnant. Flannery O'Connor's tone is more serious and judgmental, seeing moral failure in those who could take advantage of an innocent retarded woman. And Anne Tyler's story, narrated from the perspective of a distraught single mother having to commit her mentally disabled child to an institution, is infused with a tone of compassion and sadness.

In contrast, the third section finds most of the women narrators telling their own stories, giving extraordinary insights into their feelings, thoughts, and reactions to experiences. Since many of these characters have been silenced in their own contexts, have not been listened to or understood, their narrations give them a voice, effective at least for the readers. In Charlotte Perkins Gilman's "The Yellow Wallpaper," the narrator is so dominated by her physician-husband that she can break free of that prison only by escaping into madness. We hear her voice as she gradually moves into a realm where he cannot control her. The New Zealand writer, Janet Frame, in her novel based on her own life, describes the complete powerlessness of submitting to electroshock therapy. Nobody listens to her fears or questions. She has no way out. Anne Sexton also writes from within the "madhouse," where "there are no knives for cutting your throat." In a persecuted persona's voice, she says, "The world is full of enemies. / There is no safe place." Emily Dickinson, in a depressed mood, feels "a funeral in my brain." But in a more philosophical spirit, she comments that madness and sanity are defined by the majority. If you do not go along with the majority, if you deviate from their norm, "you're straightway dangerous— / and handled with a Chain." In this poem, she sounds like several of the writers in Part 1.

This third section also shows how women's experiences with mental anxieties translate across cultural and ethnic lines. Linda Hogan and Joy Harjo describe stresses in the experiences of Native American women; Maxine Hong Kingston gives a Chinese American perspective on "No Name Woman"; Laura Esquivel speaks from a Mexican American point of view. Some of their characters seem uprooted, suffering a loss of meaning and identity, as if they are not sure who they are or where they are going.

None of the Post Traumatic Stress Disorder and other anxiety stories in the fourth section is told in the first person, although almost all have an omniscient third-person narrator who gets inside the head of the disturbed man and describes what he is thinking and feeling. Such a narrative position allows both an outside, somewhat "objective" look at the character and an inside appreciation of his panics and depressions. It also prevents the careful reader from adopting a single perspective and assuming it to be accurate and sufficient. In Toni Morrison's *Sula,* for example, the narrator describes Shadrack as having been "blasted and permanently astonished by the events of 1917." Inside Shadrack's hallucination, the narrator describes the sick man's hands as growing like some giant beanstalk all over the bed and terrorizing him so much he could not look at them, let alone feed himself. This double perspective gives insight into the character's feelings but also keeps a distance and watches him from the outside. Leslie Marmon Silko's narrator gets inside Tayo's nightmares about endless torrential rains in his jungle war experiences; the narrator is also outside watching this Laguna man trying not to blame himself for the severe drought back home in the American southwest. Virginia Woolf watches Septimus from the perspectives of his wife, his doctors, and other characters as well as from within the suicidal veteran, effectively emphasizing the vast differences in how they see and interpret what is happening. Tim O'Brien moves from an external report of a platoon marching at night in Vietnam into the thoughts and fears of a young soldier who has just seen a colleague die of fright. And Wilfred Owen, in a sensitive and challenging portrait of "Mental Cases," sees them rocking in their chairs as they reexperience endlessly "the batter of guns and shatter of flying muscles . . . rucked too thick for these men's extrication."

Contrast these multiple perspectives in this section with the psychotic hallucinating narrator of Poe's "Tell-Tale Heart" in section five. The narrator hears the dead man's heart beating so loudly under the floorboards that he is driven to confess to the murder. That first-person narration crucially determines the power of Poe's story. Not so wild but perhaps even more unreliable is the narrator of Landolfi's "Gogol's Wife." This so-called historically accurate biographer describes in a matter-of-fact voice an unbelievable story about Gogol's wife being a balloon—one who could talk and contract syphilis among other non-balloonlike behaviors. In another firsthand account, the schizophrenic narrator of *The Notebooks of Malte Laurids Brigge* describes his regression back into his childhood, with all of its fears and anxieties renewed. Philip Booth's narrator tells of his panic trying to "make it" at a halfway house, as he fights "the one / with hair like old vines / who steps out of / nowhere, trying to / take you over." Desperation, hunger, and alcohol combine in Ralph Ellison's story to make his "King of the Bingo Game" unable to let go of the control button—in a temporary but devastating break with reality.

Sometimes, in section five, the first-person narrator is not the disturbed man but a relative or friend trying to cope with or to understand a mentally ill loved one. Cash, for instance, in Faulkner's *As I Lay Dying*, ponders whether his brother Darl is really insane or whether it just looks that way in the crazy context of this family carrying the rotting corpse of their mother on a nine-day wagon journey. (Cash's question resembles Dickinson's comment about the majority defining sanity and insanity. Darl's madness makes "divine sense" in this context.)

In the section on Alzheimer's and dementia, one of the most unusual first-person narrations is that of Robert Davis, an Alzheimer's patient who was able in the early days of his disease to describe what he was going through. According to professionals working with Alzheimer's, Davis gives one of the very few reliable firsthand accounts of the experience. The other descriptions of Alzheimer's and dementia in this section come from family members or friends trying to understand what is happening to the identity of a loved one. Hale Chatfield gives a heartbreaking tribute to his mother "lost in time." Joyce Dyer's account is a particularly sensitive and humble portrayal of her mother's dementia and of her own emotional reactions to losing the person she knew and loved while trying to cope with what her mother was becoming. In a more playful mood, Jean Wood describes the comic awkwardness of eating in a restaurant with her husband who suffers from Alzheimer's. Gene Hirsch's poems give both an internal and external perspective on the experience of dementia.

These literary works put us into worlds different from our ordinary ones and make us aware of other people in ways that can keep us from rejecting or trivializing them. In its powerful images and metaphors, in its plots where behavior has causes and effects, good literature requires us readers to make judgments about choice and value. It gives us alternative worlds with different norms and rival experiences. It can serve as a hedge against prejudice and fear and can open us up to understanding, especially of those who inhabit mental worlds different from our own.

Children & Adolescents with Mental Disorders

ॐ

Silent Snow, Secret Snow

CONRAD AIKEN

I

JUST WHY it should have happened, or why it should have happened just when it did, he could not, of course, possibly have said; nor perhaps would it even have occurred to him to ask. The thing was above all a secret, something to be preciously concealed from Mother and Father; and to that very fact it owed an enormous part of its deliciousness. It was like a peculiarly beautiful trinket to be carried unmentioned in one's trouser pocket—a rare stamp, an old coin, a few tiny gold links found trodden out of shape on the path in the park, a pebble of carnelian, a seashell distinguishable from all others by an unusual spot or stripe—and, as if it were any one of these, he carried around with him everywhere a warm and persistent and increasingly beautiful sense of possession. Nor was it only a sense of possession—it was also a sense of protection. It was as if, in some delightful way, his secret gave him a fortress, a wall behind which he could retreat into heavenly seclusion. This was almost the first thing he had noticed about it—apart from the oddness of the thing itself—and it was this that now again, for the fiftieth time, occurred to him, as he sat in the little school room. It was the half-hour for geography. Miss Buell was revolving with one finger, slowly, a huge terrestrial globe which had been placed on her desk. The green and yellow continents passed and repassed, questions were asked and answered, and now the little girl in front of him, Deirdre, who had a funny little constellation of freckles on the back of her neck, exactly like the Big Dipper, was standing up and telling Miss Buell that the equator was the line that ran round the middle.

Miss Buell's face, which was old and grayish and kindly, with gray stiff curls beside the cheeks, and eyes that swam very brightly, like little minnows, behind thick glasses, wrinkled itself into a complication of amusements.

"Ah! I see. The earth is wearing a belt, or a sash. Or someone drew a line round it!"

"Oh no—not that—I mean—"

In the general laughter, he did not share, or only a very little. He was thinking about the Arctic and Antarctic regions, which of course, on the globe,
were white. Miss Buell was now telling them about the tropics, the jungles, the
steamy heat of equatorial swamps, where the birds and butterflies, and even the
snakes, were like living jewels. As he listened to these things, he was already,
with a pleasant sense of half-effort, putting his secret between himself and the
words. Was it really an effort at all? For effort implied something voluntary, and
perhaps even something one did not especially want; whereas this was distinctly pleasant, and came almost of its own accord. All he needed to do was to
think of that morning, the first one, and then of all the others—

But it was all so absurdly simple! It had amounted to so little. It was nothing,
just an idea—and just why it should have become so wonderful, so permanent,
was a mystery—a very pleasant one, to be sure, but also, in an amusing way,
foolish. However, without ceasing to listen to Miss Buell, who had now moved
up to the north temperate zones, he deliberately invited his memory of the first
morning. It was only a moment or two after he had waked up—or perhaps
the moment itself. But was there, to be exact, an exact moment? Was one awake
all at once? or was it gradual? Anyway, it was after he had stretched a lazy hand
up toward the headrail, and yawned, and then relaxed again among his warm
covers, all the more grateful on a December morning, that the thing had happened. Suddenly, for no reason, he had thought of the postman, he remembered the postman. Perhaps there was nothing so odd in that. After all, he heard
the postman almost every morning in his life—his heavy boots could be heard
clumping round the corner at the top of the little cobbled hill-street, and then,
progressively nearer, progressively louder, the double knock at each door, the
crossings and re-crossings of the street, till finally the clumsy steps came stumbling across to the very door, and the tremendous knock came which shook the
house itself.

(Miss Buell was saying, "Vast wheat-growing areas in North America and
Siberia."

Deirdre had for the moment placed her left hand across the back of her
neck.)

But on this particular morning, the first morning, as he lay there with his
eyes closed, he had for some reason *waited* for the postman. He wanted to hear
him come round the corner. And that was precisely the joke—he never did.
He never came. He never had come—*round the corner*—again. For when at
last the steps *were* heard, they had already, he was quite sure, come a little down
the hill, to the first house; and even so, the steps were curiously different—they
were softer, they had a new secrecy about them, they were muffled and indistinct; and while the rhythm of them was the same, it now said a new thing—it

said peace, it said remoteness, it said cold, it said sleep. And he had understood the situation at once—nothing could have seemed simpler—there had been snow in the night, such as all winter he had been longing for; and it was this which had rendered the postman's first footsteps inaudible, and the later ones faint. Of course! How lovely! And even now it must be snowing—it was going to be a snowy day—the long white ragged lines were drifting and sifting across the street, across the faces of the old houses, whispering and hushing, making little triangles of white in the corners between cobblestones, seething a little when the wind blew them over the ground to a drifted corner; and so it would be all day, getting deeper and deeper and silenter and silenter.

(Miss Buell was saying, "Land of perpetual snow.")

All this time, of course (while he lay in bed), he had kept his eyes closed, listening to the nearer progress of the postman, the muffled footsteps thumping and slipping on the snow-sheathed cobbles; and all the other sounds—the double knocks, a frosty far-off voice or two, a bell ringing thinly and softly as if under a sheet of ice—had the same slightly abstracted quality, as if removed by one degree from actuality—as if everything in the world had been insulated by snow. But when at last, pleased, he opened his eyes, and turned them toward the window, to see for himself this long-desired and now so clearly imagined miracle—what he saw instead was brilliant sunlight on a roof; and when, astonished, he jumped out of bed and stared down into the street, expecting to see the cobbles obliterated by the snow, he saw nothing but the bare bright cobbles themselves.

Queer, the effect this extraordinary surprise had had upon him—all the following morning he had kept with him a sense as of snow falling about him, a secret screen of new snow between himself and the world. If he had not dreamed such a thing—and how could he have dreamed it while awake?—how else could one explain it? In any case, the delusion had been so vivid as to affect his entire behavior. He could not now remember whether it was on the first or the second morning—or was it even the third?—that his mother had drawn attention to some oddness in his manner.

"But my darling"—she had said at the breakfast table—"what has come over you? You don't seem to be listening. . . ."

And how often that very thing had happened since!

(Miss Buell was now asking if anyone knew the difference between the North Pole and the Magnetic Pole. Deirdre was holding up her flickering brown hand, and he could see the four white dimples that marked the knuckles.)

Perhaps it hadn't been either the second or third morning—or even the fourth or fifth. How could he be sure? How could he be sure just when the delicious *progress* had become clear? Just when it had really *begun?* The intervals weren't very precise. . . . All he now knew was, that at some point or other—perhaps the second day, perhaps the sixth—he had noticed that the presence of the snow was a little more insistent, the sound of it clearer; and, conversely, the sound of the postman's footsteps more indistinct. Not only could he not hear the steps come round the corner, he could not even hear them at the first house. It was below the first house that he heard them; and then, a few days later, it was below the second house that he heard them; and a few days later again, below the third. Gradually, gradually, the snow was becoming heavier, the sound of its seething louder, the cobblestones more and more muffled. When he found, each morning, on going to the window, after the ritual of listening, that the roofs and cobbles were as bare as ever, it made no difference. This was, after all, only what he had expected. It was even what pleased him, what rewarded him: the thing was his own, belonged to no one else. No one else knew about it, not even his mother and father. There, outside were the bare cobbles; and here, inside, was the snow. Snow growing heavier each day, muffling the world, hiding the ugly, and deadening increasingly—above all—the steps of the postman.

"But, my darling"—she had said at the luncheon table—"what has come over you? You don't seem to listen when people speak to you. That's the third time I've asked you to pass your plate. . . ."

How was one to explain this to Mother? or to Father? There was, of course, nothing to be done about it: nothing. All one could do was to laugh embarrassedly, pretend to be a little ashamed, apologize, and take a sudden and somewhat disingenuous interest in what was being done or said. The cat had stayed out all night. He had a curious swelling on his left cheek—perhaps somebody had kicked him, or a stone had struck him. Mrs. Kempton was or was not coming to tea. The house was going to be housecleaned, or "turned out," on Wednesday instead of Friday. A new lamp was provided for his evening work—perhaps it was eyestrain which accounted for this new and so peculiar vagueness of his—Mother was looking at him with amusement as she said this, but with something else as well. A new lamp? A new lamp. Yes, Mother, No, Mother, Yes, Mother. School is going very well. The geometry is very easy. The history is very dull. The geography is very interesting—particularly when it takes one to the North Pole. Why the North Pole? Oh, well, it would be fun to be an explorer. Another Perry or Scott or Shackleton. And then abruptly he found his interest in the talk at an end, stared at the pudding on his plate, listened, waited, and began once more—ah, how heavenly, too, the first beginnings—to hear or feel—for could he actually hear it?—the silent snow, the secret snow.

(Miss Buell was telling them about the search for the Northwest Passage, about Henrik Hudson, the *Half Moon.*)

This had been, indeed, the only distressing feature of the new experience; the fact that it so increasing had brought him into a kind of mute misunderstanding, or even conflict, with his father and mother. It was as if he were trying to lead a double life. On the one hand, he had to be Paul Hasleman, and keep up the appearance of being that person—dress, wash, and answer intelligently when spoken to—; on the other, he had to explore this new world which had been opened to him. Nor could there be the slightest doubt—not the slightest—that the new world was the profounder and more wonderful of the two. It was irresistible. It was miraculous. Its beauty was simply beyond anything—beyond speech as beyond thought—utterly incommunicable. But how then, between the two worlds, of which he was thus constantly aware, was he to keep a balance? One must get up, one must go to breakfast, one must talk with Mother, go to school, do one's lessons—and, in all this, try not to appear too much of a fool. But if all the while one was also trying to extract the full deliciousness of another and quite separate existence, one which could not easily (if at all) be spoken of—how was one to manage? How was one to explain? Would it be safe to explain? Would it be absurd? Would it merely mean that he would get into some obscure kind of trouble?

These thoughts came and went, came and went, as softly and secretly as the snow; they were not precisely a disturbance, perhaps they were even a pleasure; he liked to have them; their presence was something almost palpable, something he could stroke with his hand, without closing his eyes, and without ceasing to see Miss Buell and the schoolroom and the globe and the freckles on Deirdre's neck; nevertheless he did in a sense cease to see, or to see the obvious external world, and substituted for this vision the vision of snow, the sound of snow, and the slow, almost soundless, approach of the postman. Yesterday, it had been only at the sixth house that the postman had become audible; the snow was much deeper now, it was falling more swiftly and heavily, the sound of its seething was more distinct, more soothing, more persistent. And this morning, it had been—as nearly as he could figure—just above the seventh house—perhaps only a step or two above; at most, he had heard two or three footsteps before the knock had sounded. . . . And with each such narrowing of the sphere, each nearer approach of the limit at which the postman was first audible, it was odd how sharply was increased the amount of illusion which had to be carried into the ordinary business of daily life. Each day, it was harder to get out of bed, to go to the window, to look out at the—as always—perfectly empty and snowless street. Each day it was more difficult to go through the perfunctory motions of greeting Mother and Father at breakfast, to reply to their questions, to put his books together and go to school. And at school, how extraordinarily hard to conduct with success simultaneously the public life and the life that was secret! There were times when he longed—positively ached—to tell everyone about it—to burst out with it—only to be checked almost at once by a far-off feeling as of some faint absurdity which was inherent in it—but *was* it absurd?—and more importantly by a sense of mysterious power in his very secrecy. Yes; it must be kept secret. That, more and more, became clear. At whatever cost to himself, whatever pain to others—

(Miss Buell looked straight at him, smiling, and said, "Perhaps we'll ask Paul. I'm sure Paul will come out of his daydream long enough to be able to tell us. Won't you, Paul?" He rose slowly from his chair, resting one hand on the brightly varnished desk, and deliberately stared through the snow toward the blackboard. It was an effort, but it was amusing to make it. "Yes," he said slowly, "it was what we now call the Hudson River. This he thought to be the Northwest Passage. He was disappointed." He sat down again, and as he did so Deirdre half turned in her chair and gave him a shy smile, of approval and admiration.)

At whatever pain to others.

This part of it was very puzzling, very puzzling. Mother was very nice, and so was Father. Yes, that was all true enough. He wanted to be nice to them, to tell them everything—and yet, was it really wrong of him to want to have a secret place of his own?

At bed-time, the night before, Mother had said, "If this goes on, my lad, we'll have to see a doctor, we will! We can't have our boy—" But what was it she had said? "Live in another world"? "Live so far away"? The word "far" had been in it, he was sure, and then Mother had taken up a magazine again and laughed a little, but with an expression which wasn't mirthful. He had felt sorry for her. . . .

The bell rang for dismissal. The sound came to him through long curved parallels of falling snow. He saw Deirdre rise, and had himself risen almost as soon—but not quite as soon—as she.

II

On the walk homeward, which was timeless, it pleased him to see through the accompaniment, or counterpoint, of snow, the items of mere externality on his way. There were many kinds of brick in the sidewalks, and laid in many kinds of pattern. The garden walls, too, were various, some of wooden palings, some of plaster, some of stone. Twigs of bushes leaned over the walls: the little hard green winter-buds of lilac, on gray stems, sheathed and fat; other branches very thin and fine and black and desiccated. Dirty sparrows huddled in the bushes, as dull in color as dead fruit left in leafless trees. A single starling creaked on a weather vane. In the gutter, beside a drain, was a scrap of torn and dirty newspaper, caught in a little delta of filth; the word ECZEMA appeared in large capitals, and below it was a letter from Mrs. Amelia D. Cravath, 2100 Pine Street, Fort Worth, Texas, to the effect that after being a sufferer for years she had been cured by Caley's Ointment. In the little delta, beside the fan-shaped and deeply runneled continent of brown mud, were lost twigs, descended from their parent trees, dead matches, a rusty horse-chestnut burr, a small concentration of eggshell, a streak of yellow sawdust which had been wet and now was dry and congealed, a brown pebble, and a broken feather. Farther on was a cement sidewalk, ruled into geometrical parallelograms, with a brass inlay at one end commemorating the contractors who had laid it, and, halfway across, an irregular and random series of dog-tracks, immortalized in synthetic stone. He knew these well, and always stepped on them; to cover the little hollows with his own foot had always been a queer pleasure; today he did it once more, but perfunctorily and detachedly, all the while thinking of something else. That was a dog, a long time ago, who had made a mistake and walked on the cement while it was still wet. He had probably wagged his tail, but that hadn't been recorded. Now, Paul Hasleman, aged twelve, on his way home from school, crossed the same river, which in the meantime had frozen into rock. Homeward through the snow, the snow falling in bright sunshine. Homeward?

Then came the gateway with the two posts surmounted by egg-shaped stones which had been cunningly balanced on their ends, as if by Columbus, and mortared in the very act of balance; a source of perpetual wonder. On the brick wall just beyond, the letter H had been stenciled, presumably for some purpose. H? H.

The green hydrant, with a little green-painted chain attached to the brass screw-cap.

The elm tree, with the great gray wound in the bark, kidney-shaped, into which he always put his hand—to feel the cold but living wood. The injury, he had been sure, was due to the gnawings of a tethered horse. But now it deserved only a passing palm, a merely tolerant eye. There were more important things. Miracles. Beyond the thoughts of trees, mere elms. Beyond the thoughts of sidewalks, mere stone, mere brick, mere cement. Beyond the thoughts even of his own shoes, which trod these sidewalks obediently, bearing a burden—far above—of elaborate mystery. He watched them. They were not very well polished; he had neglected them, for a very good reason: they were one of the many parts of the increasing difficulty of the daily return to daily life, the morning struggle. To get up, having at last opened one's eyes, to go to the window, and discover no snow, to wash, to dress, to descend the curving stairs to breakfast—

At whatever pain to others, nevertheless, one must persevere in severance, since the incommunicability of the experience demanded it. It was desirable, of course, to be kind to Mother and Father, especially as they seemed to be worried, but it was also desirable to be resolute. If they should decide—as appeared likely—to consult the doctor, Doctor Howells, and have Paul inspected, his heart listened to through a kind of dictaphone, his lungs, his stomach—well, that was all right. He would go through with it. He would give them answer for question, too—perhaps such answers as they hadn't expected? No. That would never do. For the secret world must, at all costs, be preserved.

The bird-house in the apple tree was empty—it was the wrong time of year for wrens. The little round black door had lost its pleasure. The wrens were enjoying other houses, other nests, remoter trees. But this too was a notion which he only vaguely and grazingly entertained—as if, for the moment, he merely touched an edge of it; there was something further on, which was already assuming a sharper importance; something which already teased at the corners of his eyes, teasing also at the corner of his mind. It was funny to think that he so wanted this, so awaited it—and yet found himself enjoying this momentary dalliance with the bird-house, as if for a quite deliberate postponement and enhancement of the approaching pleasure. He was aware of his delay, of his smiling and detached and now almost uncomprehending gaze at the little bird-house; he knew what he was going to look at next: it was his own little cobbled hill-street, his own house, the little river at the bottom of the hill, the grocer's shop with the cardboard man in the window—and now, thinking of all this, he turned his head, still smiling, and looking quickly right and left through the snow-laden sunlight.

And the mist of snow, as he had foreseen, was still on it—a ghost of snow falling in the bright sunlight, softly and steadily floating and turning and pausing, soundlessly meeting the snow that covered, as with a transparent mirage, the bare bright cobbles. He loved it—he stood still and loved it. Its beauty was paralyzing—beyond all words, all experience, all dream. No fairy story he had ever read could be compared with it—none had ever given him this extraordinary combination of ethereal loveliness with a something else, unnameable, which was just faintly and deliciously terrifying. What was this thing? As he thought of it, he looked upward toward his own bedroom window, which was open—and it was as if he looked straight into the room and saw himself lying half awake in his bed. There he was—at this very instant he was still perhaps actually there—more truly there than standing here at the edge of the cobbled hill-street, with one hand lifted to shade his eyes against the snow-sun. Had he indeed ever left his room, in all this time? since that very first morning? Was the whole progress still being enacted there, was it still the same morning, and himself not yet wholly awake? And even now, had the postman not yet come round the corner? . . .

This idea amused him, and automatically, as he thought of it, he turned his head and looked toward the top of the hill. There was, of course, nothing there—nothing and no one. The street was empty and quiet. And all the more because of its emptiness it occurred to him to count the houses—a thing which, oddly enough, he hadn't before thought of doing. Of course, he had known there weren't many—many, that is, on his own side of the street, which were the ones that figured in the postman's progress—but nevertheless it came as something of a shock to find that there were precisely *six,* above his own house—his own house was the seventh.

Six!

Astonished, he looked at his own house—looked at the door, on which was the number thirteen—and then realized that the whole thing was exactly and logically and absurdly what he ought to have known. Just the same, the realization gave him abruptly, and even a little frighteningly, a sense of hurry. He was being hurried—he was being rushed. For—he knit his brow—he couldn't be mistaken—it was just above the *seventh* house, his *own* house, that the postman had first been audible this very morning. But in that case—in that case— did it mean that tomorrow he would hear nothing? The knock he had heard must have been the knock of their own door. Did it mean—and this was an idea which gave him a really extraordinary feeling of surprise—that he would never hear the postman again?—that tomorrow morning the postman would already have passed the house, in a snow so deep as to render his footsteps completely inaudible? That he would have made his approach down the snow-filled street so soundlessly, so secretly, that he, Paul Hasleman, there lying in bed, would not have waked in time, or waking, would have heard nothing?

But how could that be? Unless even the knocker should be muffled in the snow—frozen tight, perhaps? . . . But in that case—

A vague feeling of disappointment came over him; a vague sadness as if he felt himself deprived of something which he had long looked forward to, something much prized. After all this, all this beautiful progress, the slow delicious advance of the postman through the silent and secret snow, the knock creeping closer each day, and the footsteps nearer, the audible compass of the world thus daily narrowed, narrowed, narrowed, as the snow soothingly and beautifully encroached and deepened, after all this, was he to be defrauded of the one thing he had so wanted—to be able to count, as it were, the last two or three solemn footsteps, as they finally approached his own door? Was it all going to happen, at the end, so suddenly? or indeed, had it already happened? with no slow and subtle gradations of menace, in which he could luxuriate?

He gazed upward again, toward his own window which flashed in the sun; and this time almost with a feeling that it would be better if he *were* still in bed, in that room; for in that case this must still be the first morning, and there would be six more mornings to come—or, for that matter, seven or eight or nine—how could he be sure?—or even more.

III

After supper, the inquisition began. He stood before the doctor, under the lamp, and submitted silently to the usual thumpings and tappings.

"Now will you please say 'Ah!'?"

"Ah!"

"Now again, please, if you don't mind."

"Ah."

"Say it slowly, and hold it if you can—"

"Ah-h-h-h-h-h—"

"Good."

How silly all this was. As if it had anything to do with his throat! Or his heart, or lungs!

Relaxing his mouth, of which the corners, after all this absurd stretching, felt uncomfortable, he avoided the doctor's eyes, and stared toward the fireplace, past his mother's feet (in gray slippers) which projected from the green chair, and his father's feet (in brown slippers) which stood neatly side by side on the hearth rug.

"Hm. There is certainly nothing wrong there . . . ?"

He felt the doctor's eyes fixed upon him, and, as if merely to be polite, returned the look, but with a feeling of justifiable evasiveness.

"Now, young man, tell me—do you feel all right?"

"Yes, sir, quite all right."

"No headaches? no dizziness?"

"No, I don't think so."

"Let me see. Let's get a book, if you don't mind—yes, thank you, that will do splendidly—and now, Paul, if you'll just read it, holding it as you would normally hold it—"

He took the book and read:

"And another praise have I to tell for this the city our mother, the gift of a great god, a glory of the land most high; the might of horses, the might of young horses, the might of the sea. . . . For thou, son of Cronus, our lord Poseidon, hath throned herein this pride, since in these roads first thou didst show forth the curb that cures the rage of steeds. And the shapely oar, apt to men's hands, hath a wondrous speed on the brine, following the hundred-footed Nereids. . . . O land that art praised above all lands, now is it for thee to make those bright praises seen in deeds."

He stopped, tentatively, and lowered the heavy book.

"No—as I thought—there is certainly no superficial sign of eyestrain."

Silence thronged the room, and he was aware of the focused scrutiny of the three people who confronted him. . . .

"We could have his eyes examined—but I believe it is something else."

"What could it be?" That was his father's voice.

"It's only this curious absent-mindedness—" This was his mother's voice.

In the presence of the doctor, they both seemed irritatingly apologetic.

"I believe it is something else. Now Paul—I would like very much to ask you a question or two. You will answer them, won't you—you know I'm an old, old friend of yours, eh? That's right! . . ."

His back was thumped twice by the doctor's fat fist—then the doctor was grinning at him with false amiability, while with one fingernail he was scratching the top button of his waistcoat. Beyond the doctor's shoulder was the fire, the fingers of flame making light prestidigitation against the sooty fireback, the soft sound of their random flutter the only sound.

"I would like to know—is there anything that worries you?"

The doctor was again smiling, his eyelids low against the little black pupils, in each of which was a tiny white bead of light. Why answer him? why answer him at all? "At whatever pain to others"—but it was all a nuisance, this necessity for resistance, this necessity for attention; it was as if one had been stood up on a brilliantly lighted stage, under a great round blaze of spotlight; as if one were merely a trained seal, or a performing dog, or a fish, dipped out of an aquarium and held up by the tail. It would serve them right if he were merely to bark or growl. And meanwhile, to miss these last few precious hours, these hours of which each minute was more beautiful than the last, more menacing—! He still looked, as if from a great distance, at the beads of light in the doctor's eyes, at the fixed false smile, and then, beyond, once more at his mother's slippers, his father's slippers, the soft flutter of the fire. Even here, even amongst these hostile presences, and in this arranged light, he could see the snow, he could hear it—it was in the corners of the room, where the shadow was deepest, under the sofa, behind the half-opened door which led to the dining room. It was gentler here, softer, its seethe the quietest of whispers, as if, in deference to a drawing room, it had quite deliberately put on its "manners"; it kept itself out of sight, obliterated itself, but distinctly with an air of saying, "Ah, but just wait! Wait till we are alone together! Then I will begin to tell you something new! Something white! something cold! something sleepy! something of cease, and peace, and the long bright curve of space! Tell them to go away. Banish them. Refuse to speak. Leave them, go upstairs to your room, turn out the light and get into bed—I will go with you, I will be waiting for you, I will tell you a better story than Little Kay of the Skates, or

The Snow Ghost—I will surround your bed, I will close the windows, pile a deep drift against the door, so that none will ever again be able to enter. Speak to them! . . ." It seemed as if the little hissing voice came from a slow white spiral of falling flakes in the corner by the front window—but he could not be sure. He felt himself smiling, then, and said to the doctor, but without looking at him, looking beyond him still—

"Oh no, I think not—"

"But are you sure, my boy?"

His father's voice came softly and coldly then—the familiar voice of silken warning.

"You needn't answer at once, Paul—remember we're trying to help you— think it over and be quite sure, won't you?"

He felt himself smiling again, at the notion of being quite sure. What a joke! As if he weren't so sure that reassurance was no longer necessary, and all this cross-examination a ridiculous farce, a grotesque parody! What could they know about it? these gross intelligences, these humdrum minds so bound to the usual, the ordinary? Impossible to tell them about it! Why, even now, even now, with the proof so abundant, so formidable, so imminent, so appallingly present here in this very room, could they believe it?—could even his mother believe it? No—it was only too plain that if anything were said about it, the merest hint given, they would be incredulous—they would laugh—they would say "Absurd!"—think things about him which weren't true. . . .

"Why no, I'm not worried—why should I be?"

He looked then straight at the doctor's low-lidded eyes, looked from one of them to the other, from one bead of light to the other, and gave a little laugh.

The doctor seemed to be disconcerted by this. He drew back in his chair, resting a fat white hand on either knee. The smile faded slowly from his face.

"Well, Paul!" he said, and paused gravely, "I'm afraid you don't take this quite seriously enough. I think you perhaps don't quite realize—don't quite realize—" He took a deep quick breath, and turned, as if helplessly, at a loss for words, to the others. But Mother and Father were both silent—no help was forthcoming.

"You must surely know, be aware, that you have not been quite yourself, of late? Don't you know that? . . ."

It was amusing to watch the doctor's renewed attempt at a smile, a queer disorganized look, as of confidential embarrassment.

"I feel all right, sir," he said, and again gave the little laugh.

"And we're trying to help you." The doctor's tone sharpened.

"Yes, sir, I know. But why? I'm all right. I'm just *thinking* that's all."

His mother made a quick movement forward, resting a hand on the back of the doctor's chair.

"Thinking?" she said. "But my dear, about what?"

This was a direct challenge—and would have to be directly met. But before he met it, he looked again into the corner by the door, as if for reassurance. He smiled again at what he saw, at what he heard. The little spiral was still there, still softly whirling, like the ghost of a white kitten chasing the ghost of a white tail, and making as it did so the faintest of whispers. It was all right! If only he could remain firm, everything was going to be all right.

"Oh, about anything, about nothing—*you* know the way you do!"

"You mean—daydreaming?"

"Oh, no—thinking!"

"But thinking about *what?*"

"Anything."

He laughed a third time—but this time, happening to glance upward toward his mother's face, he was appalled at the effect his laughter seemed to have upon her. Her mouth had opened in an expression of horror. . . . This was too bad! Unfortunate! He had known it would cause pain, of course—but he hadn't expected it to be quite so bad as this. Perhaps—perhaps if he just gave them a tiny gleaming hint—?

"About the snow," he said.

"What on earth?" This was his father's voice. The brown slippers came a step nearer on the hearth-rug.

"But my dear, what do you mean?" This was his mother's voice.

The doctor merely stared.

"Just *snow,* that's all. I like to think about it."

"Tell us about it, my boy."

"But that's all it is. There's nothing to tell. *You* know what snow is?"

This he said almost angrily, for he felt that they were trying to corner him. He turned sideways so as no longer to face the doctor, and the better to see the inch of blackness between the window-sill and the lowered curtain—the cold inch of beckoning and delicious night. At once he felt better, more assured.

"Mother—can I go to bed, now, please? I've got a headache."

"But I thought you said—"

"It's just come. It's all these questions—! Can I, mother?"

"You can go as soon as the doctor has finished."

"Don't you think this thing ought to be gone into thoroughly, and *now?*" This was Father's voice. The brown slippers again came a step nearer, the voice was the well-known "punishment" voice, resonant and cruel.

"Oh, what's the use, Norman—"

Quite suddenly, everyone was silent. And without precisely facing them, nevertheless he was aware that all three of them were watching him with an extraordinary intensity—staring hard at him—as if he had done something monstrous, or was himself some kind of monster. He could hear the soft irregular flutter of the flames; the cluck-click-cluck-click of the clock; far and faint, two sudden spurts of laughter from the kitchen, as quickly cut off as begun; a murmur of water in the pipes; and then, the silence seemed to deepen, to spread out, to become world-long and world-wide, to become timeless and shapeless, and to center inevitably and rightly, with a slow and sleepy but enormous concentration of all power, on the beginning of a new sound. What this new sound was going to be, he knew perfectly well. It might begin with a hiss, but it would end with a roar—there was no time to lose—he must escape. It mustn't happen here—

Without another word, he turned and ran up the stairs.

IV

Not a moment too soon. The darkness was coming in long white waves. A prolonged sibilance filled the night—a great seamless seethe of wild influence went abruptly across it—a cold low humming shook the windows. He shut the door and flung off his clothes in the dark. The bare black floor was like a little raft tossed in waves of snow, almost overwhelmed, washed under whitely, up again, smothered in curled billows of feather. The snow was laughing; it spoke from all sides at once; it pressed closer to him as he ran and jumped exulting into his bed.

"Listen to us!" it said. "Listen! We have come to tell you the story we told you about. You remember? Lie down. Shut your eyes, now—you will no longer see much—in this white darkness who could see, or want to see? We will take the place of everything. . . . Listen—"

A beautiful varying dance of snow began at the front of the room, came forward and then retreated, flattened out toward the floor, then rose fountain-like to the ceiling, swayed, recruited itself from a new stream of flakes which poured laughing in through the humming window, advanced again, lifted long white arms. It said peace, it said remoteness, it said cold—it said—

But then a gash of horrible light fell brutally across the room from the opening door—the snow drew back hissing—something alien had come into the room—something hostile. This thing rushed at him, clutched at him, shook him—and he was not merely horrified, he was filled with such a loathing as he had never known. What was this? this cruel disturbance? this act of anger and hate? It was as if he had to reach up a hand toward another world for any understanding of it—an effort of which he was only barely capable. But of that other world he still remembered just enough to know the exorcising words. They tore themselves from his other life suddenly—

"Mother! Mother! Go away! I hate you!"

And with that effort, everything was solved, everything became all right: the seamless hiss advanced once more, the long white wavering lines rose and fell like enormous whispering sea-waves, the whisper becoming louder, the laughter more numerous.

"Listen!" it said. "We'll tell you the last, the most beautiful and secret story—shut your eyes—it is a very small story—a story that gets smaller and smaller—it comes inward instead of opening like a flower—it is a flower becoming a seed—a little cold seed—do you hear? we are leaning closer to you—"

The hiss was now becoming a roar—the whole world was a vast moving screen of snow—but even now it said peace, it said remoteness, it said cold, it said sleep.

The End of the Party

GRAHAM GREENE

PETER MORTON woke with a start to face the first light. Rain tapped against the glass. It was January the fifth.

He looked across a table on which a night-light had guttered into a pool of water, at the other bed. Francis Morton was still asleep, and Peter lay down again with his eyes on his brother. It amused him to imagine it was himself whom he watched, the same hair, the same eyes, the same lips and line of cheek. But the thought palled, and the mind went back to the fact which lent the day importance. It was the fifth of January. He could hardly believe a year had passed since Mrs Henne-Falcon had given her last children's party.

Francis turned suddenly upon his back and threw an arm across his face, blocking his mouth. Peter's heart began to beat fast, not with pleasure now but with uneasiness. He sat up and called across the table, 'Wake up.' Francis's shoulders shook and he waved a clenched fist in the air, but his eyes remained closed. To Peter Morton the whole room seemed to darken, and he had the impression of a great bird swooping. He cried again, 'Wake up,' and once more there was silver light and the touch of rain on the windows. Francis rubbed his eyes. 'Did you call out?' he asked.

'You are having a bad dream,' Peter said. Already experience had taught him how far their minds reflected each other. But he was the elder, by a matter of minutes, and that brief extra interval of light, while his brother still struggled in pain and darkness, had given him self-reliance and an instinct of protection towards the other who was afraid of so many things.

'I dreamed that I was dead,' Francis said.

'What was it like?' Peter asked.

'I can't remember,' Francis said.

'You dreamed of a big bird.'

'Did I?'

The two lay silent in bed facing each other, the same green eyes, the same nose tilting at the tip, the same firm lips, and the same premature modelling of the chin. The fifth of January, Peter thought again, his mind drifting idly from the image of cakes to the prizes which might be won. Egg-and-spoon races, spearing apples in basins of water, blind man's bluff.

'I don't want to go,' Francis said suddenly. 'I suppose Joyce will be there . . .
Mabel Warren.' Hateful to him, the thought of a party shared with those two.
They were older than he. Joyce was eleven and Mabel Warren thirteen. Their
long pigtails swung superciliously to a masculine stride. Their sex humiliated
him, as they watched him fumble with his egg, from under lowered scornful
lids. And last year . . . he turned his face away from Peter, his cheeks scarlet.

'What's the matter?' Peter asked.

'Oh, nothing. I don't think I'm well. I've got a cold. I oughtn't to go to the
party.' Peter was puzzled. 'But Francis, is it a bad cold?'

'It will be a bad cold if I go to the party. Perhaps I shall die.'

'Then you mustn't go,' Peter said, prepared to solve all difficulties with
one plain sentence, and Francis let his nerves relax, ready to leave everything to
Peter. But though he was grateful he did not turn his face towards his brother.
His cheeks still bore the badge of a shameful memory, of the game of hide and
seek last year in the darkened house, and of how he had screamed when Mabel
Warren put her hand suddenly upon his arm. He had not heard her coming.
Girls were like that. Their shoes never squeaked. No boards whined under the
tread. They slunk like cats on padded claws.

When the nurse came in with hot water Francis lay tranquil leaving everything to Peter. Peter said, 'Nurse, Francis has got a cold.'

The tall starched woman laid the towels across the cans and said, without
turning, 'The washing won't be back till tomorrow. You must lend him some of
your handkerchiefs.'

'But, Nurse,' Peter asked, 'hadn't he better stay in bed?'

'We'll take him for a good walk this morning,' the nurse said. 'Wind'll blow
away the germs. Get up now, both of you,' and she closed the door behind her.

'I'm sorry,' Peter said. 'Why don't you just stay in bed? I'll tell mother you felt
too ill to get up.' But rebellion against destiny was not in Francis's power. If he
stayed in bed they would come up and tap his chest and put a thermometer in
his mouth and look at his tongue, and they would discover he was malingering.
It was true he felt ill, a sick empty sensation in his stomach and a rapidly beating heart, but he knew the cause was only fear, fear of the party, fear of being
made to hide by himself in the dark, uncompanioned by Peter and with no
night-light to make a blessed breach.

'No, I'll get up,' he said, and then with sudden desperation, 'But I won't
go to Mrs Henne-Falcon's party. I swear on the Bible I won't.' Now surely
all would be well, he thought. God would not allow him to break so solemn an
oath. He would show him a way. There was all the morning before him and all
the afternoon until four o'clock. No need to worry when the grass was still
crisp with the early frost. Anything might happen. He might cut himself or
break his leg or really catch a bad cold. God would manage somehow.

He had such confidence in God that when at breakfast his mother said, 'I hear you have a cold, Francis,' he made light of it. 'We should have heard more about it,' his mother said with irony, 'if there was not a party this evening,' and Francis smiled, amazed and daunted by her ignorance of him. His happiness would have lasted longer if, out for a walk that morning, he had not met Joyce. He was alone with his nurse, for Peter had leave to finish a rabbit-hutch in the woodshed. If Peter had been there he would have cared less; the nurse was Peter's nurse also, but now it was as though she were employed only for his sake, because he could not be trusted to go for a walk alone. Joyce was only two years older and she was by herself.

She came striding towards them, pigtails flapping. She glanced scornfully at Francis and spoke with ostentation to the nurse. 'Hello, Nurse. Are you bringing Francis to the party this evening? Mabel and I are coming.' And she was off again down the street in the direction of Mabel Warren's home, consciously alone and self-sufficient in the long empty road. 'Such a nice girl,' the nurse said. But Francis was silent, feeling again the jump-jump of his heart, realizing how soon the hour of the party would arrive. God had done nothing for him, and the minutes flew.

They flew too quickly to plan any evasion, or even to prepare his heart for the coming ordeal. Panic nearly overcame him when, all unready, he found himself standing on the doorstep, with coat-collar turned up against a cold wind, and the nurse's electric torch making a short trail through the darkness. Behind him were the lights of the hall and the sound of a servant laying the table for dinner, which his mother and father would eat alone. He was nearly overcome by the desire to run back into the house and call out to his mother that he would not go to the party, that he dared not go. They could not make him go. He could almost hear himself saying those final words, breaking down for ever the barrier of ignorance which saved his mind from his parents' knowledge. 'I'm afraid of going. I won't go. I daren't go. They'll make me hide in the dark, and I'm afraid of the dark. I'll scream and scream and scream.' He could see the expression of amazement on his mother's face, and then the cold confidence of a grown-up's retort.

'Don't be silly. You must go. We've accepted Mrs Henne-Falcon's invitation.' But they couldn't make him go; hesitating on the doorstep while the nurse's feet crunched across the frost-covered grass to the gate, he knew that. He would answer: 'You can say I'm ill. I won't go. I'm afraid of the dark.' And his mother: 'Don't be silly. You know there's nothing to be afraid of in the dark.' But he knew the falsity of that reasoning; he knew how they taught also that there was nothing to fear in death, and how fearfully they avoided the idea of it. But they couldn't make him go to the party. 'I'll scream. I'll scream.'

'Francis, come along.' He heard the nurse's voice across the dimly phospho-rescent lawn and saw the yellow circle of her torch wheel from tree to shrub. 'I'm coming,' he called with despair; he couldn't bring himself to lay bare his last secrets and end reserve between his mother and himself, for there was still in the last resort a further appeal possible to Mrs Henne-Falcon. He comforted himself with that, as he advanced steadily across the hall, very small, towards her enormous bulk. His heart beat unevenly, but he had control now over his voice, as he said with meticulous accent, 'Good evening, Mrs Henne-Falcon. It was very good of you to ask me to your party.' With his strained face lifted towards the curve of her breasts, and his polite set speech, he was like an old withered man. As a twin he was in many ways an only child. To address Peter was to speak to his own image in a mirror, an image a little altered by a flaw in the glass, so as to throw back less a likeness of what he was than of what he wished to be, what he would be without his unreasoning fear of darkness, foot-steps of strangers, the flight of bats in dusk-filled gardens.

'Sweet child,' said Mrs Henne-Falcon absentmindedly, before, with a wave of her arms, as though the children were a flock of chickens, she whirled them into her set programme of entertainments: egg-and-spoon races, three-legged races, the spearing of apples, games which held for Francis nothing worse than humiliation. And in the frequent intervals when nothing was required of him and he could stand alone in corners as far removed as possible from Mabel Warren's scornful gaze, he was able to plan how he might avoid the approach-ing terror of the dark. He knew there was nothing to fear until after tea, and not until he was sitting down in a pool of yellow radiance cast by the ten candles on Colin Henne-Falcon's birthday cake did he become fully conscious of the im-minence of what he feared. He heard Joyce's high voice down the table, 'After tea we are going to play hide and seek in the dark.'

'Oh, no,' Peter said, watching Francis's troubled face, 'don't let's. We play that every year.'

'But it's in the programme,' cried Mabel Warren. 'I saw it myself. I looked over Mrs Henne-Falcon's shoulder. Five o'clock tea. A quarter to six to half past, hide and seek in the dark. It's all written down in the programme.'

Peter did not argue, for if hide and seek had been inserted in Mrs Henne-Falcon's programme, nothing which he could say would avert it. He asked for another piece of birthday cake and sipped his tea slowly. Perhaps it might be possible to delay the game for a quarter of an hour, allow Francis at least a few extra minutes to form a plan, but even in that Peter failed, for children were al-ready leaving the table in twos and threes. It was his third failure, and again he saw a great bird darken his brother's face with its wings. But he upbraided him-self silently for his folly, and finished his cake encouraged by the memory of that adult refrain, 'There's nothing to fear in the dark.' The last to leave the table, the brothers came together to the hall to meet the mustering and impatient eyes of Mrs Henne-Falcon.

'And now,' she said, 'we will play hide and seek in the dark.'

Peter watched his brother and saw the lips tighten. Francis, he knew, had feared this moment from the beginning of the party, had tried to meet it with courage and had abandoned the attempt. He must have prayed for cunning to evade the game, which was now welcomed with cries of excitement by all the other children. 'Oh, do let's.' 'We must pick sides.' 'Is any of the house out of bounds?' 'Where shall home be?'

'I think,' said Francis Morton, approaching Mrs Henne-Falcon, his eyes focused unwaveringly on her exuberant breasts, 'it will be no use my playing. My nurse will be calling for me very soon.'

'Oh, but your nurse can wait, Francis,' said Mrs Henne-Falcon, while she clapped her hands together to summon to her side a few children who were already straying up the wide staircase to upper floors. 'Your mother will never mind.'

That had been the limit of Francis's cunning. He had refused to believe that so well-prepared an excuse could fail. All that he could say now, still in the precise tone which other children hated, thinking it a symbol of conceit, was, 'I think I had better not play.' He stood motionless, retaining, though afraid, unmoved features. But the knowledge of his terror, or the reflection of the terror itself, reached his brother's brain. For the moment, Peter Morton could have cried aloud with the fear of bright lights going out, leaving him alone in an island of dark surrounded by the gentle lappings of strange footsteps. Then he remembered that the fear was not his own, but his brother's. He said impulsively to Mrs Henne-Falcon, 'Please, I don't think Francis should play. The dark makes him jump so.' They were the wrong words. Six children began to sing, 'Cowardy cowardy custard,' turning torturing faces with the vacancy of wide sunflowers towards Francis Morton.

Without looking at his brother, Francis said, 'Of course I'll play. I'm not afraid, I only thought . . .' But he was already forgotten by his human tormentors. The children scrambled round Mrs Henne-Falcon, their shrill voices pecking at her with questions and suggestions. 'Yes, anywhere in the house. We will turn out all the lights. Yes, you can hide in the cupboards. You must stay hidden as long as you can. There will be no home.'

Peter stood apart, ashamed of the clumsy manner in which he had tried to help his brother. Now he could feel, creeping in at the corners of his brain, all Francis's resentment of his championing. Several children ran upstairs, and the lights on the top floor went out. Darkness came down like the wings of a bat and settled on the landing. Others began to put out the lights at the edge of the hall, till the children were all gathered in the central radiance of the chandelier, while the bats squatted round on hooded wings and waited for that, too, to be extinguished.

'You and Francis are on the hiding side,' a tall girl said, and then the light was gone, and the carpet wavered under his feet with the sibilance of footfalls, like small cold draughts, creeping away into corners.

'Where's Francis?' he wondered. 'If I join him he'll be less frightened of all these sounds.' 'These sounds' were the casing of silence: the squeak of a loose board, the cautious closing of a cupboard door, the whine of a finger drawn along polished wood.

Peter stood in the centre of the dark deserted floor, not listening but waiting for the idea of his brother's whereabouts to enter his brain. But Francis crouched with fingers on his ears, eyes uselessly closed, mind numbed against impressions, and only a sense of strain could cross the gap of dark. Then a voice called 'Coming,' and as though his brother's self-possession had been shattered by the sudden cry, Peter Morton jumped with his fear. But it was not his own fear. What in his brother was a burning panic was in him an altruistic emotion that left the reason unimpaired. 'Where, if I were Francis, should I hide?' And because he was, if not Francis himself, at least a mirror to him, the answer was immediate. 'Between the oak bookcase on the left of the study door, and the leather settee.' Between the twins there could be no jargon of telepathy. They had been together in the womb, and they could not be parted.

Peter Morton tiptoed towards Francis's hiding-place. Occasionally a board rattled, and because he feared to be caught by one of the soft questers through the dark, he bent and untied his laces. A tag struck the floor and the metallic sound set a host of cautious feet moving in his direction. But by that time he was in his stockings and would have laughed inwardly at the pursuit had not the noise of someone stumbling on his abandoned shoes made his heart trip. No more boards revealed Peter Morton's progress. On stockinged feet he moved silently and unerringly towards his object. Instinct told him he was near the wall, and, extending a hand, he laid the fingers across his brother's face.

Francis did not cry out, but the leap of his own heart revealed to Peter a proportion of Francis's terror. 'It's all right,' he whispered, feeling down the squatting figure until he captured a clenched hand. 'It's only me. I'll stay with you.' And grasping the other tightly, he listened to the cascade of whispers his utterance had caused to fall. A hand touched the book-case close to Peter's head and he was aware of how Francis's fear continued in spite of his presence. It was less intense, more bearable, he hoped, but it remained. He knew that it was his brother's fear and not his own that he experienced. The dark to him was only an absence of light; the groping hand that of a familiar child. Patiently he waited to be found.

He did not speak again, for between Francis and himself was the most intimate communion. By way of joined hands thought could flow more swiftly than lips could shape themselves round words. He could experience the whole progress of his brother's emotion, from the leap of panic at the unexpected contact to the steady pulse of fear, which now went on and on with the regularity of a heart-beat. Peter Morton thought with intensity, 'I am here. You needn't be afraid. The lights will go on again soon. That rustle, that movement is nothing to fear. Only Joyce, only Mabel Warren.' He bombarded the drooping form with thoughts of safety, but he was conscious that the fear continued. 'They are beginning to whisper together. They are tired of looking for us. The lights will go on soon. We shall have won. Don't be afraid. That was only someone on the stairs. I believe it's Mrs Henne-Falcon. Listen. They are feeling for the lights.' Feet moving on a carpet, hands brushing a wall, a curtain pulled apart, a clicking handle, the opening of a cupboard door. In the case above their heads a loose book shifted under a touch. 'Only Joyce, only Mabel Warren, only Mrs Henne-Falcon,' a crescendo of reassuring thought before the chandelier burst, like a fruit-tree, into bloom.

The voices of the children rose shrilly into the radiance. 'Where's Peter?' 'Have you looked upstairs?' 'Where's Francis?' but they were silenced again by Mrs Henne-Falcon's scream. But she was not the first to notice Francis Morton's stillness, where he had collapsed against the wall at the touch of his brother's hand. Peter continued to hold the clenched fingers in an arid and puzzled grief. It was not merely that his brother was dead. His brain, too young to realize the full paradox, wondered with an obscure self-pity why it was that the pulse of his brother's fear went on and on, when Francis was now where he had always been told there was no more terror and no more darkness.

From Girl, Interrupted

SUSANNA KAYSEN

McLean Hospital   F49

INTER OFFICE MEMORANDUM

TO *Record Room*   Date *June 15, 1967*
                                                          Dr.

FROM Dr. ——

SUBJECT Susanna Kaysen

Susanna Kaysen was seen by me on April 27, 1967; following my evaluation which extended over three hours, I referred her to McLean Hospital for
admission.

My decision was based on:

1. The chaotic unplanned life of the patient at present with progressive decompensation and reversal of sleep cycle.
2. Severe depression and hopelessness and suicidal ideas.
3. History of suicidal attempts.
4. No therapy and no plan at present. Immersion in fantasy, progressive with-
   drawal and isolation.

The patient had been seen in psychotherapy by Dr. ——. At no time did I
have her in therapy, and the patient knew that I was not a potential therapist.

Etiology

This person is (pick one):

1. on a perilous journey from which we can learn much when he or she returns;
2. possessed by (pick one):
   a) the gods,
   b) God (that is, a prophet),
   c) some bad spirits, demons, or devils,
   d) the Devil;
3. a witch;
4. bewitched (variant of 2);

5. bad, and must be isolated and punished;
6. ill, and must be isolated and treated by (pick one):
   a) purging and leeches,
   b) removing the uterus if the person has one,
   c) electric shock to the brain,
   d) cold sheets wrapped tight around the body,
   e) Thorazine or Stelazine;
7. ill, and must spend the next seven years talking about it;
8. a victim of society's low tolerance for deviant behavior;
9. sane in an insane world;
10. on a perilous journey from which he or she may never return.

FIRE

One girl among us had set herself on fire. She used gasoline. She was too young to drive at the time. I wondered how she'd gotten hold of it. Had she walked to her neighborhood garage and told them her father's car had run out of gas? I couldn't look at her without thinking about it.

I think the gasoline had settled in her collarbones, forming pools there beside her shoulders, because her neck and cheeks were scarred the most. The scars were thick ridges, alternating bright pink and white, in stripes up from her neck. They were so tough and wide that she couldn't turn her head, but had to swivel her entire upper torso if she wanted to see a person standing next to her.

Scar tissue has no character. It's not like skin. It doesn't show age or illness or pallor or tan. It has no pores, no hair, no wrinkles. It's like a slipcover. It shields and disguises what's beneath. That's why we grow it; we have something to hide.

Her name was Polly. This name must have seemed ridiculous to her in the days—or months—when she was planning to set herself on fire, but it suited her well in her slipcovered, survivor life. She was never unhappy. She was kind and comforting to those who were unhappy. She never complained. She always had time to listen to other people's complaints. She was faultless, in her impermeable tight pink-and-white casing. Whatever had driven her, whispered "Die!" in her once-perfect, now-scarred ear, she had immolated it.

Why did she do it? Nobody knew. Nobody dared to ask. Because—what courage! Who had the courage to burn herself? Twenty aspirin, a little slit alongside the veins of the arm, maybe even a bad half hour standing on a roof: We've all had those. And somewhat more dangerous things, like putting a gun in your mouth. But you put it there, you taste it, it's cold and greasy, your finger is on the trigger, and you find that a whole world lies between this moment and the moment you've been planning, when you'll pull the trigger. That world defeats you. You put the gun back in the drawer. You'll have to find another way.

What was that moment like for her? The moment she lit the match. Had she already tried roofs and guns and aspirin? Or was it just an inspiration?

I had an inspiration once. I woke up one morning and I knew that today I had to swallow fifty aspirin. It was my task: my job for the day. I lined them up on my desk and took them one by one, counting. But it's not the same as what she did. I could have stopped, at ten, or at thirty. And I could have done what I did do, which was go onto the street and faint. Fifty aspirin is a lot of aspirin, but going onto the street and fainting is like putting the gun back in the drawer.

She lit the match.

Where? In the garage at home, where she wouldn't set anything else on fire? Out in a field? In the high school gym? In an empty swimming pool?

Somebody found her, but not for a while.

Who would kiss a person like that, a person with no skin?

She was eighteen before this thought occurred to her. She'd spent a year with us. Other people stormed and screamed and cringed and cried; Polly watched and smiled. She sat by people who were frightened, and her presence calmed them. Her smile wasn't mean, it was understanding. Life was hellish, she knew that. But, her smile hinted, she'd burned all that out of her. Her smile was a little bit superior: We wouldn't have the courage to burn it out of ourselves—but she understood that too. Everyone was different. People just did what they could.

One morning somebody was crying, but mornings were often noisy: fights about getting up on time and complaints about nightmares. Polly was so quiet, so unobtrusive a presence, that we didn't notice she wasn't at breakfast. After breakfast, we could still hear crying.

"Who's crying?"

Nobody knew.

And at lunch, there was still crying.

"It's Polly," said Lisa, who knew everything.

"Why?"

But even Lisa didn't know why.

At dusk the crying changed to screaming. Dusk is a dangerous time. At first she screamed, "Aaaaaah!" and "Eeeeeh!" Then she started to scream words.

"My face! My face! *My face!*"

We could hear other voices shushing her, murmuring comfort, but she continued to scream her two words long into the night.

Lisa said, "Well, I've been expecting this for a while."

And then I think we all realized what fools we'd been.

We might get out sometime, but she was locked up forever in that body.

My Suicide

Suicide is a form of murder—premeditated murder. It isn't something you do the first time you think of doing it. It takes getting used to. And you need the means, the opportunity, the motive. A successful suicide demands good organization and a cool head, both of which are usually incompatible with the suicidal state of mind.

It's important to cultivate detachment. One way to do this is to practice imagining yourself dead, or in the process of dying. If there's a window, you must imagine your body falling out the window. If there's a knife, you must imagine the knife piercing your skin. If there's a train coming, you must imagine your torso flattened under its wheels. These exercises are necessary to achieving the proper distance.

The motive is paramount. Without a strong motive, you're sunk.

My motives were weak: an American-history paper I didn't want to write and the question I'd asked months earlier, Why not kill myself? Dead, I wouldn't have to write the paper. Nor would I have to keep debating the question.

The debate was wearing me out. Once you've posed that question, it won't go away. I think many people kill themselves simply to stop the debate about whether they will or they won't.

Anything I thought or did was immediately drawn into the debate. Made a stupid remark—why not kill myself? Missed the bus—better put an end to it all. Even the good got in there. I liked that movie—maybe I shouldn't kill myself.

Actually, it was only part of myself I wanted to kill: the part that wanted to kill herself, that dragged me into the suicide debate and made every window, kitchen implement, and subway station a rehearsal for tragedy.

I didn't figure this out, though, until after I'd swallowed the fifty aspirin.

I had a boyfriend named Johnny who wrote me love poems—good ones. I called him up, said I was going to kill myself, left the phone off the hook, took my fifty aspirin, and realized it was a mistake. Then I went out to get some milk, which my mother had asked me to do before I took the aspirin.

Johnny called the police. They went to my house and told my mother what I'd done. She turned up in the A&P on Mass. Ave. just as I was about to pass out over the meat counter.

As I walked the five blocks to the A&P I was gripped by humiliation and regret. I'd made a mistake and I was going to die because of it. Perhaps I even deserved to die because of it. I began to cry about my death. For a moment, I felt compassion for myself and all the unhappiness I contained. Then things started to blur and whiz. By the time I reached the store, the world had been reduced to a narrow, throbbing tunnel. I'd lost my peripheral vision, my ears were ringing, my pulse was pounding. The bloody chops and steaks straining against their plastic wrappings were the last things I saw clearly.

Having my stomach pumped brought me around. They took a long tube and put it slowly up my nose and down the back of my throat. That was like being choked to death. Then they began to pump. That was like having blood drawn on a massive scale—the suction, the sense of tissue collapsing and touching itself in a way it shouldn't, the nausea as all that was inside was pulled out. It was a good deterrent. Next time, I decided, I certainly wouldn't take aspirin.

But when they were done, I wondered if there would be a next time. I felt good. I wasn't dead, yet something was dead. Perhaps I'd managed my peculiar objective of partial suicide. I was lighter, airier than I'd been in years.

My airiness lasted for months. I did some of my homework. I stopped seeing Johnny and took up with my English teacher, who wrote even better poems, though not to me. I went to New York with him; he took me to the Frick to see the Vermeers.

The only odd thing was that suddenly I was a vegetarian.

I associated meat with suicide, because of passing out at the meat counter. But I knew there was more to it.

The meat was bruised, bleeding, and imprisoned in a tight wrapping. And, though I had a six-month respite from thinking about it, so was I.

Elementary Topography

Perhaps it's still unclear how I ended up in there. It must have been something more than a pimple. I didn't mention that I'd never seen that doctor before, that he decided to put me away after only fifteen minutes. Twenty, maybe. What about me was so deranged that in less than half an hour a doctor would pack me off to the nuthouse? He tricked me, though: a couple of weeks. It was closer to two years. I was eighteen.

I signed myself in. I had to, because I was of age. It was that or a court order, though they could never have gotten a court order against me. I didn't know that, so I signed myself in.

I wasn't a danger to society. Was I a danger to myself? The fifty aspirin—but I've explained them. They were metaphorical. I wanted to get rid of a certain aspect of my character. I was performing a kind of self-abortion with those aspirin. It worked for a while. Then it stopped; but I had no heart to try again.

Take it from his point of view. It was 1967. Even in lives like his, professional lives lived out in the suburbs behind shrubbery, there was a strange undertow, a tug from the other world—the drifting, drugged-out, no-last-name youth universe—that knocked people off balance. One could call it "threatening," to use his language. What are these kids *doing*? And then one of them walks into his office wearing a skirt the size of a napkin, with a mottled chin and speaking in monosyllables. Doped up, he figures. He looks again at the name jotted on the notepad in front of him. Didn't he meet her parents at a party two years ago? Harvard faculty—or was it MIT? Her boots are worn down but her coat's a good one. It's a mean world out there, as Lisa would say. He can't in good conscience send her back into it, to become flotsam on the subsocietal tide that washes up now and then in his office, depositing others like her. A form of preventive medicine.

Am I being too kind to him? A few years ago I read he'd been accused of sexual harassment by a former patient. But that's been happening a lot these days; it's become fashionable to accuse doctors. Maybe it was just too early in the morning for him as well as for me, and he couldn't think of what else to do. Maybe, most likely, he was just covering his ass.

My point of view is harder to explain. I went. First I went to his office, then I got into the taxi, then I walked up the stone steps to the Administration Building of McLean Hospital, and, if I remember correctly, sat in a chair for fifteen minutes waiting to sign my freedom away.

Several preconditions are necessary if you are going to do such a thing.

I was having a problem with patterns. Oriental rugs, tile floors, printed curtains, things like that. Supermarkets were especially bad, because of the long, hypnotic checkerboard aisles. When I looked at these things, I saw other things within them. That sounds as though I was hallucinating, and I wasn't. I knew I was looking at a floor or a curtain. But all patterns seemed to contain potential representations, which in a dizzying array would flicker briefly to life. That could be . . . a forest, a flock of birds, my second-grade class picture. Well, it wasn't—it was a rug, or whatever it was, but my glimpses of the other things it might be were exhausting. Reality was getting too dense.

Something also was happening to my perceptions of people. When I looked at someone's face, I often did not maintain an unbroken connection to the concept of a face. Once you start parsing a face, it's a peculiar item: squishy, pointy, with lots of air vents and wet spots. This was the reverse of my problem with patterns. Instead of seeing too much meaning, I didn't see any meaning.

But I wasn't simply going nuts, tumbling down a shaft into Wonderland. It was my misfortune—or salvation—to be at all times perfectly conscious of my misperceptions of reality. I never "believed" anything I saw or thought I saw. Not only that, I correctly understood each new weird activity.

Now, I would say to myself, you are feeling alienated from people and unlike other people, therefore you are projecting your discomfort onto them. When you look at a face, you see a blob of rubber because you are worried that your face is a blob of rubber.

This clarity made me able to behave normally, which posed some interesting questions. Was everybody seeing this stuff and acting as though they weren't? Was insanity just a matter of dropping the act? If some people didn't see these things, what was the matter with them? Were they blind or something? These questions had me unsettled.

Something had been peeled back, a covering or shell that works to protect us. I couldn't decide whether the covering was something on me or something attached to everything in the world. It didn't matter, really; wherever it had been, it wasn't there anymore.

And this was the main precondition, that anything might be something else. Once I'd accepted that, it followed that I might be mad, or that someone might think me mad. How could I say for certain that I wasn't, if I couldn't say for certain that a curtain wasn't a mountain range?

I have to admit, though, that I knew I wasn't mad.

It was a different precondition that tipped the balance: the state of contrariety. My ambition was to negate. The world, whether dense or hollow, provoked only my negations. When I was supposed to be awake, I was asleep; when I was supposed to speak, I was silent; when a pleasure offered itself to me, I avoided it. My hunger, my thirst, my loneliness and boredom and fear were all weapons aimed at my enemy, the world. They didn't matter a whit to the world, of course, and they tormented me, but I got a gruesome satisfaction from my sufferings. They proved my existence. All my integrity seemed to lie in saying No.

So the opportunity to be incarcerated was just too good to resist. It was a very big No—the biggest No this side of suicide.

Perverse reasoning. But back of that perversity, I knew I wasn't mad and that they wouldn't keep me there, locked up in a loony bin.

McLean Hospital

F-90

No. 22201   Name   Kaysen, Susanna N.

1967 |ABSTRACT FROM VOLUNTARY APPLICATION: Patient withdrew to her room, ate very little, did not work or study and contemplated jumping into the river. She signed this voluntary application fully realizing the nature of her act.

———M.D./h

Director

April 27

From Equus

PETER SHAFFER

SCENE 18

DYSART: This boy, with his stare. He's trying to save himself through me.

HESTHER: I'd say so.

DYSART: What am I trying to do to him?

HESTHER: Restore him, surely?

DYSART: To what?

HESTHER: A normal life.

DYSART: Normal?

HESTHER: It still means something.

DYSART: Does it?

HESTHER: Of course.

DYSART: You mean a normal boy has one head: a normal head has two ears?

HESTHER: You know I don't.

DYSART: Then what else?

HESTHER: [*lightly*] Oh, stop it.

DYSART: No, what? You tell me.

HESTHER: [*rising: smiling*] I won't be put on the stand like this, Martin. You're really disgraceful! . . . [*Pause*] You know what I mean by a normal smile in a child's eyes, and one that isn't—even if I can't exactly define it. Don't you?

DYSART: Yes.

HESTHER: Then we have a duty to that, surely? Both of us.

DYSART: Touché. . . . I'll talk to you.

HESTHER: Dismissed?

DYSART: You said you had to go.

HESTHER: I do . . . [*she kisses his cheek*]. Thank you for what you're doing. . . . You're going through a rotten patch at the moment. I'm sorry . . . I suppose one of the few things one can do is simply hold on to priorities.

DYSART: Like what?

HESTHER: Oh—children before grown-ups. Things like that.

He contemplates her.

DYSART: You're really quite splendid.

HESTHER: Famous for it. Goodnight.

She leaves him.

DYSART: [*to himself—or to the audience*] Normal! . . . Normal!

SCENE 19

Alan rises and enters the square. He is subdued.

DYSART: Good afternoon.

ALAN: Afternoon.

DYSART: I'm sorry about our row yesterday.

ALAN: It was stupid.

DYSART: It was.

ALAN: What I said, I mean.

DYSART: How are you sleeping?

Alan shrugs.

You're not feeling well, are you?

ALAN: All right.

DYSART: Would you like to play a game? It could make you feel better.

ALAN: What kind?

DYSART: It's called *Blink*. You have to fix your eyes on something: say, that little stain over there on the wall—and I tap this pen on the desk. The first time I tap it, you close your eyes. The next time you open them. And so on. Close, open, close, open, till I say Stop.

ALAN: How can that make you feel better?

DYSART: It relaxes you. You'll feel as though you're talking to me in your sleep.

ALAN: It's stupid.

DYSART: You don't have to do it, if you don't want to.

ALAN: I didn't say I didn't want to.

DYSART: Well?

ALAN: I don't mind.

DYSART: Good. Sit down and start watching that stain. Put your hands by your sides, and open the fingers wide.

He opens the left bench and Alan sits on the end of it.

The thing is to feel comfortable, and relax absolutely . . . Are you looking at the stain?

ALAN: Yes.

DYSART: Right. Now try and keep your mind as blank as possible.

ALAN: That's not difficult.

DYSART: Ssh. Stop talking . . . On the first tap, close. On the second, open. Are you ready?

Alan nods. Dysart taps his pen on the wooden rail. Alan shuts his eyes. Dysart taps again. Alan opens them. The taps are evenly spaced. After four of them the sound cuts out, and is replaced by a louder, metallic sound, on tape. Dysart talks through this, to the audience—the light changes to cold—while the boy sits in front of him, staring at the wall, opening and shutting his eyes.

The Normal is the good smile in a child's eyes—all right. It is also the dead stare in a million adults. It both sustains and kills—like a God. It is the Ordinary made beautiful: it is also the Average made lethal. The Normal is the indispensable, murderous God of Health, and I am his Priest. My tools are very delicate. My compassion is honest. I have honestly assisted children in this room. I have talked away terrors and relieved many agonies. But also—beyond question—I have cut from them parts of individuality repugnant to this God, in both his aspects. Parts sacred to rarer and more wonderful Gods. And at what length . . . Sacrifices to Zeus took at the most surely, sixty seconds each. Sacrifices to the Normal can take as long as sixty months.

The natural sound of the pencil resumes.
Light changes back.

[*to Alan*] Now your eyes are feeling heavy. You want to sleep, don't you? You want a long, deep sleep. Have it. Your head is heavy. Very heavy. Your shoulder are heavy. Sleep.

The pencil stops. Alan's eyes remain shut and his head has sunk on his chest.

Can you hear me?

ALAN: Mmm.

DYSART: You can speak normally. Say Yes, if you can.

ALAN: Yes.

DYSART: Good boy. Now raise your head, and open your eyes.

He does so.

Now, Alan, you're going to answer questions I'm going to ask you. Do you understand?

ALAN: Yes.

DYSART: And when you wake up, you are going to remember everything you tell me. All right?

ALAN: Yes.

DYSART: Good. Now I want you to think back in time. You are on that beach you told me about. The tide has gone out, and you're making sandcastles. Above you, staring down at you, is that great horse's head, and the cream dropping from it. Can you see that?

ALAN: Yes.

DYSART: You ask him a question. 'Does the chain hurt?'

ALAN: Yes.

DYSART: Do you ask him aloud?

ALAN: No.

DYSART: And what does the horse say back?

ALAN: 'Yes.'

DYSART: Then what do you say?

ALAN: 'I'll take it out for you.'

DYSART: And he says?

ALAN: 'It never comes out. They have me in chains.'

DYSART: Like Jesus?

ALAN: Yes!

DYSART: Only his name isn't Jesus, is it?

ALAN: No.

DYSART: What is it?

ALAN: No one knows but him and me.

DYSART: You can tell me, Alan. Name him.

ALAN: Equus.

DYSART: Thank you. Does he live in all horses or just some?

ALAN: All.

DYSART: Good boy. Now: you leave the beach. You're in your bedroom at home. You're twelve years old. You're in front of the picture. You're looking at Equus from the foot of your bed. Would you like to kneel down?

ALAN: Yes.

DYSART: [*encouragingly*] Go on, then.

Alan kneels.

Now tell me. Why is Equus in chains?

ALAN: For the sins of the world.

DYSART: What does he say to you?

ALAN: 'I see you.' 'I will save you.'

DYSART: How?

ALAN: 'Bear you away. Two shall be one.'

DYSART: Horse and rider shall be one beast?

ALAN: One person!

DYSART: Go on.

ALAN: 'And my chinkle-chankle shall be in thy hand.'

DYSART: Chinkle-chankle? That's his mouth chain?

ALAN: Yes.

DYSART: Good. You can get up . . . Come on.

Alan rises.

Now: think of the stable. What is the stable? His Temple? His Holy of Holies?

ALAN: Yes.

DYSART: Where you wash him? Where you tend him, and brush him with many brushes?

ALAN: Yes.

DYSART: And there he spoke to you, didn't he? He looked at you with his gentle eyes, and spake unto you?

ALAN: Yes.

DYSART: What did he say? 'Ride me? Mount me, and ride me forth at night?'

ALAN: Yes.

DYSART: And you obeyed?

ALAN: Yes.

DYSART: How did you learn? By watching others?

ALAN: Yes.

DYSART: It must have been difficult. You bounced about?

ALAN: Yes.

DYSART: But he showed you, didn't he? Equus showed you the way.

ALAN: No!

DYSART: He didn't?

ALAN: He showed me nothing! He's a mean bugger! Ride—or fall! That's Straw Law.

DYSART: Straw Law?

ALAN: He was born in the straw, and this is his law.

DYSART: But you managed? You mastered him?

ALAN: Had to!

DYSART: And then you rode in secret?

ALAN: Yes.

DYSART: How often?

ALAN: Every three weeks. More, people would notice.

DYSART: On a particular horse?

ALAN: No.

DYSART: How did you get into the stable?

ALAN: Stole a key. Had it copied at Bryson's.
DYSART: Clever boy.

Alan smiles.

> Then you'd slip out of the house?

ALAN: Midnight! On the stroke!
DYSART: How far's the stable?
ALAN: Two miles.

Pause.

DYSART: Let's do it! Let's go riding! . . . Now!

He stands up, and pushes in his bench.

> You are there now, in front of the stable door.

Alan turns upstage.

> That key's in your hand. Go and open it.

. . . .

From Scene 25

DYSART: [*quietly*] Can you think of anything worse one can do to anybody than take away their worship?
HESTHER: Worship?
DYSART: Yes, that word again!
HESTHER: Aren't you being a little extreme?
DYSART: Extremity's the point.
HESTHER: Worship isn't destructive, Martin. I know that.
DYSART: I don't. I only know it's the core of his life. What else has he got? Think about him. He can hardly read. He knows no physics or engineering to make the world real for him. No paintings to show him how others have enjoyed it. No music except television jingles. No history except tales from a desperate mother. No friends. Not one kid to give him a joke, or make him know himself more moderately. He's a modern citizen for whom society doesn't exist. He lives *one hour* every three weeks—howling in a mist. And after the service kneels to a slave who stands over him obviously and unthrowably his master. With my body I thee worship! . . . Many men have less vital with their wives.

Pause.

HESTHER: All the same, they don't usually blind their wives, do they?

DYSART: Oh, come on!

HESTHER: Well, do they?

DYSART: [*sarcastically*] You mean he's dangerous? A violent, dangerous mad-man who's going to run round the country doing it again and again?

HESTHER: I mean he's in pain, Martin. He's been in pain for most of his life. That much, at least, you *know*.

DYSART: Possibly.

HESTHER: *Possibly*?! . . . That cut-off little figure you just described must have been in pain for years.

DYSART: [*doggedly*] Possibly.

HESTHER: And you can take it away.

DYSART: Still—possibly.

HESTHER: Then that's enough. That simply has to be enough for you, surely?

DYSART: No!

HESTHER: Why not?

DYSART: Because it's his.

HESTHER: I don't understand.

DYSART: His pain. His own. He made it.

Pause.

[*earnestly*] Look . . . to go through life and call it yours—*your life*—you first have to get your own pain. Pain that's unique to you. You can't just dip into the common bin and say 'That's enough!' . . . He's done that. All right, he's sick. He's full of misery and fear. He was dangerous, and could be again, though I doubt it. But that boy has known a passion more ferocious than I have felt in any second of my life. And let me tell you something: I envy it.

HESTHER: You can't.

DYSART: [*vehemently*] Don't you see? That's the Accusation! That's what his stare has been saying to me all the time. *'At least I galloped! When did you?'* . . . [*simply*] I'm jealous, Hesther. Jealous of Alan Strang.

HESTHER: That's absurd.

DYSART: Is it? . . . I go on about my wife. That smug woman by the fire. Have you thought of the fellow on the other side of it? The finicky, critical hus-band looking through his art books on mythical Greece. What worship has *he* ever known? Real worship! Without worship you shrink, it's as brutal as that . . . I shrank my *own* life. No one can do it for you. I settled for being pallid and provincial, out of my own eternal timidity. The old story of blus-ter, and do bugger-all . . . I imply that we can't have children: but actually, it's only me. I had myself tested behind her back. The lowest sperm count you could find. And I never told her. That's all I need—her sympathy mixed with resentment . . . I tell everyone Margaret's the puritan, I'm the pagan. Some pagan! Such wild returns I make to the womb of civilization. Three weeks a year in the Peleponnese, every bed booked in advance, every meal paid for by vouchers, cautious jaunts in hired Fiats, suitcase crammed with Kao-Pectate! Such a fantastic surrender to the primitive. And I use that word endlessly: 'primitive'. 'Oh, the primitive world.' I say. 'What instinctual truths were lost with it!' And while I sit there, baiting a poor unimaginative woman with the word, that freaky boy tries to conjure the reality! I sit looking at pages of centaurs trampling the soil of Argos—and outside my window he is trying to *become one,* in a Hampshire field! . . . I watch that woman knitting, night after night—a woman I haven't *kissed* in six years—and he stands in the dark for an hour, sucking the sweat off his God's hairy cheek! [*pause*] Then in the morning, I put away my books on the cultural shelf, close up the kodachrome snaps of Mount Olympus, touch my reproduction statue of Dionysus for luck—and go off to hospital to treat him for insanity. Do you see?

HESTHER: The boy's in pain, Martin. That's all I see. In the end . . . I'm sorry.

He looks at her. Alan gets up from his bench and stealthily places an envelope in the left-hand entrance of the square, then goes back and sits with his back to the audience, as if watching television.
Hesther rises.

HESTHER: That stare of his. Have you thought it might not be accusing you at all?
DYSART: What then?
HESTHER: Claiming you.
DYSART: For what?
HESTHER: [*mischievously*] A new God.

Pause.

DYSART: Too conventional, for him. Finding a religion in Psychiatry is really for very ordinary patients.

She laughs.

HESTHER: Maybe he just wants a new Dad. Or is that too conventional too? . . . Since you're questioning your profession anyway, perhaps you ought to try it and see.
DYSART: [*amused*] I'll talk to you.
HESTHER: Goodbye.

She smiles, and leaves him.

FROM SCENE 35

The boy's breath is drawn into his body with a harsh rasping sound, which slowly grows less. Dysart puts the blanket over him.

Keep it going . . .That's a good boy . . . Very good boy. . . It's all over now, Alan. It's all over. He'll go away now. You'll never see him again, I promise. You'll have no more bad dreams. No more awful nights. Think of that! . . .You are going to be well. I'm going to make you well, I promise you. . . .You'll be here for a while, but I'll be here too, so it won't be so bad. Just trust me . . .

He stands upright. The boy lies still.

Sleep now. Have a good long sleep. You've earned it . . . Sleep. Just sleep. . . . I'm going to make you well.

He steps backwards into the centre of the square. The light brightens some more. A pause.

DYSART: I'm lying to you, Alan. He won't really go that easily. Just clop away from you like a nice old nag. Oh, no! When Equus leaves—if he leaves at all—it will be with your intestines in his teeth. And I don't stock replacements . . . If you knew anything, you'd get up this minute and run from me fast as you could.

Hesther speaks from her place.

HESTHER: The boy's in pain, Martin.
DYSART: Yes.
HESTHER: And you can take it away.
DYSART: Yes.
HESTHER: Then that has to be enough for you, surely? . . . In the end!
DYSART: [*crying out*] All right! *I'll take it away!* He'll be delivered from madness. *What then?* He'll feel himself acceptable! *What then?* Do you think feelings like his can be simply re-attached, like plasters? Stuck on to other objects we select? *Look at him!* . . . My desire might be to make this boy an ardent husband—a caring citizen—a worshipper of abstract and unifying God. My achievement, however, is more likely to make a ghost! . . . Let me tell you exactly what I'm going to do to him!

He steps out of the square and walks round the upstage end of it, storming at the audience.

I'll heal the rash on his body. I'll erase the welts cut into his mind by flying manes. When that's done, I'll set him on a nice mini-scooter and send him puttering off into the Normal world where animals are treated *properly:* made extinct, or put into servitude, or tethered all their lives in dim light, just to feed it! I'll give him the good Normal world where we're tethered beside them—blinking our nights away in a nonstop drench of cathode-ray over our shrivelling heads! I'll take away his Field of Ha Ha, and give him Normal places for his ecstasy—multi-lane highways driven through the guts of cities, extinguishing Place altogether, *even the idea of Place!* He'll trot on his metal pony tamely through the concrete evening—and one thing I promise you: he will never touch hide again! With any luck his private parts will come to feel as plastic to him as the products of the factory to which he will almost certainly be sent. Who knows? He may even come to find sex funny. Smirky funny. Bit of grunt funny. Trampled and furtive and entirely in control. Hopefully, he'll feel nothing at his fork but Approved Flesh. *I doubt, however, with much passion!* . . . Passion, you see, can be destroyed by a doctor. It cannot be created.

He addresses Alan directly, in farewell.

You won't gallop any more, Alan. Horses will be quite safe. You'll save your pennies every week, till you can change that scooter in for a car, and put the odd fifty P on the gee-gees, quite forgetting that they were ever anything more to you than bearers of little profits and little losses. You will, however, be without pain. More or less completely without pain.

Pause.
He speaks directly to the theatre, standing by the motionless body of Alan Strang, under the blanket.

And now for me it never stops: that voice of Equus out of the cave—'Why Me? . . . Why Me? . . . Account for Me!' . . . All right—I surrender! I say it . . . In an ultimate sense I cannot know what I do in this place—yet I do ultimate things. Essentially I cannot know what I do—yet I do essential things. Irreversible, terminal things. I stand in the dark with a pick in my hand, striking at heads!

He moves away from Alan, back to the downstage bench, and finally sits.

I need—more desperately than my children need me—a way of seeing in the dark. What way is this? . . . *What dark is this?* . . . I cannot call it ordained of God: I can't get that far. I will however pay it so much homage. There is now, in my mouth, this sharp chain. And it never comes out.

A long pause.
Dysart sits staring.

Blackout

SECTION TWO

*Mental Disability
(Retardation)*

§

Two Stick Drawings

SEAMUS HEANEY

1

Claire O'Reilly used her granny's stick—
A crook-necked one—to snare the highest briars
That always grew the ripest blackberries.
When it came to gathering, Persephone
Was in the halfpenny place compared to Claire.
She'd trespass and climb gates and walk the railway
Where sootflakes blew into convolvulus
And the train tore past with the stoker yelling
Like a balked king from his iron chariot.

2

With its drover's canes and blackthorns and ash plants,
The ledge of the back seat of my father's car
Had turned into a kind of stick-shop window,
But the only one who ever window-shopped
Was Jim of the hanging jaw, for Jim was simple
And rain or shine he'd make his desperate rounds
From windscreen to back window, hands held up
To both sides of his face, peering and groaning.
So every now and then the sticks would be
Brought out for him and stood up one by one
Against the front mudguard; and one by one
Jim would take the measure of them, sight
And wield and slice and poke and parry
The unhindering air; until he found
The true extension of himself in one
That made him jubilant. He'd run and crow,

Stooped forward, with his right elbow stuck out
And the stick held horizontal to the ground,
Angled across in front of him, as if
He were leashed to it and it drew him on
Like a harness rod of the inexorable.

From Joe Egg

PETER NICHOLS

FROM ACT ONE:

JOE: Aaah!

BRI: What's the matter, crackpot?

JOE: Aaah!

BRI: Language? You think this is language! I'll introduce you to Scanlon. He'll
let you hear some language. (*Aside.*) What a madam! Well. Let's see what
she's left for tea.

JOE: Aaah!

(*Makes revving noises and pushes her chair off to the kitchen. Going out, he
struggles with the cats.*)

BRI: Get back, you flea-bitten whores! Get back! (*Shuts door behind him.*)

(*Pause. At least five seconds.*)
(SHEILA *comes on from a corner downstage of the set. She has changed into a
dress and is brushing her hair.*)

SHEILA: One of these days I'll hit him. Honestly. (*Brushes hair, looks at audience.*) He thinks because he throws a tantrum I'm going to stay home
comforting him and miss the rehearsal and let them all down. He thinks he's
only got to cry to get what he wants. I blame his mother. She gave him the
kind of suffocating love that makes him think the world revolves around
him but because he's too intelligent to believe it really, he gets into these pad-
dies and depressions. And when he's in one of those, he'll do anything to
draw attention to himself. That beetle on his face—you saw that. And all
this stuff about Freddie. And yet it was Brian made me join these amateurs
in the first place, he said I needed to get out more, have a rest from Joe. But
she's no trouble. It's Brian. I don't know which is the greatest baby. Watching
somebody as limited as Joe over ten years, I've begun to feel she's only one
kind of cripple. Everybody's damaged in some way. There's a limit to what
we can do. Brian, for instance, he goes so far—and hits the ceiling. Just can't

fly any higher. Then he drops to the floor and we get self-pity again . . . despair. I'm sure, though, if he could go farther—he could be a marvelous painter. That's another reason I said I'd join the amateurs: the thought that he'd be forced to go upstairs several nights a week and actually put paint on canvas. And even if he *isn't* any good, he seems to need some work he can be proud of. Something to take his mind off his jealousy of anyone or anything I take to . . . relatives, friends, pets . . . even pot-plants. I'm sure it's because they take up time he thinks I could be devoting to him. And Joe, most of all, poor love . . . *(She puts brush on table or chair. A thought brings her back.)* Look, you mustn't assume I feel like this in the ordinary way. And even when I *am* a bit down, I shouldn't normally talk about it to a lot of complete strangers. But all this childish temper over Freddie—showing-off—it's more than I can stand, it makes me boil, honestly! Wouldn't you feel the same? *(Checks her appearance in imaginary full-length glass.)* That's why I'm telling you all this. A lot of total strangers. But wouldn't it make *you* boil? Honestly! A grown man jealous of poor Joe—

(Breaks off as she sees BRI *coming from downstage corner.)*
(They look at each other in silence).

BRI: What are you telling them?
SHEILA: What?
BRI: I heard you talking.

*(*SHEILA *picks threads from her clothes.)*

I heard you mention Joe.

(No answer. BRI *speaks to audience.)*

Sheila's got a theory about Joe's birth. She doesn't blame the doctors. She blames herself.
SHEILA: I don't say that. I say it wasn't *entirely* the doctors.
BRI *(nodding)*: It was because she choked it back.
SHEILA: It was partly that.
BRI: Because she'd slept around.
SHEILA: I think it was partly because I'd been promiscuous, yes, and my sub-conscious was making me shrink or withdraw from motherhood, all right!

(Pause. He looks away. She goes on titivating.)

BRI: The vicar told us it was the devil's doing. Why don't you believe *that?* It's about as brilliant.
SHEILA *(shrugs)*: It comes down in the end to what you believe.
BRI: I'll tell you what *I* believe.

SHEILA: I *know* what you believe.

BRI (*points at audience*): They don't. (*To audience.*) I believe the doctor botched it. There was no other cause. (*To SHEILA.*) That specialist said as much, he said it had nothing at all to do with the way you'd lived or whether there was a nut in the family . . . or what kind of fags you smoked.

SHEILA: He didn't say the doctor did it either.

(*Pause. He looks at her.*)

BRI: No. You've got a good point there. He didn't mention that, quite true. He didn't say, "Yes, he's a shoddy midwife, my colleague, always was, I'll see he get struck off the register." Very true. Weakens my argument, that.

SHEILA: Oh, you're so *clever!*

BRI: He'd only say for certain that it was a chance in a million it could happen again.

SHEILA: Mmm. We haven't had an opportunity yet to check on that.

(*Both pause.*)

BRI: It's due to this that Joe lives at home with us.

SHEILA: She's our daughter.

BRI (*to audience*): She was on the way before we married. That feeds the furnace of guilt.

SHEILA: No need to tell them everything.

BRI: It was a white wedding.

SHEILA: For my dad's sake. He was a bell-ringer and always looked forward to the day he'd lead the peal as I left the church. You said you didn't mind.

BRI: I didn't. At the reception afterwards the ringers were the only people worth talking to. All twisted and crippled. Picture them bouncing up and down at the end of their ropes.

(*And he tries to guess at it.*)

SHEILA: We might have taken them for an omen. The baby came six months later. I'd done my exercises and read the antenatal books—mostly the ones that made it seem as simple as having a tooth filled.

BRI: But more spiritual.

SHEILA: Oh, yes, a lot about you sitting by the bed holding my hand and looking sincere.

(*BRI does it*)

BRI: Giving the lead with shallow breathing. (*Does it.*)

SHEILA (*to audience*): I don't know whether any of you are like me, but I half-expected to hear snatches of the Hallelujah Chorus.

BRI: I was sympathetic but queasy. The idea of sharing the birth seemed irrefutable *qua idea* . . . but not so gay when it came to the blood and fluid.

SHEILA: As it happened, you needn't have worried.

BRI: No. (*To audience*) How long do *your* labours last? Two, three hours? A day? Dilettantes! (*Points at* SHEILA.) Five days!

SHEILA: Yes. From the first show on the sheets to the last heave of the forceps. Five days.

BRI: You'll all be saying, "He should have *done* something," but I didn't *know* at the time. You don't, do you?

SHEILA: You'd know *now*.

BRI: Oh, yeah. It was all good experience.

SHEILA: (*To audience*): This doctor kept on drugging me.

BRI: You were stoned.

SHEILA: I join in these jokes to please him. If it helps him live with her, I can't see the harm, can you? He hasn't any faith she's ever going to improve. Where I have, you see . . . I believe, even if she *showed* improvement, Bri wouldn't notice. He's dense about faith—faith isn't believing in fairy-tales, it's being in a receptive state of mind. I'm always on the look-out for some sign . . . (*Looks off again to wings to make sure* BRI's *not coming.*) One day she was—what?—about a twelve month old, I suppose, she was lying on the floor kicking her legs about and I was doing the flat. I'd made a little tower of four coloured bricks—plastic bricks—on a rug near her head. I got on with my dusting and when I looked again I saw she'd knocked it down. I put the four bricks up again and this time watched her. First her eyes, usually moving in all directions, must have glanced in passing at this bright tower. Then the arm that side began to show real signs of intention . . . and her fist started clenching and—spreading with the effort. The other arm—held there like that—(*raises one bent arm to shoulder level*) didn't move. You see the importance—she was using for the first time one arm instead of both. She'd seen something, touched it and found that when she touched it whatever-it-was was changed. Fell down. Now her bent arm started twitching towards the bricks. Must have taken—I should think—ten minutes'—strenuous labor—to reach them with her fingers . . . then her hand jerked in a spasm and she pulled down the tower. (*Reliving the episode, she puts her hands over her face to regain composure.*) I can't tell you what that was like. But you can imagine, can't you? Several times the hand very nearly touched and got jerked away by spasm . . . and she'd try again. That was the best of it—she had a will, she had a mind of her own. Soon as Bri came home, I told him. I think he said something stupid like—you know—"That's great, put her down for piano lessons." But when he tested her—putting piles of bricks all along the circle of her reach—both arms—and even sometimes out of reach so that she had to stretch to get there—well, of course, he saw it was true. It wasn't *much* to wait for—one arm movement completed—and even that wasn't sure. She'd fall asleep, the firelight would distract her, sometimes the effort would bring on a fit. But more often than not she'd manage . . . and a vegetable couldn't have done that. Visitors never believed it. They hadn't the patience to watch so long. And it amazed me—I remember being stunned—when I realized they thought I shouldn't deceive myself. For one thing, it wasn't deception . . . and, anyway, what else could I do? We got very absorbed in the daily games. Found her coloured balls and bells and a Kelly—those clowns that won't lie down. Then she caught some bug and was very sick . . . had fit and fit—the Grand Mal, not the others—what amounted to a complete relapse. When she was over it, we tried the bricks again, but she couldn't even seem to see them. That was when Bri lost interest in her. I still try, though of course I don't bother telling him. I'll tell him when something happens. It seems to me only common sense. If she did it once, she could again. I think while there's life there's hope, don't you? (*Looks to wings again.*) I wish he'd talk more seriously about her. I wonder if he ever imagines what she'd be like if her brain worked. *I* do. And Bri's mother always says, "Wouldn't she be lovely if she was running about?" which makes Bri hoot with laughter. But I think of it too. Perhaps it's being a woman. (*Lights off* SHEILA. *Lights on set upstage, very strong like a continuous lightning flash.*)

JOE: Mrs. D, Mrs. I, Mrs. FFI, Mrs. C, Mrs. U, Mrs. LTY, Mrs. D, Mrs. I, Mrs. FFI, Mrs. C, Mrs. U, Mrs. LTY. (*Stops skipping.*)

Ladies and gentlemen, there will now be an interval. Afterwards the ordinary play, with which we began the performance, will continue and we shall try to show you what happens when Sheila returns home with their mutual friends, Freddie and Pam.

(*She bows and resumes skipping.*)

FROM ACT TWO:

BRI: That kind of thing certainly gives legalized killing a bad name, but—what about the other forms? The bomb-aimer gets decorated but anyone who lets Joe die gets ten years.

FREDDIE: The case are different. A rational intelligence can distinguish between the different cases.

BRI: So I've noticed.

FREDDIE: Put it this way. You don't agree with killing?

BRI (*shrugs*): No.

FREDDIE: But if a madman breaks in here and tries to rape your wife, what d'you do?

BRI: Kill him.

FREDDIE: Exactly. Killing is sometimes unavoidable.

BRI: Thou shalt not kill unless it's absolutely necessary.

FREDDIE (*doubtfully*): Yes.

BRI (*to audience*): Whose side is he on?

(*BRI smokes. Pause. The singing has ceased.*)

PAM: Darling—it's half past ten.

FREDDIE (*suddenly*): You're like a blasted speaking clock. On the third stroke— peep-peep-peep.

(*Walks away.*)

PAM: Oh, charming.

(*Looks at both men, ignoring her and now each other. Complete separation of all three people on the stage.* PAM *comes to audience.*)

It wasn't my idea coming back here in the first place. But once Freddie's set eyes on a lame dog, you might as well talk to the moon. I keep looking at that door and thinking she's going to come through it any moment with that poor weirdie. I know it's awful but it's one of my—you know— THINGS. We're none of us perfect . . . I can't stand anything N.P.A. Non-Physically Attractive. Old women in bathing suits—and skin diseases—and cripples . . . Rowton House-looking men who spit and have hair growing out of their ears . . . . No good, I just can't look at them. I know Freddie's right about Hitler and of course that's horrid. Still, I can't help sympathizing with Brian, can you? I don't mean the way he described. I think it should be done by the state. And so should charity. Then we might have an end of all those hideous dolls in shop-doorways with irons on their legs. . . . Freddie won't hear of it, of course. But then he loves a lame dog. Every year he buys so many tickets for the spastic raffle he wins the TV set and every year he gives it to an old folks' home. He used to try taking me along on his visits but I said it wasn't me at all and he gave up. One-place—we went, there were these poor freaks with—oh, you know—enormous heads and so on— and you just feel: oh, put them out of their misery. Well, they wouldn't have survived in nature, it's only modern medicine, so modern medicine should be allowed to do away with them. A committee of doctors and do-gooders, naturally, to make sure there's no funny business and then—if I say gas-chamber that makes it sound horrid—but I do mean put to sleep. When Freddie gets all mealy-mouthed about it, I say, look, darling, if one of our kids was dying and they had a cure and you knew it had been discovered in the Nazi laboratories, would you refuse to let them use it? I certainly wouldn't. I love my own immediate family and that's the lot. Can't manage any more. I want to go home and see them again. They may not be the most hard-working, well-behaved geniuses on earth, but no one in their right mind could say they were N.P.A. (*Turns back.*) Freddie, I'm going. You can get a taxi and—

(*SHEILA carries JOE in, in her nightdress and dressing-gown.*)

SHEILA: Aaaah! The carols have stopped.
BRI: They've stopped, yes.
FREDDIE: This little Josephine?
SHEILA: This is Joe. Say hullo to Uncle Freddie.
FREDDIE (*shakes her hand*): Hullo, Joe, what do you know?
SHEILA: Not much, I'm afraid.
SHEILA: And Auntie Pamela.

The Life You Save May Be Your Own

FLANNERY O'CONNOR

THE OLD WOMAN and her daughter were sitting on their porch when Mr. Shiftlet came up their road for the first time. The old woman slid to the edge of her chair and leaned forward, shading her eyes from the piercing sunset with her hand. The daughter could not see far in front of her and continued to play with her fingers. Although the old woman lived in this desolate spot with only her daughter and she had never seen Mr. Shiftlet before, she could tell, even from a distance, that he was a tramp and no one to be afraid of. His left coat sleeve was folded up to show there was only half an arm in it and his gaunt figure listed slightly to the side as if the breeze were pushing him. He had on a black town suit and a brown felt hat that was turned up in the front and down in the back and he carried a tin tool box by a handle. He came on, at an amble, up her road, his face turned toward the sun which appeared to be balancing itself on the peak of a small mountain.

The old woman didn't change her position until he was almost into her yard; then she rose with one hand fisted on her hip. The daughter, a large girl in a short blue organdy dress, saw him all at once and jumped up and began to stamp and point and make excited speechless sounds.

Mr. Shiftlet stopped just inside the yard and set his box on the ground and tipped his hat at her as if she were not in the least afflicted; then he turned toward the old woman and swung the hat all the way off. He had long black slick hair that hung flat from a part in the middle to beyond the tips of his ears on either side. His face descended in forehead for more than half its length and ended suddenly with his features just balanced over a jutting steel-trap jaw. He seemed to be a young man but he had a look of composed dissatisfaction as if he understood life thoroughly.

"Good evening," the old woman said. She was about the size of a cedar fence post and she had a man's gray hat pulled down low over her head.

The tramp stood looking at her and didn't answer. He turned his back and faced the sunset. He swung both his whole and his short arm up slowly so that they indicated an expanse of sky and his figure formed a crooked cross. The old woman watched him with her arms folded across her chest as if she were the owner of the sun, and the daughter watched, her head thrust forward and her fat helpless hands hanging at the wrists. She had long pink-gold hair and eyes as blue as a peacock's neck.

He held the pose for almost fifty seconds and then he picked up his box and came on to the porch and dropped down on the bottom step. "Lady," he said in a firm nasal voice, "I'd give a fortune to live where I could see me a sun do that every evening."

"Does it every evening," the old woman said and sat back down. The daughter sat down too and watched him with a cautious sly look as if he were a bird that had come up very close. He leaned to one side, rooting in his pants pocket, and in a second he brought out a package of chewing gum and offered her a piece. She took it and unpeeled it and began to chew without taking her eyes off him. He offered the old woman a piece but she only raised her upper lip to indicate she had no teeth.

Mr. Shiftlet's pale sharp glance had already passed over everything in the yard—the pump near the corner of the house and the big fig tree that three or four chickens were preparing to roost in—and had moved to a shed where he saw the square rusted back of an automobile. "You ladies drive?" he asked.

"That car ain't run in fifteen year," the old woman said. "The day my husband died, it quit running."

"Nothing is like it used to be, lady," he said. "The world is almost rotten."

"That's right," the old woman said. "You from around here?"

"Name Tom T. Shiftlet," he murmured, looking at the tires.

"I'm pleased to meet you," the old woman said. "Name Lucynell Crater and daughter Lucynell Crater. What you doing around here, Mr. Shiftlet?"

He judged the car to be about a 1928 or '29 Ford. "Lady," he said, and turned and gave her his full attention, "lemme tell you something. There's one of these doctors in Atlanta that's taken a knife and cut the human heart—the human heart," he repeated, leaning forward, "out of a man's chest and held it in his hand," and he held his hand out, palm up, as if it were slightly weighted with the human heart, "and studied it like it was a day-old chicken, and lady," he said, allowing a long significant pause in which his head slid forward and his clay-colored eyes brightened, "he don't know no more about it than you or me."

"That's right," the old woman said.

"Why, if he was to take that knife and cut into every corner of it, he still wouldn't know no more than you or me. What you want to bet?"

"Nothing," the old woman said wisely. "Where you come from, Mr. Shiftlet?"

He didn't answer. He reached into his pocket and brought out a sack of tobacco and a package of cigarette papers and rolled himself a cigarette, expertly with one hand, and attached it in a hanging position to his upper lip. Then he took a box of wooden matches from his pocket and struck one on his shoe. He held the burning match as if he were studying the mystery of flame while it traveled dangerously toward his skin. The daughter began to make loud noises and to point to his hand and shake her finger at him, but when the flame was just before touching him, he leaned down with his hand cupped over it as if he were going to set fire to his nose and lit the cigarette.

He flipped away the dead match and blew a stream of gray into the evening. A sly look came over his face. "Lady," he said, "nowadays, people'll do anything anyways. I can tell you my name is Tom T. Shiftlet and I come from Tarwater, Tennessee, but you never have seen me before: how you know I ain't lying? How you know my name ain't Aaron Sparks, lady, and I come from Single-berry, Georgia, or how you know it's not George Speeds and I come from Lucy, Alabama, or how you know I ain't Thompson Bright from Toolafalls, Mis-sissippi?"

"I don't know nothing about you," the old woman muttered, irked.

"Lady," he said, "people don't care how they lie. Maybe the best I can tell you is, I'm a man; but listen lady," he said and paused and made his tone more omi-nous still, "what is a man?"

The old woman began to gum a seed. "What you carry in that tin box, Mr. Shiftlet?" she asked.

"Tools," he said, put back. "I'm a carpenter."

"Well, if you come out here to work, I'll be able to feed you and give you a place to sleep but I can't pay. I'll tell you that before you begin," she said.

There was no answer at once and no particular expression on his face. He leaned back against the two-by-four that helped support the porch roof. "Lady," he said slowly, "there's some men that some things mean more to them than money." The old woman rocked without comment and the daughter watched the trigger that moved up and down in his neck. He told the old woman then that all most people were interested in was money, but he asked what a man was made for. He asked her if a man was made for money, or what. He asked her what she thought she was made for but she didn't answer, she only sat rocking and wondered if a one-armed man could put a new roof on her garden house. He asked a lot of questions that she didn't answer. He told her that he was twenty-eight years old and had lived a varied life. He had been a gospel singer, a foreman on the railroad, an assistant in an undertaking parlor, and he come over the radio for three months with Uncle Roy and his Red Creek Wranglers. He said he had fought and bled in the Arm Service of his coun-try and visited every foreign land and that everywhere he had seen people that didn't care if they did a thing one way or another. He said he hadn't been raised thataway.

A fat yellow moon appeared in the branches of the fig tree as if it were going to roost there with the chickens. He said that a man had to escape to the country to see the world whole and that he wished he lived in a desolate place like this where he could see the sun go down every evening like God made it to do.

"Are you married or are you single?" the old woman asked.

There was a long silence. "Lady," he asked finally, "where would you find you an innocent woman today? I wouldn't have any of this trash I could just pick up."

The daughter was leaning very far down, hanging her head almost between her knees watching him through a triangular door she had made in her overturned hair; and she suddenly fell in a heap on the floor and began to whimper. Mr. Shiftlet straightened her out and helped her get back in the chair.

"Is she your baby girl?" he asked.

"My only," the old woman said "and she's the sweetest girl in the world. I would give her up for nothing on earth. She's smart too. She can sweep the floor, cook, wash, feed the chickens, and hoe. I wouldn't give her up for a casket of jewels."

"No," he said kindly, "don't ever let any man take her away from you."

"Any man come after her," the old woman said, " he'll have to stay around the place."

Mr. Shiftlet's eye in the darkness was focused on a part of the automobile bumper that glittered in the distance. "Lady," he said, jerking his short arm up as if he could point with it to her house and yard and pump, "there ain't a broken thing on this plantation that I couldn't fix for you, one-arm jackleg or not. I'm a man," he said with a sullen dignity, "even if I ain't a whole one. I got," he said, tapping his knuckles on the floor to emphasize the immensity of what he was going to say, "a moral intelligence!" and his face pierced out of the darkness into a shaft of doorlight and he stared at her as if he were astonished himself at this impossible truth.

The old woman was not impressed with the phrase. "I told you you could hang around and work for food," she said, "if you don't mind sleeping in that car yonder."

"Why listen, lady," he said with a grin of delight, "the monks of old slept in their coffins!"

"They wasn't as advanced as we are," the old woman said.

The next morning he began on the roof of the garden house while Lucynell, the daughter, sat on a rock and watched him work. He had not been around a week before the change he had made in the place was apparent. He had patched the front and back steps, built a new hog pen, restored a fence, and taught Lucynell, who was completely deaf and had never said a word in her life, to say the word "bird." The big rosy-faced girl followed him everywhere, saying "Burrttddt ddbirrrttdt," and clapping her hands. The old woman watched from a distance, secretly pleased. She was ravenous for a son-in-law.

Mr. Shiftlet slept on the hard narrow back seat of the car with his feet out the side window. He had his razor and a can of water on a crate that served him as a bedside table and he put up a piece of mirror against the back glass and kept his coat neatly on a hanger that he hung over one of the windows.

In the evenings he sat on the steps and talked while the old woman and Lucynell rocked violently in their chairs on either side of him. The old woman's three mountains were black against the dark blue sky and were visited off and on by various planets and by the moon after it had left the chickens. Mr. Shift-let pointed out that the reason he had improved this plantation was because he had taken a personal interest in it. He said he was even going to make the auto-mobile run.

He had raised the hood and studied the mechanism and he said he could tell that the car had been built in the days when cars were really built. You take now, he said, one man puts in one bolt and another man puts in another bolt and another man puts in another bolt so that it's a man for a bolt. That's why you have to pay so much for a car: you're paying all those men. Now if you didn't have to pay but one man, you could get you a cheaper car and one that had had a personal interest taken in it, and it would be a better car. The old woman agreed with him that this was so.

Mr. Shiftlet said that the trouble with the world was that nobody cared, or stopped and took any trouble. He said he never would have been able to teach Lucynell to say a word if he hadn't cared and stopped long enough.

"Teach her to say something else," the old woman said.

"What you want her to say next?" Mr. Shiftlet asked.

The old woman's smile was broad and toothless and suggestive. "Teach her to say 'sugarpie,' " she said.

Mr. Shiftlet already knew what was on her mind.

The next day he began to tinker with the automobile and that evening he told her that if she would buy a fan belt, he would be able to make the car run.

The old woman said she would give him the money. "You see that girl yonder?" she asked, pointing to Lucynell who was sitting on the floor a foot away, watching him, her eyes blue even in the dark. "If it was ever a man wanted to take her away, I would say, 'No man on earth is going to take that sweet girl of mine away from me!' but if he was to say, 'Lady, I don't want to take her away, I want her right here,' I would say, 'Mister, I don't blame you none. I wouldn't pass up a chance to live in a permanent place and get the sweetest girl in the world myself. You ain't no fool,' I would say."

"How old is she?" Mr. Shiftlet asked casually.

"Fifteen, sixteen," the old woman said. The girl was nearly thirty but because of her innocence it was impossible to guess.

"It would be a good idea to paint it too," Mr. Shiftlet remarked. "You don't want it to rust out."

"We'll see about that later," the old woman said.

The next day he walked into town and returned with the parts he needed and a can of gasoline. Late in the afternoon, terrible noises issued from the shed and the old woman rushed out of the house, thinking Lucynell was somewhere having a fit. Lucynell was sitting on a chicken crate, stamping her feet and screaming, "Burrddttt! bddurrddtttt!" but her fuss was drowned out by the car. With a volley of blasts it emerged from the shed, moving in a fierce and stately way. Mr. Shiftlet was in the driver's seat, sitting very erect. He had an expression of serious modesty on his face as if he had just raised the dead.

That night, rocking on the porch, the old woman began her business, at once. "You want you an innocent woman, don't you?" she asked sympathetically. "You don't want none of this trash."

"No'm, I don't," Mr. Shiftlet said.

"One that can't talk," she continued, "can't sass you back or use foul language. That's the kind for you to have. Right there," and she pointed to Lucynell sitting cross-legged in her chair, holding both feet in her hands.

"That's right," he admitted. "She wouldn't give me any trouble."

"Saturday," the old woman said, "you and her and me can drive into town and get married."

Mr. Shiftlet eased his position on the steps.

"I can't get married right now," he said. "Everything you want to do takes money and I ain't got any."

"What you need with money?" she asked.

"It takes money," he said. "Some people'll do anything anyhow these days, but the way I think, I wouldn't marry no woman that I couldn't take on a trip like she was somebody. I mean take her to a hotel and treat her. I wouldn't marry the Duchesser Windsor," he said firmly, "unless I could take her to a hotel and giver something good to eat.

"I was raised thataway and there ain't a thing I can do about it. My old mother taught me how to do."

"Lucynell don't even know what a hotel is," the old woman muttered. "Listen here, Mr. Shiftlet," she said, sliding forward in her chair, "you'd be getting a permanent house and a deep well and the most innocent girl in the world. You don't need no money. Lemme tell you something: there ain't any place in the world for a poor disabled friendless drifting man."

The ugly words settled in Mr. Shiftlet's head like a group of buzzards in the top of a tree. He didn't answer at once. He rolled himself a cigarette and lit it and then he said in an even voice, "Lady, a man is divided into two parts, body and spirit."

The old woman clamped her gums together.

"A body and a spirit," he repeated. "The body, lady, is like a house: it don't go anywhere; but the spirit, lady, is like a automobile: always on the move, always . . ."

"Listen, Mr. Shiftlet," she said, "my well never goes dry and my house is always warm in the winter and there's no mortgage on a thing about this place. You can go to the courthouse and see for yourself. And yonder under that shed is a fine automobile." She laid the bait carefully. "You can have it painted by Saturday. I'll pay for the paint."

In the darkness, Mr. Shiftlet's smile stretched like a weary snake waking up by a fire. After a second he recalled himself and said, "I'm only saying a man's spirit means more to him than anything else. I would have to take my wife off for the weekend without no regards at all for cost. I got to follow where my spirit says to go."

"I'll give you fifteen dollars for a weekend trip," the old woman said in a crabbed voice. "That's the best I can do."

"That wouldn't hardly pay for more than the gas and the hotel," he said. "It wouldn't feed her."

"Seventeen-fifty," the old woman said. "That's all I got so it isn't any use you trying to milk me. You can take a lunch."

Mr. Shiftlet was deeply hurt by the word "milk." He didn't doubt that she had more money sewed up in her mattress but he had already told her he was not interested in her money. "I'll make that do," he said and rose and walked off without treating with her further.

On Saturday the three of them drove into town in the car that the paint had barely dried on and Mr. Shiftlet and Lucynell were married in the Ordinary's office while the old woman witnessed. As they came out of the courthouse, Mr. Shiftlet began twisting his neck in his collar. He looked morose and bitter as if he had been insulted while someone held him. "That didn't satisfy me none," he said. "That was just something a woman in an office did, nothing but paper work and blood tests. What do they know about my blood? If they was to take my heart and cut it out," he said, "they wouldn't know a thing about me. It didn't satisfy me at all."

"It satisfied the law," the old woman said sharply.

"The law," Mr. Shiftlet said and spit. "It's the law that don't satisfy me."

He had painted the car dark green with a yellow band around it just under the windows. The three of them climbed in the front seat and the old woman said, "Don't Lucynell look pretty? Looks like a baby doll." Lucynell was dressed up in a white dress that her mother had uprooted from a trunk and there was a Panama hat on her head with a bunch of red wooden cherries on the brim. Every now and then her placid expression was changed by a sly isolated little thought like a shoot of green in the desert. "You got a prize!" the old woman said.

Mr. Shiftlet didn't even look at her.

They drove back to the house to let the old woman off and pick up the lunch. When they were ready to leave, she stood staring in the window of the car, with her fingers clenched around the glass. Tears began to seep sideways out of her eyes and run along the dirty creases in her face. "I ain't ever been parted with her for two days before," she said.

Mr. Shiftlet started the motor.

"And I wouldn't let no man have her but you because I seen you would do right. Good-by, Sugarbaby," she said, clutching at the sleeve of the white dress. Lucynell looked straight at her and didn't seem to see her there at all. Mr. Shiftlet eased the car forward so that she had to move her hands.

The early afternoon was clear and open and surrounded by pale blue sky. Although the car would go only thirty miles an hour, Mr. Shiftlet imagined a terrific climb and dip and swerve that went entirely to his head so that he forgot his morning bitterness. He had always wanted an automobile but he had never been able to afford one before. He drove very fast because he wanted to make Mobile by nightfall.

Occasionally he stopped his thoughts long enough to look at Lucynell in the seat beside him. She had eaten the lunch as soon as they were out of the yard and now she was pulling the cherries off the hat one by one and throwing them out the window. He became depressed in spite of the car. He had driven about a hundred miles when he decided that she must be hungry again and at the next small town they came to, he stopped in front of an aluminum-painted eating place called The Hot Spot and took her in and ordered her a plate of ham and grits. The ride had made her sleepy and as soon as she got up on the stool, she rested her head on the counter and shut her eyes. There was no one in The Hot Spot but Mr. Shiftlet and the boy behind the counter, a pale youth with a greasy rag hung over his shoulder. Before he could dish up the food, she was snoring gently.

"Give it to her when she wakes up," Mr. Shiftlet said. "I'll pay for it now."

The boy bent over her and stared at the long pink-gold hair and the half-shut sleeping eyes. Then he looked up and stared at Mr. Shiftlet. "She looks like an angel of Gawd," he murmured.

"Hitchhiker," Mr. Shiftlet explained. "I can't wait. I got to make Tuscaloosa."

The boy bent over again and very carefully touched his finger to a strand of the golden hair and Mr. Shiftlet left.

He was more depressed than ever as he drove on by himself. The late afternoon had grown hot and sultry and the country had flattened out. Deep in the sky a storm was preparing very slowly and without thunder as if it meant to drain every drop of air from the earth before it broke. There were times when Mr. Shiftlet preferred not to be alone. He felt too that a man with a car had a responsibility to others and he kept his eye out for a hitchhiker. Occasionally he saw a sign that warned: "Drive carefully. The life you save may be your own."

The narrow road dropped off on either side into dry fields and here and there a shack or a filling station stood in a clearing. The sun began to set directly in front of the automobile. It was a reddening ball that through his windshield was slightly flat on the bottom and top. He saw a boy in overalls and a gray hat standing on the edge of the road and he slowed the car down and stopped in front of him. The boy didn't have his hand raised to thumb the ride, he was only standing there, but he had a small cardboard suitcase and his hat was set on his head in a way to indicate that he had left somewhere for good. "Son," Mr. Shiftlet said, "I see you want a ride."

The boy didn't say he did or he didn't but he opened the door of the car and got in, and Mr. Shiftlet started driving again. The child held the suitcase on his lap and folded his arms on top of it. He turned his head and looked out the window away from Mr. Shiftlet. Mr. Shiftlet felt oppressed. "Son," he said after a minute, "I got the best old mother in the world so I reckon you only got the second best."

The boy gave him a quick dark glance and then turned his face back out the window.

"It's nothing so sweet," Mr. Shiftlet continued, "as a boy's mother. She taught him his first prayers at her knee, she give him love when no other would, she told him what was right and what wasn't, and she seen that he done the right thing. Son," he said, "I never rued a day in my life like the one I rued when I left that old mother of mine."

The boy shifted in his seat but he didn't look at Mr. Shiftlet. He unfolded his arms and put one hand on the door handle.

"My mother was a angel of Gawd," Mr. Shiftlet said in a very strained voice. "He took her from heaven and giver to me and I left her." His eyes were instantly clouded over with a mist of tears. The car was barely moving.

The boy turned angrily in the seat. "You go to the devil!" he cried. "My old woman is a flea bag and yours is a stinking pole cat!" and with that he flung the door open and jumped out with his suitcase into the ditch.

Mr. Shiftlet was so shocked that for about a hundred feet he drove along slowly with the door still open. A cloud, the exact color of the boy's hat and shaped like a turnip, had descended over the sun, and another, worse looking, crouched behind the car. Mr. Shiftlet felt that the rottenness of the world was about to engulf him. He raised his arm and let it fall again to his breast. "Oh Lord!" he prayed. "Break forth and wash the slime from this earth!"

The turnip continued slowly to descend. After a few minutes there was a guffawing peal of thunder from behind and fantastic raindrops, like tin-can tops, crashed over the rear of Mr. Shiftlet's car. Very quickly he stepped on the gas and with his stump sticking out the window he raced the galloping shower into Mobile.

From Of Mice and Men

JOHN STEINBECK

ACT ONE

Scene 1

Thursday night.
A sandy bank of the Salinas River sheltered with willows—one giant sycamore
right, upstage.
The stage is covered with dry leaves. The feeling of the stage is sheltered and quiet.
Stage is lit by a setting sun.
Curtain rises on an empty stage. A sparrow is singing. There is a distant sound of
ranch dogs barking aimlessly and one clear quail call. The quail call turns to a
warning call and there is a beat of the flock's wings. Two figures are seen entering
the stage in single file, with GEORGE, *the short man, coming in ahead of* LENNIE.
Both men are carrying blanket rolls. They approach the water. The small man
throws down his blanket roll, the large man follows and then falls down and
drinks from the river, snorting as he drinks.

GEORGE (*irritably*). Lennie, for God's sake, don't drink so much. (*Leans over*
   and shakes LENNIE.) Lennie, you hear me! You gonna be sick like you was
   last night.
LENNIE (*dips his whole head under, hat and all. As he sits upon the bank, his*
   hat drips down the back). That's good. You drink some, George. You drink
   some too.
GEORGE (*kneeling and dipping his finger in the water*). I ain't sure it's good
   water. Looks kinda scummy to me.
LENNIE (*imitates, dipping his finger also*). Look at them wrinkles in the water,
   George. Look what I done.
GEORGE (*drinking from his cupped palm*). Tastes all right. Don't seem to be
   runnin' much, though. Lennie, you oughtn' to drink water when it ain't
   running. (*Hopelessly.*) You'd drink water out of a gutter if you was thirsty.
   (*He throws a scoop of water into his face and rubs it around with his hand,*
   pushes himself back and embraces his knees. LENNIE, *after watching him, imi-*
   tates him in every detail.)

GEORGE (*beginning tiredly and growing angry as he speaks*). God damn it, we could just as well of rode clear to the ranch. That bus driver didn't know what he was talkin' about. "Just a little stretch down the highway," he says. "Just a little stretch"—damn near four miles. I bet he didn't want to stop at the ranch gate. . . . I bet he's too damn lazy to pull up. Wonder he ain't too lazy to stop at Soledad at all! (*Mumbling.*) Just a little stretch down the road.

LENNIE (*timidly*). George?

GEORGE. Yeh . . . what you want?

LENNIE. Where we goin', George?

GEORGE (*jerks down his hat furiously*). So you forgot that already, did you? So I got to tell you again! Jeez, you're a crazy bastard!

LENNIE (*softly*). I forgot. I tried not to forget, honest to God, I did!

GEORGE. Okay, okay, I'll tell you again. . . . (*With sarcasm.*) I ain't got nothin' to do. Might just as well spen' all my time tellin' you things. You forgit 'em and I tell you again.

LENNIE (*continuing on from his last speech*). I tried and tried, but it didn't do no good. I remember about the rabbits, George!

GEORGE. The hell with the rabbits! You can't remember nothing but them rabbits. You remember settin' in that gutter on Howard Street and watchin' that blackboard?

LENNIE (*delightedly*). Oh, sure! I remember that . . . but . . . wha'd we do then? I remember some girls come by, and you says—

GEORGE. The hell with what I says! You remember about us goin' in Murray and Ready's and they give us work cards and bus tickets?

LENNIE (*confidently*). Oh, sure, George . . . I remember that now. (Puts his hand into his side *coat-pocket; his confidence vanishes. Very gently.*) . . . George?

GEORGE. Huh?

LENNIE (*staring at the ground in despair*). I ain't got mine. I musta lost it.

GEORGE. You never had none. I got both of 'em here. Think I'd let you carry your own work card?

LENNIE (*with tremendous relief*). I thought I put it in my side pocket. (*Puts his hand in his pocket again.*)

GEORGE (*looking sharply at him; and as he looks, LENNIE brings his hand out of his pocket*). Wha'd you take out of that pocket?

LENNIE (*cleverly*). Ain't a thing in my pocket.

GEORGE. I know there ain't. You got it in your hand now. What you got in your hand?

LENNIE. I ain't got nothing, George! Honest!

GEORGE. Come on, give it here!

LENNIE (*holds his closed hand away from GEORGE*). It's on'y a mouse!

GEORGE. A mouse? A live mouse?

LENNIE. No . . . just a dead mouse. (*Worriedly.*) I didn't kill it. Honest. I found it. I found it dead.

GEORGE. Give it here!

LENNIE. Leave me have it, George.

GEORGE (*sternly*). Give it here! (*LENNIE reluctantly gives him the mouse.*) What do you want of a dead mouse, anyway?

LENNIE (*in a propositional tone*). I was petting it with my thumb while we walked along.

GEORGE. Well, you ain't pettin' no mice while you walk with me. Now let's see if you can remember where we're going. (*GEORGE throws it across the water into the brush.*)

LENNIE (*looks startled and then in embarrassment hides his face against his knees*). I forgot again.

GEORGE. Jesus Christ! (*Resignedly.*) Well, look, we are gonna work on a ranch like the one we come from up north.

LENNIE. Up north?

GEORGE. In Weed!

LENNIE. Oh, sure I remember—in Weed.

GEORGE (*still with exaggerated patience*). That ranch we're goin' to is right down there about a quarter mile. We're gonna go in and see the boss.

LENNIE (*repeats as a lesson*). And see the boss!

GEORGE. Now, look! I'll give him the work tickets, but you ain't gonna say a word. You're just gonna stand there and not say nothing.

LENNIE. Not say nothing!

GEORGE. If he finds out what a crazy bastard you are, we won't get no job. But if he sees you work before he hears you talk, we're set. You got that?

LENNIE. Sure, George . . . sure, I got that.

GEORGE. Okay. Now when we go in to see the boss, what you gonna do?

LENNIE (*concentrating*). I . . . I . . . I ain't gonna say nothing . . . jus' gonna stand there.

GEORGE (*greatly relieved*). Good boy, that's swell! Now say that over two or three times so you sure won't forget it.

LENNIE (*drones softly under his breath*). I ain't gonna say nothing . . . I ain't gonna say nothing . . . (*Trails off into a whisper.*)

GEORGE. And you ain't gonna do no bad things like you done in Weed neither.

LENNIE (*puzzled*). Like I done in Weed?

GEORGE. So you forgot that too, did you?

LENNIE (*triumphantly*). They run us out of Weed!

GEORGE (*disgusted*). Run us out, hell! We run! They was lookin' for us, but they didn't catch us.

LENNIE (*happily*). I didn't forget that, you bet.

GEORGE (*lies back on the sand, crosses his hands under his head. And again LENNIE imitates him*). God, you're a lot of trouble! I could get along so easy and nice, if I didn't have you on my tail. I could live so easy!

LENNIE (*hopefully*). We gonna work on a ranch, George.

GEORGE. All right, you got that. But we're gonna sleep here tonight, because . . . I want to. I want to sleep out.

(*The light is going fast, dropping into evening. A little wind whirls into the clearing and blows leaves. A dog howls in the distance.*)

LENNIE. Why ain't we goin' on to the ranch to get some supper? They got supper at the ranch.

GEORGE. No reason at all. I just like it here. Tomorrow we'll be goin' to work. I seen thrashing machines on the way down; that means we'll be buckin' grain bags. Bustin' a gut liftin' up them bags. Tonight I'm gonna lay right here an' look up! Tonight there ain't a grain bag or a boss in the world. Tonight, the drinks is on the . . . house. Nice house we got here, Lennie.

LENNIE (*gets up on his knees and looks down at GEORGE, plaintively*). Ain't we gonna have no supper?

GEORGE. Sure we are. You gather up some dead willow sticks. I got three cans of beans in my bindle. I'll open 'em up while you get a fire ready. We'll eat 'em cold.

LENNIE (*companionably*). I like beans with ketchup.

GEORGE. Well, we ain't got no ketchup. You go get the wood, and don't you fool around none. Be dark before long. (*LENNIE lumbers to his feet and disappears into the brush. GEORGE gets out the bean cans, opens two of them, suddenly turns his head and listens. A little sound of splashing comes from the direction that LENNIE has taken. GEORGE looks after him; shakes his head. LENNIE comes back carrying a few small willow sticks in his hand.*) All right, give me that mouse.

LENNIE (*with elaborate pantomime of innocence*). What, George? I ain't got no mouse.

GEORGE (*holding out his hand*). Come on! Give it to me! You ain't puttin' nothing over. (*LENNIE hesitates, backs away, turns and looks as if he were going to run. Coldly*). You gonna give me that mouse or do I have to take a sock at you?

LENNIE. Give you what, George?

GEORGE. You know goddamn well, what! I want that mouse!

LENNIE (*almost in tears*). I don't know why I can't keep it. It ain't nobody's mouse. I didn't steal it! I found it layin' right beside the road. (*GEORGE *snaps his fingers sharply, and* LENNIE *lays the mouse in his hand.*) I wasn't doin' nothing bad with it. Just stroking it. That ain't bad.

GEORGE (*stands up and throws the mouse as far as he can into the brush, then he steps to the pool, and washes his hands*). You crazy fool! Thought you could get away with it, didn't you? Don't you think I could see your feet was wet where you went in the water to get it? (LENNIE *whimpers like a puppy.*) Blubbering like a baby. Jesus Christ, a big guy like you! (LENNIE *tries to control himself, but his lips quiver and his face works with an effort.* GEORGE *puts his hand on* LENNIE's *shoulder for a moment.*) Aw, Lennie, I ain't takin' it away just for meanness. That mouse ain't fresh. Besides, you broke it pettin' it. You get a mouse that's fresh and I'll let you keep it a little while.

LENNIE. I don't know where there is no other mouse. I remember a lady used to give 'em to me. Ever' one she got she used to give it to me, but that lady ain't here no more.

GEORGE. Lady, huh! . . . Give me them sticks there. . . . Don't even remember who that lady was. That was your own Aunt Clara. She stopped givin' 'em to you. You always killed 'em.

LENNIE (*sadly and apologetically*). They was so little. I'd pet 'em and pretty soon they bit my fingers and then I pinched their head a little bit and then they was dead . . . because they was so little. I wish we'd get the rabbits pretty soon, George. They ain't so little.

GEORGE. The hell with the rabbits! Come on, let's eat. (*The light has continued to go out of the scene so that when* GEORGE *lights the fire, it is the major light on the stage.* GEORGE *hands one of the open cans of beans to* LENNIE.) There's enough beans for four men.

LENNIE (*sitting on the other side of the fire, speaks patiently*). I like 'em with ketchup.

GEORGE (*explodes*). Well, we ain't got any. Whatever we ain't got, that's what you want. God Almighty, if I was alone, I could live so easy. I could go get a job of work and no trouble. No mess . . . and when the end of the month come, I could take my fifty bucks and go into town and get whatever I want. Why, I could stay in a cat-house all night. I could eat any place I want. Order any damn thing.

LENNIE (*plaintively, but softly*). I didn't want no ketchup.

GEORGE (*continuing violently*). I could do that every damn month. Get a gallon of whiskey or set in a pool room and play cards or shoot pool. (LENNIE *gets up to his knees and looks over the fire, with frightened face.*) And what have I got? (*Disgustedly.*) I got *you*. You can't keep a job and you lose me every job I get!

LENNIE (*in terror*). I don't mean nothing, George.

GEORGE. Just keep me shovin' all over the country all the time. And that ain't the worst—you get in trouble. You do bad things and I got to get you out. It ain't bad people that raises hell. It's dumb ones. (*He shouts.*) You crazy son-of-a-bitch, you keep me in hot water all the time. (LENNIE *is trying to stop* GEORGE's *flow of words with his hands. Sarcastically.*) You just wanta feel that girl's dress. Just wanta pet it like it was a mouse. Well, how the hell'd she know you just wanta feel her dress? How'd she know you'd just hold onto it like it was a mouse?

LENNIE (*in panic*). I didn't mean to, George!

GEORGE. Sure you didn't mean to. You didn't mean for her to yell bloody hell, either. You didn't mean for us to hide in the irrigation ditch all day with guys out lookin' for us with guns. Alla time it's something you didn't mean. God damn it, I wish I could put you in a cage with a million mice and let them pet *you.* (GEORGE's *anger leaves him suddenly. For the first time he seems to see the expression of terror on* LENNIE's *face. He looks down ashamedly at the fire, and maneuvers some beans onto the blade of his pocket-knife and puts them into his mouth.*)

LENNIE (*after a pause*). George! (GEORGE *purposely does not answer him.*) George?

GEORGE. What do you want?

LENNIE. I was only foolin', George. I don't want no ketchup. I wouldn't eat no ketchup if it was right here beside me.

GEORGE (*with a sullenness of shame*). If they was some here you could have it. And if I had a thousand bucks I'd buy ya a bunch of flowers.

LENNIE. I wouldn't eat no ketchup, George. I'd leave it all for you. You could cover your beans so deep with it, and I wouldn't touch none of it.

GEORGE (*refusing to give in from his sullenness, refusing to look at* LENNIE). When I think of the swell time I could have without you, I go nuts. I never git no peace!

LENNIE. You want I should go away and leave you alone?

GEORGE. Where the hell could you go?

LENNIE. Well, I could . . . I could go off in the hills there. Some place I could find a cave.

GEORGE. Yeah, how'd ya eat? You ain't got sense enough to find nothing to eat.

LENNIE. I'd find things. I don't need no nice food with ketchup. I'd lay out in the sun and nobody would hurt me. And if I found a mouse—why, I could keep it. Wouldn't nobody take it away from me.

GEORGE (*at last he looks up*). I been mean, ain't I?

LENNIE (*presses his triumph*). If you don't want me, I can go right in them hills, and find a cave. I can go away any time.

GEORGE. No. Look! I was just foolin' ya. 'Course I want you to stay with me. Trouble with mice is you always kill 'em. (*He pauses.*) Tell you what I'll do, Lennie. First chance I get I'll find you a pup. Maybe you wouldn't kill it. That would be better than mice. You could pet it harder.

LENNIE (*still avoiding being drawn in*). If you don't want me, you only gotta say so. I'll go right up on them hills and live by myself. And I won't get no mice stole from me.

GEORGE. I want you to stay with me. Jesus Christ, somebody'd shoot you for a coyote if you was by yourself. Stay with me. Your Aunt Clara wouldn't like your runnin' off by yourself, even if she is dead.

LENNIE. George?

GEORGE. Huh?

LENNIE (*craftily*). Tell me—like you done before.

GEORGE. Tell you what?

LENNIE. About the rabbits.

GEORGE (*near to anger again*). You ain't gonna put nothing over on me!

LENNIE (*pleading*). Come on, George . . . tell me! Please! Like you done before.

GEORGE. You get a kick out of that, don't you? All right, I'll tell you. And then we'll lay out our beds and eat our dinner.

LENNIE. Go on, George. (*Unrolls his bed and lies on his side, supporting his head on one hand.* GEORGE *lays out his bed and sits cross-legged on it.* GEORGE *repeats the next speech rhythmically, as though he had said it many times before.*)

GEORGE. Guys like us that work on ranches is the loneliest guys in the world. They ain't got no family. They don't belong no place. They come to a ranch and work up a stake and then they go in to town and blow their stake. And then the first thing you know they're poundin' their tail on some other ranch. They ain't got nothin' to look ahead to.

LENNIE (*delightedly*). That's it, that's it! Now tell how it is with us.

GEORGE (*still almost chanting*). With us it ain't like that. We got a future. We got somebody to talk to that gives a damn about us. We don't have to sit in no barroom blowin' in our jack, just because we got no place else to go. If them other guys gets in jail, they can rot for all anybody gives a damn.

LENNIE (*who cannot restrain himself any longer. Bursts into speech.*). But not us! And why? Because . . . because I got you to look after me . . . and you got me to look after you . . . and that's why! (*He laughs.*) Go on, George!

GEORGE. You got it by heart. You can do it yourself.

LENNIE. No, no. I forget some of the stuff. Tell about how it's gonna be.

GEORGE. Some other time.

LENNIE. No, tell how it's gonna be!

GEORGE. Okay. Some day we're gonna get the jack together and we're gonna have a little house, and a couple of acres and a cow and some pigs and . . .

LENNIE (*shouting*). And live off the fat of the land! And have rabbits. Go on, George! Tell about what we're gonna have in the garden. And about the rabbits in the cages. Tell about the rain in the winter . . . and about the stove and how thick the cream is on the milk, you can hardly cut it. Tell about that, George!

GEORGE. Why don't you do it yourself—you know all of it!

LENNIE. It ain't the same if I tell it. Go on now. How I get to tend the rabbits.

GEORGE (*resignedly*). Well, we'll have a big vegetable patch and a rabbit hutch and chickens. And when it rains in the winter we'll just say to hell with goin' to work. We'll build up a fire in the stove, and set around it and listen to the rain comin' down on the roof—Nuts! (*Begins to eat with his knife.*) I ain't got time for no more. (*He falls to eating. LENNIE imitates him, spilling a few beans from his mouth with every bite. GEORGE, gesturing with his knife.*) What you gonna say tomorrow when the boss asks you questions?

LENNIE (*stops chewing in the middle of a bite, swallows painfully. His face contorts with thought*). I . . . I ain't gonna say a word.

GEORGE. Good boy. That's fine. Say, maybe you're gettin' better. I bet I can let you tend the rabbits . . . specially if you remember as good as that!

LENNIE (*choking with pride*). I can remember, by God!

GEORGE (*as though remembering something, points his knife at LENNIE's chest*). Lennie, I want you to look around here. Think you can remember this place? The ranch is 'bout a quarter mile up that way. Just follow the river and you can get here.

LENNIE (*looking around carefully*). Sure, I can remember here. Didn't I remember 'bout not gonna say a word?

GEORGE. 'Course you did. Well, look, Lennie, if you just happen to get in trouble, I want you to come right here and hide in the brush.

LENNIE (*slowly*). Hide in the brush.

GEORGE. Hide in the brush until I come for you. Think you can remember that?

LENNIE. Sure I can, George. Hide in the brush till you come for me!

GEORGE. But you ain't gonna get in no trouble. Because if you do I won't let you tend the rabbits.

LENNIE. I won't get in no trouble. I ain't gonna say a word.

GEORGE. You got it. Anyways, I hope so. (*GEORGE stretches out on his blankets. The light dies slowly out of the fire until only the faces of the two men can be seen. GEORGE is still eating from his can of beans.*) It's gonna be nice sleeping here. Lookin' up . . . and the leaves . . . Don't build no more fire. We'll let her die. Jesus, you feel free when you ain't got a job—if you ain't hungry.

(*They sit silently for a few moments. A night owl is heard far off. From across the river there comes the sound of a coyote howl and on the heels of the howl all the dogs in the country start to bark.*)

LENNIE (*from almost complete darkness*). George?

GEORGE. What do you want?

LENNIE. Let's have different color rabbits, George.

GEORGE. Sure. Red rabbits and blue rabbits and green rabbits. Millions of 'em!

LENNIE. Furry ones, George. Like I seen at the fair in Sacramento.

GEORGE. Sure. Furry ones.

LENNIE. 'Cause I can jus' as well go away, George, and live in a cave.

GEORGE (*amiably*). Aw, shut up.

LENNIE (*after a long pause*). George?

GEORGE. What is it?

LENNIE. I'm shutting up, George.

(*A coyote howls again.*)

Curtain

Average Waves in Unprotected Waters

ANNE TYLER

AS SOON AS it got light, Bet woke him and dressed him, and then she walked him over to the table and tried to make him eat a little cereal. He wouldn't, though. He could tell something was up. She pressed the edge of the spoon against his lips till she heard it click on his teeth, but he just looked off at a corner of the ceiling—a knobby child with great glassy eyes and her own fair hair. Like any other nine-year-old, he wore a striped shirt and jeans, but the shirt was too neat and the jeans too blue, unpatched and unfaded, and would stay that way till he outgrew them. And his face was elderly—pinched, strained, tired—though it should have looked as unused as his jeans. He hardly ever changed his expression.

She left him in his chair and went to make the beds. Then she raised the yellowed shade, rinsed a few spoons in the bathroom sink, picked up some bits of magazines he'd torn the night before. This was a rented room in an ancient, crumbling house, and nothing you could do to it would lighten its cluttered look. There was always that feeling of too many lives layered over other lives, like the layers of brownish wallpaper her child had peeled away in the corner by his bed.

She slipped her feet into flat-heeled loafers and absently patted the front of her dress, a worn beige knit she usually saved for Sundays. Maybe she should take it in a little; it hung from her shoulders like a sack. She felt too slight and frail, too wispy for all she had to do today. But she reached for her coat anyhow, and put it on and tied a blue kerchief under her chin. Then she went over to the table and slowly spun, modeling the coat. "See, Arnold?" she said. "We're going out."

Arnold went on looking at the ceiling, but his gaze turned wild and she knew he'd heard.

She fetched his jacket from the closet—brown corduroy, with a hood. It had set her back half a week's salary. But Arnold didn't like it; he always wanted his old one, a little red duffel coat he'd long ago outgrown. When she came toward him, he started moaning and rocking and shaking his head. She had to struggle to stuff his arms in the sleeves. Small though he was, he was strong, wiry; he was getting to be too much for her. He shook free of her hands and ran over to his bed. The jacket was on, though. It wasn't buttoned, the collar was askew, but never mind; that just made him look more real. She always felt bad at how he stood inside his clothes, separate from them, passive, unaware of all the buttons and snaps she'd fastened as carefully as she would a doll's.

She gave a last look around the room, checked to make sure the hot plate was off, and then picked up her purse and Arnold's suitcase. "Come along, Arnold," she said.

He came, dragging out every step. He looked at the suitcase suspiciously, but only because it was new. It didn't have any meaning for him. "See?" she said. "It's yours. It's Arnold's. It's going on the train with us."

But her voice was all wrong. He would pick it up, for sure. She paused in the middle of locking the door and glanced over at him fearfully. Anything could set him off nowadays. He hadn't noticed, though. He was too busy staring around the hallway, goggling at a freckled, walnut-framed mirror as if he'd never seen it before. She touched his shoulder. "Come, Arnold," she said.

They went down the stairs slowly, both of them clinging to the sticky mahogany railing. The suitcase banged against her shins. In the entrance hall, old Mrs. Puckett stood waiting outside her door—a huge, soft lady in a black crêpe dress and orthopedic shoes. She was holding a plastic bag of peanut-butter cookies, Arnold's favorites. There were tears in her eyes. "Here, Arnold," she said, quavering. Maybe she felt to blame that he was going. But she'd done the best she could: babysat him all these years and only given up when he'd grown too strong and wild to manage. Bet wished Arnold would give the old lady some sign—hug her, make his little crowing noise, just take the cookies, even. But he was too excited. He raced on out the front door, and it was Bet who had to take them. "Well, thank you, Mrs. Puckett," she said. "I know he'll enjoy them later."

"Oh, no . . ." said Mrs. Puckett, and she flapped her large hands and gave up, sobbing.

They were lucky and caught a bus first thing. Arnold sat by the window. He must have thought he was going to work with her; when they passed the red-and-gold Kresge's sign, he jabbered and tried to stand up. "No, honey," she said, and took hold of his arm. He settled down then and let his hand stay curled in hers awhile. He had very small, cool fingers, and nails as smooth as thumbtack heads.

At the train station, she bought the tickets and then a pack of Wrigley's spearmint gum. Arnold stood gaping at the vaulted ceiling, with his head flopped back and his arms hanging limp at his sides. People stared at him. She would have liked to push their faces in. "Over here, honey," she said, and she nudged him toward the gate, straightening his collar as they walked.

He hadn't been on a train before and acted a little nervous, bouncing up and down in his seat and flipping the lid of his ashtray and craning forward to see the man ahead of them. When the train started moving, he crowed and pulled at her sleeve. "That's right, Arnold. Train. We're taking a trip," Bet said. She unwrapped a stick of chewing gum and gave it to him. He loved gum. If she didn't watch him closely, he sometimes swallowed it—which worried her a little because she'd heard it clogged your kidneys; but at least it would keep him busy. She looked down at the top of his head. Through the blond prickles of his hair, cut short for practical reasons, she could see his skull bones moving as he chewed. He was so thin-skinned, almost transparent; sometimes she imagined she could see the blood traveling in his veins.

When the train reached a steady speed, he grew calmer, and after a while he nodded over against her and let his hands sag on his knees. She watched his eyelashes slowly drooping—two colorless, fringed crescents, heavier and heavier, every now and then flying up as he tried to fight off sleep. He had never slept well, not ever, not even as a baby. Even before they'd noticed anything wrong, they'd wondered at his jittery, jerky catnaps, his tiny hands clutching tight and springing open, his strange single wail sailing out while he went right on sleeping. Avery said it gave him the chills. And after the doctor talked to them Avery wouldn't have anything to do with Arnold anymore—just walked in wide circles around the crib, looking stunned and sick. A few weeks later, he left. She wasn't surprised. She even knew how he felt, more or less. Halfway, he blamed her; halfway, he blamed himself. You can't believe a thing like this will just fall on you out of nowhere.

She'd had moments herself of picturing some kind of evil gene in her husband's ordinary, stocky body—a dark little egg like a black jelly bean, she imagined it. All his fault. But other times she was sure the gene was hers. It seemed so natural; she never could do anything as well as most people. And then other times she blamed their marriage. They'd married too young, against her parents' wishes. All she'd wanted was to get away from home. Now she couldn't remember why. What was wrong with home? She thought of her parents' humped green trailer, perched on cinder blocks near a forest of masts in Salt Spray, Maryland. At this distance (parents dead, trailer rusted to bits, even Salt Spray changed past recognition), it seemed to her that her old life had been beautifully free and spacious. She closed her eyes and saw wide gray skies. Everything had been ruled by the sea. Her father (who'd run a fishing boat for tourists) couldn't arrange his day till he'd heard the marine forecast—the wind, the tides, the small-craft warnings, the height of average waves in unprotected waters. He loved to fish, offshore and on, and he swam every chance he could get. He'd tried to teach her to bodysurf, but it hadn't worked out. There was something about the breakers: she just gritted her teeth and stood staunch and let them slam into her. As if standing staunch were a virtue, really. She couldn't explain it. Her father thought she was scared, but it wasn't that at all.

She'd married Avery against their wishes and been sorry ever since—sorry to move so far from home, sorrier when her parents died within a year of each other, sorriest of all when the marriage turned grim and cranky. But she never would have thought of leaving him. It was Avery who left; she would have stayed forever. In fact, she did stay on in their apartment for months after he'd gone, though the rent was far too high. It wasn't that she expected him back. She just took some comfort from enduring.

Arnold's head snapped up. He looked around him and made a gurgling sound. His chewing gum fell onto the front of his jacket. "Here, honey," she told him. She put the gum in her ashtray. "Look out the window. See the cows?"

He wouldn't look. He began bouncing in his seat, rubbing his hands together rapidly.

"Arnold? Want a cookie?"

If only she'd brought a picture book. She'd meant to and then forgot. She wondered if the train people sold magazines. If she let him get too bored, he'd go into one of his tantrums, and then she wouldn't be able to handle him. The doctor had given her pills just in case, but she was always afraid that while he was screaming he could choke on them. She looked around the car. "Arnold," she said, "see the . . . see the hat with feathers on? Isn't it pretty? See the red suitcase? See the, um . . ."

The car door opened with a rush of clattering wheels and the conductor burst in, singing "Girl of my dreams, I love you." He lurched down the aisle, plucking pink tickets from the back of each seat. Just across from Bet and Arnold, he stopped. He was looking down at a tiny black lady in a purple coat, with a fox fur piece biting its own tail around her neck. "You!" he said.

The lady stared straight ahead.

"You, I saw you. You're the one in the washroom."

A little muscle twitched in her cheek.

"You got on this train in Beulah, didn't you. Snuck in the washroom. Darted back like you thought you could put something over on me. I saw that bit of purple! Where's your ticket gone to?"

She started fumbling in a blue cloth purse. The fumbling went on and on. The conductor shifted his weight.

"Why!" she said finally. "I must've left it back in my other seat."

"What other seat?"

"Oh, the one back . . ." She waved a spidery hand.

The conductor sighed. "Lady," he said, "you owe me money."

"I do no such thing!" she said. "Viper! Monger! Hitler! Her voice screeched up all at once; she sounded like a parrot. Bet winced and felt herself flushing, as if *she* were the one. But then at her shoulder she heard a sudden, rusty clang, and she turned and saw that Arnold was laughing. He had his mouth wide open and his tongue curled, the way he did when he watched "Sesame Street." Even after the scene had worn itself out, and the lady had paid and the conductor had moved on, Arnold went on chortling and la-la-ing, and Bet looked gratefully at the little black lady, who was settling her fur piece fussily and muttering under her breath.

From the Parkinsville Railroad Station, which they seemed to be tearing down or else remodeling—she couldn't tell which—they took a taxicab to Parkins State Hospital. "Oh, I been out there many and many a time," said the driver. "Went out there just the other—"

But she couldn't stop herself; she had to tell him before she forgot. "Listen," she said, "I want you to wait for me right in the driveway. I don't want you to go on away."

"Well, fine," he said.

"Can you do that? I want you to be sitting right by the porch or the steps or whatever, right where I come out of, ready to take me back to the station. Don't just go off and—"

"I *got* you, I got you," he said.

She sank back. She hoped he understood.

Arnold wanted a peanut-butter cookie. He was reaching and whimpering. She didn't know what to do. She wanted to give him anything he asked for, anything; but he'd get it all over his face and arrive not looking his best. She couldn't stand it if they thought he was just ordinary and unattractive. She wanted them to see how small and neat he was, how somebody cherished him. But it would be awful if he went into one of his rages. She broke off a little piece of cookie from the bag. "Here," she told him. "Don't mess, now."

He flung himself back in the corner and ate it, keeping one hand flattened across his mouth while he chewed.

The hospital looked like someone's great, pillared mansion, with square brick buildings all around it. "Here we are," the driver said.

"Thank you," she said. "Now you wait here, please. Just wait till I get—"

"*Lady*," he said. "I'll wait."

She opened the door and nudged Arnold out ahead of her. Lugging the suitcase, she started toward the steps. "Come on, Arnold," she said.

He hung back.

"Arnold?"

Maybe he wouldn't allow it, and they would go on home and never think of this again.

But he came, finally, climbing the steps in his little hobbled way. His face was clean, but there were a few cookie crumbs on his jacket. She set down the suitcase to brush them off. Then she buttoned all his buttons and smoothed his shirt collar over his jacket collar before she pushed open the door.

In the admitting office, a lady behind a wooden counter showed her what papers to sign. Secretaries were clacketing typewriters all around. Bet thought Arnold might like that, but instead he got lost in the lights—chilly, hanging ice-cube tray lights with a little flicker to them. He gazed upward, looking astonished. Finally a flat-fronted nurse came in and touched his elbow. "Come along, Arnold. Come, Mommy. We'll show you where Arnold is staying." she said.

They walked back across the entrance hall, then up wide marble steps with hollows worn in them. Arnold clung to the bannister. There was a smell Bet hated, pine-oil disinfectant, but Arnold didn't seem to notice. You never knew; sometimes smells could just put him in a state.

The nurse unlocked a double door that had chicken-wired windows. They walked through a corridor, passing several fat, ugly women in shapeless gray dresses and ankle socks. "Ha!" one of the women said, and fell giggling into the arms of a friend. The nurse said, "*Here* we are." She led them into an enormous hallway lined with little white cots. Nobody else was in it; there wasn't a sign that children lived here except for a tiny cardboard clown picture hanging on one vacant wall. "This one is your bed, Arnold," said the nurse. Bet laid the suitcase on it. It was made up so neatly, the sheets might have been painted on. A steely-gray blanket was folded across the foot. She looked over at Arnold, but he was pivoting back and forth to hear how his new sneakers squeaked on the linoleum.

"Usually," said the nurse, "we like to give new residents six months before the family visits. That way they settle in quicker, don't you see." She turned away and adjusted the clown picture, though as far as Bet could tell it was fine the way it was. Over her shoulder, the nurse said, "You can tell him goodbye now, if you like."

"Oh," Bet said. "All right." She set her hands on Arnold's shoulders. Then she laid her face against his hair, which felt warm and fuzzy. "Honey," she said. But he went on pivoting. She straightened and told the nurse, "I brought his special blanket."

"Oh, fine," said the nurse, turning toward her again. "We'll see that he gets it."

"He always likes to sleep with it; he has ever since he was little."

"All right."

"Don't wash it. He hates if you wash it."

"Yes. Say goodbye to Mommy now, Arnold."

"A lot of times he'll surprise you. I mean there's a whole lot to him. He's not just—"

"We'll take very good care of him, Mrs. Blevins, don't worry."

"Well," she said. "Bye, Arnold."

She left the ward with the nurse and went down the corridor. As the nurse was unlocking the doors for her, she heard a single, terrible scream, but the nurse only patted her shoulder and pushed her gently on through.

In the taxi, Bet said, "Now, I've just got fifteen minutes to get to the station. I wonder if you could hurry?"

"Sure thing," the driver said.

She folded her hands and looked straight ahead. Tears seemed to be coming down her face in sheets.

Once she'd reached the station, she went to the ticket window. "Am I in time for the twelve-thirty-two?" she asked.

"Easily," said the man. "It's twenty minutes late."

"What?"

"Got held up in Norton somehow."

"But you can't!" she said. The man looked startled. She must be a sight, all swollen-eyed and wet-cheeked. "Look," she said, in a lower voice. "I figured this on purpose. I chose the one train from Beulah that would let me catch another one back without waiting. I do not want to sit and wait in this station."

"Twenty *minutes,* lady. That's all it is."

"What am I going to do?" she asked him.

He turned back to his ledgers.

She went over to a bench and sat down. Ladders and scaffolding towered above her, and only ten or twelve passengers were dotted through the rest of the station. The place looked bombed out—nothing but a shell. "Twenty minutes!" she said aloud. "What am I going to do?"

Through the double glass doors at the far end of the station, a procession of gray-suited men arrived with briefcases. More men came behind them, dressed in work clothes, carrying folding chairs, black trunk like boxes with silver hinges, microphones, a wooden lectern and an armload of bunting. They set the lectern down in the center of the floor, not six feet from Bet. They draped the bunting across it—an arc of red, white, and blue. Wires were connected, floodlights were lit. A microphone screeched. One of the workmen said, "Try her, Mayor." He held the microphone out to a fat man in a suit, who cleared his throat and said, "Ladies and gentlemen, on the occasion of the expansion of this fine old railway station—"

"Sure do get an echo here," the workman said. "Keep on going."

The Mayor cleared his throat again. "If I may," he said, "I'd like to take about twenty minutes of your time, friends."

He straightened his tie. Bet blew her nose, and then she wiped her eyes and smiled. They had come just for her sake, you might think. They were putting on a sort of private play. From now on, all the world was going to be like that—just something on a stage, for her to sit back and watch.

Lily Daw and the Three Ladies

EUDORA WELTY

MRS. WATTS and Mrs. Carson were both in the post office in Victory when the letter came from the Ellisville Institute for the Feeble-Minded of Mississippi. Aimee Slocum, with her hand still full of mail, ran out in front and handed it straight to Mrs. Watts, and they all three read it together. Mrs. Watts held it taut between her pink hands, and Mrs. Carson underscored each line slowly with her thimbled finger. Everybody else in the post office wondered what was up now.

"What will Lily say," beamed Mrs. Carson at last, "when we tell her we're sending her to Ellisville!"

"She'll be tickled to death," said Mrs. Watts, and added in a guttural voice to a deaf lady, "Lily Daw's getting in at Ellisville!"

"Don't you all dare go off and tell Lily without me!" called Aimee Slocum, trotting back to finish putting up the mail.

"Do you suppose they'll look after her down there?" Mrs. Carson began to carry on a conversation with a group of Baptist ladies waiting in the post office. She was the Baptist preacher's wife.

"I've always heard it was lovely down there, but crowded," said one.

"Lily lets people walk over her so," said another.

"Last night at the tent show—" said another, and then popped her hand over her mouth.

"Don't mind me, I know there are such things in the world," said Mrs. Carson, looking down and fingering the tape measure which hung over her bosom.

"Oh, Mrs. Carson. Well, anyway, last night at the tent show, why, the man was just before making Lily buy a ticket to get in."

"A ticket!"

"Till my husband went up and explained she wasn't bright, and so did everybody else."

The ladies all clucked their tongues.

"Oh, it was a very nice show," said the lady who had gone. "And Lily acted so nice. She was a perfect lady—just set in her seat and stared."

"Oh, she can be a lady—she can be," said Mrs. Carson, shaking her head and turning her eyes up. "That's just what breaks your heart."

"Yes'm, she kept her eyes on—what's that thing makes all the commotion?—the xylophone," said the lady. "Didn't turn her head to the right or to the left the whole time. Set in front of me."

"The point is, what did she do after the show?" asked Mrs. Watts practically. "Lily has gotten so she is very mature for her age."

"Oh, Etta!" protested Mrs. Carson, looking at her wildly for a moment.

"And that's how come we are sending her to Ellisville," finished Mrs. Watts.

"I'm ready, you all," said Aimee Slocum, running out with white powder all over her face. "Mail's up. I don't know how good it's up."

"Well, of course, I do hope it's for the best," said several of the other ladies. They did not go at once to take their mail out of their boxes; they felt a little left out.

The three women stood at the foot of the water tank.

"To find Lily is a different thing," said Aimee Slocum.

"Where in the wide world do you suppose she'd be?" It was Mrs. Watts who was carrying the letter.

"I don't see a sign of her either on this side of the street or on the other side," Mrs. Carson declared as they walked along.

Ed Newton was stringing Redbird school tablets on the wire across the store.

"If you're after Lily, she come in here while ago and tole me she was fixin' to git married," he said.

"Ed Newton!" cried the ladies all together, clutching one another. Mrs. Watts began to fan herself at once with the letter from Ellisville. She wore widow's black, and the least thing made her hot.

"Why she is not. She's going to Ellisville, Ed," said Mrs. Carson gently. "Mrs. Watts and I and Aimee Slocum are paying her way out of our own pockets. Besides, the boys of Victory are on their honor. Lily's not going to get married, that's just an idea she's got in her head."

"More power to you, ladies," said Ed Newton, spanking himself with a tablet.

When they came to the bridge over the railroad tracks, there was Estelle Mabers, sitting on a rail. She was slowly drinking an orange Ne-Hi.

"Have you seen Lily?" they asked her.

"I'm supposed to be out here watching for her now," said the Mabers girl, as though she weren't there yet. "But for Jewel—Jewel says Lily come in the store while ago and picked out a two-ninety-eight hat and wore it off. Jewel wants to swap her something else for it."

"Oh, Estelle, Lily says she's going to get married!" cried Aimee Slocum.

"Well, I declare," said Estelle; she never understood anything.

Loralee Adkins came riding by in her Willys-Knight, tooting the horn to find out what they were talking about.

Aimee threw up her hands and ran out into the street. "Loralee, Loralee, you got to ride us up to Lily Daws'. She's up yonder fixing to get married!"

"Hop in, my land!"

"Well, that just goes to show you right now," said Mrs. Watts, groaning as she was helped into the back seat. "What we've got to do is persuade Lily it will be nicer to go to Ellisville."

"Just to think!"

While they rode around the corner Mrs. Carson was going on in her sad voice, sad as the soft noises in the hen house at twilight. "We buried Lily's poor defenseless mother. We gave Lily all her food and kindling and every stitch she had on. Sent her to Sunday school to learn the Lord's teachings, had her baptized a Baptist. And when her old father commenced beating her and tried to cut her head off with the butcher knife, why, we went and took her away from him and gave her a place to stay."

The paintless frame house with all the weather vanes was three stories high in places and had yellow and violet stained-glass windows in front and gingerbread around the porch. It leaned steeply to one side, toward the railroad, and the front steps were gone. The car full of ladies drew up under the cedar tree.

"Now Lily's almost grown up," Mrs. Carson continued. "In fact, she's grown," she concluded, getting out.

"Talking about getting married," said Mrs. Watts disgustedly. "Thanks, Loralee, you run on home."

They climbed over the dusty zinnias onto the porch and walked through the open door without knocking.

"There certainly is always a funny smell in this house. I say it every time I come," said Aimee Slocum.

Lily was there, in the dark of the hall, kneeling on the floor by a small open trunk.

When she saw them she put a zinnia in her mouth, and held still.

"Hello, Lily," said Mrs. Carson reproachfully.

"Hello," said Lily. In a minute she gave a suck on the zinnia stem that sounded exactly like a jay bird. There she sat, wearing a petticoat for a dress, one of the things Mrs. Carson kept after her about. Her milky-yellow hair streamed freely down from under a new hat. You could see the wavy scar on her throat if you knew it was there.

Mrs. Carson and Mrs. Watts, the two fattest, sat in the double rocker. Aimee Slocum sat on the wire chair donated from the drugstore that burned.

"Well, what are you doing, Lily?" asked Mrs. Watts, who led the rocking. Lily smiled.

The trunk was old and lined with yellow and brown paper, with an asterisk pattern showing in darker circles and rings. Mutely the ladies indicated to each other that they did not know where in the world it had come from. It was empty except for two bars of soap and a green washcloth, which Lily was now trying to arrange in the bottom.

"Go on and tell us what you're doing, Lily," said Aimee Slocum.

"Packing, silly," said Lily.

"Where are you going?"

"Going to get married, and I bet you wish you was me now," said Lily. But shyness overcame her suddenly, and she popped the zinnia back into her mouth.

"Talk to me, dear," said Mrs. Carson. "Tell old Mrs. Carson why you want to get married."

"No," said Lily, after a moment's hesitation.

"Well, we've thought of something that will be so much nicer," said Mrs. Carson. "Why don't you go to Ellisville!"

"Won't that be lovely?" said Mrs. Watts. "Goodness, yes."

"It's a lovely place," said Aimee Slocum uncertainly.

"You've got bumps on your face," said Lily.

"Aimee, dear, you stay out of this, if you don't mind," said Mrs. Carson anxiously. "I don't know what it is comes over Lily when you come around her."

Lily stared at Aimee Slocum meditatively.

"There! Wouldn't you like to go to Ellisville now?" asked Mrs. Carson.

"No'm," said Lily.

"Why not?" All the ladies leaned down toward her in impressive astonishment.

" 'Cause I'm goin' to get married," said Lily.

"Well, and who are you going to marry, dear?" asked Mrs. Watts. She knew how to pin people down and make them deny what they'd already said.

Lily bit her lip and began to smile. She reached into the trunk and held up both cakes of soap and wagged them.

"Tell us," challenged Mrs. Watts. "Who you're going to marry, now."

"A man last night."

There was a gasp from each lady. The possible reality of a lover descended suddenly like a summer hail over their heads. Mrs. Watts stood up and balanced herself.

"One of those show fellows! A musician!" she cried.

Lily looked up in admiration.

"Did he—did he do anything to you?" In the long run, it was still only Mrs. Watts who could take charge.

"Oh, yes'm," said Lily. She patted the cakes of soap fastidiously with the tips of her small fingers and tucked them in with the washcloth.

"What?" demanded Aimee Slocum, rising up and tottering before her scream. "What?" she called out in the hall.

"Don't ask her what," said Mrs. Carson, coming up behind. "Tell me, Lily— just yes or no—are you the same as you were?"

"He had a red coat," said Lily graciously. "He took little sticks and went *ping-pong! ding-dong!*"

"Oh, I think I'm going to faint," said Aimee Slocum, but they said, "No, you're not."

"The xylophone!" cried Mrs. Watts. "The xylophone player! Why, the coward, he ought to be run out of town on a rail!"

"Out of town? He is out of town, by now," cried Aimee. "Can't you read?— the sign in the café—Victory on the ninth, Como on the tenth? He's in Como. Como!"

"All right! We'll bring him back!" cried Mrs. Watts. "He can't get away from me!"

"Hush," said Mrs. Carson. "I don't think it's any use following that line of reasoning at all. It's better in the long run for him to be gone out of our lives for good and all. That kind of man. He was after Lily's body alone and he wouldn't ever in this world make the poor little thing happy, even if we went out and forced him to marry her like he ought—at the point of a gun."

"Still—" began Aimee, her eyes widening.

"Shut up," said Mrs. Watts. "Mrs. Carson, you're right, I expect."

"This is my hope chest—see?" said Lily politely in the pause that followed. "You haven't even looked at it. I've already got soap and a washrag. And I have my hat—on. What are you all going to give me?"

"Lily," said Mrs. Watts, starting over, "we'll give you lots of gorgeous things if you'll only go to Ellisville instead of getting married."

"What will you give me?" asked Lily.

"I'll give you a pair of hemstitched pillowcases," said Mrs. Carson.

"I'll give you a big caramel cake," said Mrs. Watts.

"I'll give you a souvenir from Jackson—a little toy bank," said Aimee Slocum. "Now will you go?"

"No," said Lily.

"I'll give you a pretty little Bible with your name on it in real gold," said Mrs. Carson.

"What if I was to give you a pink crêpe de Chine brassière with adjustable shoulder straps?" asked Mrs. Watts grimly.

"Oh, Etta."

"Well, she needs it," said Mrs. Watts. "What would they think if she ran all over Ellisville in a petticoat looking like a Fiji?"

"I wish *I* could go to Ellisville," said Aimee Slocum luringly.

"What will they have for me down there?" asked Lily softly.

"Oh! lots of things. You'll have baskets to weave, I expect. . . ." Mrs. Carson looked vaguely at the others.

"Oh, yes indeed, they will let you make all sorts of baskets," said Mrs. Watts; then her voice too trailed off.

"No'm, I'd rather get married," said Lily.

"Lily Daw! Now that's just plain stubbornness!" cried Mrs. Watts. "You almost said you'd go and then you took it back!"

"We've all asked God, Lily," said Mrs. Carson finally, "and God seemed to tell us—Mr. Carson, too—that the place where you ought to be, so as to be happy, was Ellisville."

Lily looked reverent, but still stubborn.

"We've really just got to get her there—now!" screamed Aimee Slocum all at once. "Suppose—! She can't stay here!"

"Oh, no, no, no," said Mrs. Carson hurriedly. "We mustn't think that."

They sat sunken in despair.

"Could I take my hope chest—to go to Ellisville?" asked Lily shyly, looking at them sidewise.

"Why, yes," said Mrs. Carson blankly.

Silently they rose once more to their feet.

"Oh, if I could just take my hope chest!"

"All the time it was just her hope chest," Aimee whispered.

Mrs. Watts struck her palms together. "It's settled!"

"Praise the fathers," murmured Mrs. Carson.

Lily looked up at them, and her eyes gleamed. She cocked her head and spoke out in a proud imitation of someone—someone utterly unknown.

"O.K.—Toots!"

The ladies had been nodding and smiling and backing away toward the door.

"I think I'd better stay," said Mrs. Carson, stopping in her tracks. "Where—where could she have learned that terrible expression?"

"Pack up," said Mrs. Watts. "Lily Daw is leaving for Ellisville on Number One."

In the station the train was puffing. Nearly everyone in Victory was hanging around waiting for it to leave. The Victory Civic Band had assembled without any orders and was scattered through the crowd. Ed Newton gave false signals to start on his bass horn. A crate full of baby chickens got loose on the platform. Everybody wanted to see Lily all dressed up, but Mrs. Carson and Mrs. Watts had sneaked her into the train from the other side of the tracks.

The two ladies were going to travel as far as Jackson to help Lily change trains and be sure she went in the right direction.

Lily sat between them on the plush seat with her hair combed and pinned up into a knot under a small blue hat which was Jewel's exchange for the pretty one. She wore a traveling dress made out of part of Mrs. Watts's last summer's mourning. Pink straps glowed through. She had a purse and a Bible and a warm cake in a box, all in her lap.

Aimee Slocum had been getting the outgoing mail stamped and bundled. She stood in the aisle of the coach now, tears shaking from her eyes.

"Good-bye, Lily," she said. She was the one who felt things.

"Good-bye, silly," said Lily.

"Oh, dear, I hope they get our telegram to meet her in Ellisville!" Aimee cried sorrowfully, as she thought how far away it was. "And it was so hard to get it all in ten words, too."

"Get off, Aimee, before the train starts and you break your neck," said Mrs. Watts, all settled and waving her dressy fan gaily. "I declare, it's so hot, as soon as we get a few miles out of town I'm going to slip my corset down."

"Oh, Lily, don't cry down there. Just be good, and do what they tell you—it's all because they love you." Aimee drew her mouth down. She was backing away, down the aisle.

Lily laughed. She pointed across Mrs. Carson's bosom out the window toward a man. He had stepped off the train and just stood there, by himself. He was a stranger and wore a cap.

"Look," she said, laughing softly through her fingers.

"Don't—look," said Mrs. Carson very distinctly, as if, out of all she had ever spoken, she would impress these two solemn words upon Lily's soft little brain. She added, "Don't look at anything till you get to Ellisville."

Outside, Aimee Slocum was crying so hard she almost ran into the stranger. He wore a cap and was short and seemed to have on perfume, if such a thing could be.

"Could you tell me, madam," he said, "where a little lady lives in this burg name of Miss Lily Daw?" He lifted his cap—and he had red hair.

"What do you want to know for?" Aimee asked before she knew it.

"Talk louder," said the stranger. He almost whispered, himself.

"She's gone away—she's gone to Ellisville!"

"Gone?"

"Gone to Ellisville!"

"Well, I like that!" The man stuck out his bottom lip and puffed till his hair jumped.

"What business did you have with Lily?" cried Aimee suddenly.

"We was only going to get married, that's all," said the man.

Aimee Slocum started to scream in front of all those people. She almost pointed to the long black box she saw lying on the ground at the man's feet. Then she jumped back in fright.

"The xylophone! The xylophone!" she cried, looking back and forth from the man to the hissing train. Which was more terrible? The bell began to ring hollowly, and the man was talking.

"Did you say Ellisville? That in the state of Mississippi?" Like lightning he had pulled out a red notebook entitled, "Permanent Facts & Data." He wrote down something. "I don't hear well."

Aimee nodded her head up and down, and circled around him.

Under "Ellis-Ville Miss" he was drawing a line; now he was flicking it with two little marks. "Maybe she didn't say she would. Maybe she said she wouldn't." He suddenly laughed very loudly, after the way he had whispered. Aimee jumped back. "Women!—Well, if we play anywheres near Ellisville, Miss., in the future I may look her up and I may not," he said.

The bass horn sounded the true signal for the band to begin. White steam rushed out of the engine. Usually the train stopped for only a minute in Victory, but the engineer knew Lily from waving at her, and he knew this was her big day.

"Wait!" Aimee Slocum did scream. "Wait, mister! I can get her for you. Wait, Mister Engineer! Don't go!"

Then there she was back on the train, screaming in Mrs. Carson's and Mrs. Watts's faces.

"The xylophone player! The xylophone player to marry her! Yonder he is!"

"Nonsense," murmured Mrs. Watts, peering over the others to look where Aimee pointed. "If he's there I don't see him. Where is he? You're looking at One-Eye Beasley."

"The little man with the cap—no, with the red hair! Hurry!"

"Is that really him?" Mrs. Carson asked Mrs. Watts in wonder. "Mercy! He's small, isn't he?"

"Never saw him before in my life!" cried Mrs. Watts. But suddenly she shut up her fan.

"Come on! This is a train we're on!" cried Aimee Slocum. Her nerves were all unstrung.

"All right, don't have a conniption fit, girl," said Mrs. Watts. "Come on," she said thickly to Mrs. Carson.

"Where are we going now?" asked Lily as they struggled down the aisle.

"We're taking you to get married," said Mrs. Watts. "Mrs. Carson, you'd better phone up your husband right there in the station."

"But I don't want to git married," said Lily, beginning to whimper. "I'm going to Ellisville."

"Hush, and we'll all have some ice-cream cones later," whispered Mrs. Carson.

Just as they climbed down the steps at the back end of the train, the band went into "Independence March."

The xylophone player was still there, patting his foot. He came up and said, "Hello, Toots. What's up—tricks?" and kissed Lily with a smack, after which she hung her head.

"So you're the young man we've heard so much about," said Mrs. Watts. Her smile was brilliant. "Here's your little Lily."

"What say?" asked the xylophone player.

"My husband happens to be the Baptist preacher of Victory," said Mrs. Carson in a loud, clear voice. "Isn't that lucky? I can get him here in five minutes: I know exactly where he is."

They were in a circle around the xylophone player, all going into the white waiting room.

"Oh, I feel just like crying, at a time like this," said Aimee Slocum. She looked back and saw the train moving slowly away, going under the bridge at Main Street. Then it disappeared around the curve.

"Oh, the hope chest!" Aimee cried in a stricken voice.

"And whom have we the pleasure of addressing?" Mrs. Watts was shouting, while Mrs. Carson was ringing up the telephone.

The band went on playing. Some of the people thought Lily was on the train, and some swore she wasn't. Everybody cheered, though, and a straw hat was thrown into the telephone wires.

Women's Experiences with Mental Disorders

§

Three Poems

EMILY DICKINSON

MUCH MADNESS IS DIVINEST SENSE

Much Madness is divinest Sense—
To a discerning Eye—
Much Sense—the starkest Madness—
'Tis the Majority
In this, as All, prevail—
Assent—and you are sane—
Demur—you're straightway dangerous—
And handled with a Chain—

I STARTED EARLY—TOOK MY DOG

I started Early—Took my Dog—
And visited the Sea—
The Mermaids in the Basement
Came out to look at me—

And Frigates—in the Upper Floor
Extended Hempen Hands—
Presuming Me to be a Mouse—
Aground—upon the Sands—

But no Man moved Me—till the Tide
Went past my simple Shoe—
And past my Apron—and my Belt
And past my Boddice—too—

And made as He would eat me up—
As wholly as a Dew

Upon a Dandelion's Sleeve—
And then—I started—too—

And He—He followed—close behind—
I felt His Silver Heel
Upon my Ancle—Then my Shoes
Would overflow with Pearl—

Until We met the Solid Town—
No One He seemed to know—
And bowing—with a Mighty look—
At me—The Sea withdrew—

I Felt a Funeral in My Brain

I felt a funeral in my brain,
    And mourners, to and fro,
Kept treading, treading, till it seemed
    That sense was breaking through.

And when they all were seated,
    A service like a drum
Kept beating, beating, till I thought
    My mind was going numb.

And then I heard them lift a box,
    And creak across my soul
With those same boots of lead, again.
    Then space began to toll

As all the heavens were a bell,
    And Being but an ear,
And I and silence some strange race,
    Wrecked, solitary, here.

From Like Water for Chocolate

LAURA ESQUIVEL

PREPARATION:

THE GUM ARABIC is dissolved in enough hot water to form a paste that is not too thick; when the paste is ready, the phosphorus is added and dissolved into it, and the same is done with the potassium nitrate. Then enough minium is added to color the mixture.

Tita was watching in silence as Dr. Brown completed these procedures.

She was sitting by the window of the doctor's little laboratory in the back of the patio behind his house. The light that filtered in through the window struck her shoulders and provided a faint sensation of warmth, so slight it was almost imperceptible. A chronic chill kept her from feeling warm, in spite of being covered with her heavy woolen bedspread. One of her greatest interests was still working on the bedspread each night, with yarn John had bought for her.

Of the whole house, this was the place they both like best. Tita had discovered it the week she arrived at Dr. Brown's. John, ignoring Mama Elena's order, had not put Tita in a madhouse but had taken her to live with him. Tita would never be able to thank him enough. In a madhouse she might have become truly insane. But here, with John's warmth toward her in word and manner, she felt better each day. Her arrival there was like a dream. Among the blurry images, she remembered the terrible pain she felt when the doctor had set her broken nose.

Afterward, John's large, loving hands, had taken off her clothes and bathed her and carefully removed the pigeon droppings from her body, leaving her clean and sweet-smelling. Finally, he gently brushed her hair and put her in a bed with starched sheets.

Those hands had rescued her from horror and she would never forget it.

Some day, when she felt like talking, she would tell John that; but now, she preferred silence. There were many things she needed to work out in her mind, and she could not find the words to express the feelings seething inside her since she left the ranch. She was badly shaken. The first few days she didn't even want to leave her room; her food was brought to her by Katy, a seventy-year-old woman, who besides being in charge of the kitchen also took care of Alex, the doctor's little boy, whose mother had died when he was born. Tita heard Alex laughing and running in the patio, but she felt no desire to meet him.

Sometimes Tita didn't even taste her food, which was bland and didn't appeal to her. Instead of eating, she would stare at her hands for hours on end. She would regard them like a baby, marveling that they belonged to her. She could move them however she pleased, yet she didn't know what to do with them, other than knitting. She had never taken time to stop and think about these things. At her mother's, what she had to do with her hands was strictly determined, no questions asked. She had to get up, get dressed, get the fire going in the stove, fix breakfast, feed the animals, wash the dishes, make the beds, fix lunch, wash the dishes, iron the clothes, fix dinner, wash the dishes, day after day, year after year. Without pausing for a moment, without wondering if this was what she wanted. Now, seeing her hands no longer at her mother's command, she didn't know what to ask them to do, she had never decided for herself before. They could do anything or become anything. They could turn into birds and fly into the air! She would like them to carry her far away, as far as possible. Going to the window facing the patio, she raised her hands to heaven; she wanted to escape from herself, didn't want to think about making a choice, didn't want to talk again. She didn't want her words to shriek her pain.

She yearned with all her soul to be borne off by her hands. She stood that way for a while, looking at the deep blue of the sky around her motionless hands. Tita thought the miracle was actually occurring when she saw her fingers turning into a thin cloud rising to the sky. She prepared to ascend drawn by a superior power, but nothing happened. Disappointed, she discovered that the smoke wasn't hers. . . .

From Faces in the Water

JANET FRAME

II

I WAS COLD. I tried to find a pair of long woolen ward socks to keep my feet warm in order that I should not die under the new treatment, electric shock therapy, and have my body sneaked out the back way to the mortuary. Every morning I woke in dread, waiting for the day nurse to go on her rounds and announce from the list of names in her hand whether or not I was for shock treatment, the new and fashionable means of quieting people and of making them realize that orders are to be obeyed and floors are to be polished without anyone protesting and faces are made to be fixed into smiles and weeping is a crime. Waiting in the early morning, in the black-capped frosted hours, was like waiting for the pronouncement of a death sentence.

I tried to remember the incidents of the day before. Had I wept? Had I refused to obey an order from one of the nurses? Or, becoming upset at the sight of a very ill patient, had I panicked, and tried to escape? Had a nurse threatened, "If you don't take care you'll be for treatment tomorrow?" Day after day I spent the time scanning the faces of the staff as carefully as if they were radar screens which might reveal the approach of the fate that had been prepared for me. I was cunning. "Let me mop the office," I pleaded. "Let me mop the office in the evenings, for by evening the film of germs has settled on your office furniture and report books, and if the danger is not removed you might fall prey to disease which means disquietude and fingerprints and a sewn shroud of cheap cotton."

So I mopped the office, as a precaution, and sneaked across to the sister's desk and glanced quickly at the open report book and the list of names for treatment the next morning. One time I read my name there, Istina Mavet. What had I done? I hadn't cried or spoken out of turn or refused to work the bumper with the polishing rag under it or to help set the tables for tea, or to carry out the overflowing pig-tin to the side door. There was obviously a crime which was unknown to me, which I had not included in my list because I could not track it with the swinging spotlight of my mind to the dark hinterland of unconsciousness. I knew then that I would have to be careful. I would have to wear gloves, to leave no trace when I burgled the crammed house of feeling and took for my own use exuberance depression suspicion terror.

As we watched the day nurse moving from one patient to another with the list in her hand our sick dread became more intense.

"You're for treatment. No breakfast for you. Keep on your nightgown and dressing gown and take your teeth out."

We had to be careful, calm, controlled. If our forebodings were unwarranted we experienced a dizzy lightness and relief which, if carried too far, made us liable to be given emergency treatment. If our name appeared on the fateful list we had to try with all our might, at times unsuccessfully, to subdue the rising panic. For there was no escape. Once the names were known all doors were scrupulously locked; we had to stay in the observation dormitory where the treatment was being held.

It was a time of listening—to the other patients walking along the corridor for breakfast; the silence as Sister Honey, her head bowed, her eyes watchfully open, said grace.

"For what you are about to receive the Lord make you truly thankful."

And then we heard the sudden cheerful clatter of spoons on porridge plates, the scraping of chairs, the disconcerted murmur at the end of the meal when the inevitably missing knife was being searched for while the sister warned sternly, "Let no one leave the table until the knife is found." Then further scraping and rustling following the sister's orders. "Rise, Ladies." Side doors being unlocked as the patients were ordered to their separate places of work. Laundry, Ladies. Sewing room, Ladies. Nurses' Home, Ladies. Then the pegging footsteps as the massive Matron Glass on her tiny blackshod feet approached down the corridor, unlocked the observation dormitory and stood surveying us, with a query to the nurse, like a stockman appraising head of cattle waiting in the saleyards to go by truck to the slaughterhouse. "They're all here? Make sure they have nothing to eat." We stood in small groups, waiting; or crouched in a semi-circle around the great locked fireplace where a heap of dull coal smouldered sulkily; our hands on the blackened bars of the fireguard, to warm our nipped fingers.

For in spite of the snapdragons and the dusty millers and the cherry blossoms, it was always winter. And it was always our season of peril: Electricity, the peril the wind sings to in the wires on a gray day. Time after time I thought, What safety measures must I apply to protect myself against electricity? And I listed the emergencies—lightning, riots, earthquakes, and the measures provided for the world by man's Red Cross God Safety to whom we owe allegiance or die on the separated ice floe, in double loneliness. But it would not come to my mind what to do when I was threatened by electricity, except that I thought of my father's rubber hip boots that he used for fishing and that stood in the wash house where the moth-eaten coats hung behind the door, beside the pile of old *Humor Magazines, the Finest Selections of the World's Wit,* for reading in the lavatory. Where was the wash house and the old clothes with spiders' nests and wood lice in their folds? Lost in a foreign land, take your position from the creeks flowing towards the sea, and your time from the sun.

Yes, I was cunning. I remembered once a relationship between electricity and wetness, and on the excuse of going to the lavatory I filled the admission bath and climbed in, wearing my nightgown and dressing gown, and thinking, Now they will not give me treatment, and perhaps I may have a secret influence over the sleek cream-painted machine with its knobs and meters and lights.

Do you believe in a secret influence?

There had been occasions of delirious relief when the machine broke down and the doctor emerged, frustrated, from the treatment room, and Sister Honey made the welcome proclamation, "You can all get dressed. No treatment today."

But this day when I climbed in the bath the secret influence was absence, and I was given treatment, hurried into the room as the first patient, even before the noisy people from Ward Two, the disturbed ward, were brought in for "multiples," which means they were given two treatments and sometimes three, consecutively. These excited people in their red ward dressing gowns and long gray ward stockings and bunchy striped bloomers which some took care to display to us, were called by their Christian names or nicknames, Dizzy, Goldie, Dora. Sometimes they approached us and began to confide in us or touch our sleeves, reverently, as if we were indeed what we felt ourselves to be, a race apart from them. Were we not the "sensibly" ill who did not yet substitute animal noises for speech or fling our limbs in uncontrolled motion or dissolve into secret silent hilarity? And yet when the time of treatment came and they and we were ushered or dragged into the room at the end of the dormitory all of us whether from the disturbed ward or the "good" ward uttered the same kind of stifled choking scream when the electricity was turned on and we dropped into immediate lonely unconsciousness.

It was early in my dream. The tracks of time crossed and merged and with the head-on collision of hours a fire broke out blackening the vegetation that sprouts a green memory along the side of the track. I took a thimbleful of water distilled from the sea and tried to extinguish the fire. I waved a small green flag in the face of the oncoming hours and they passed through the scarred countryside to their destination and as the faces peered from the window at me I saw they were the faces of the people awaiting shock treatment. There was

Miss Caddick, Caddie, they called her, bickering and suspicious, not knowing that she would soon die and her body be sneaked out the back way to the mortuary. And there was my own face staring from the carriageful of the nicknamed people in their ward clothes, striped smocks and gray woolen jerseys. What did it mean?

I was so afraid. When I first came to Cliffhaven and walked into the dayroom and saw the people sitting and staring, I thought, as a passerby in the street thinks when he sees someone staring into the sky, If I look up too, I will see it. And I looked but I did not see it. And the staring was not, as it is in the streets, an occasion for crowds who share the spectacle; it was an occasion of loneliness, of vision on a closed, private circuit.

And it is still winter. Why is it winter when the cherry blossom is in flower? I have been here in Cliffhaven for years now. How can I get to school by nine o'clock if I am trapped in the observation dormitory waiting for E.S.T.? It is such a long way to go to school, down Eden Street past Ribble Street and Dee Street past the doctor's house and their little girl's dollhouse standing on the lawn. I wish I had a dollhouse; I wish I could make myself small and live inside it, curled up in a matchbox with satin bed curtains and gold stars painted on the striking side, for good conduct.

There is no escape. Soon it will be time for E.S.T. Through the veranda windows I can see the nurses returning from second breakfast, and the sight of them walking in twos and threes past the border of snapdragons granny's bonnets and the cherry blossom tree brings a sick feeling of despair and finality. I feel like a child who has been forced to eat a strange food in a strange house and who must spend the night there in a strange room with a different smell in the bedclothes and different borders on the blankets, and waken in the morning to the sight of a different and terrifying landscape from the window.

The nurses enter the dormitory. They collect false teeth from the treatment patients, plunging them in water in old cracked cups and writing the names on the outside in pale blue ink from a ballpoint pen; the ink slips on the impenetrable china surface, and spreads, blurring from itself, with the edges of the letters appearing like the microfilm of flies' feet. A nurse brings two small chipped enamel bowls of methylated spirits and ethereal soap, to "rub up" our temples in order that the shock will "take."

I try to find a pair of gray woolen socks for if my feet are cold I know that I shall die. One patient is careful to put on her pants "in case I kick up my legs in front of the doctor." At the last minute, as the feel of nine o'clock surrounds us and we sit in the hard chairs, our heads tipped back, the soaked cotton wool being rubbed on our temples until the skin tears and stings and the dregs of the spirits run down into own ears making sudden blockages of sound, there is a final outbreak of screaming and panicking, attempts by some to grab leftover food from the bed patients, and as a nurse calls "Lavatory, Ladies," and the dormitory door is opened for a brief supervised visit to the doorless lavatories, with guards set in the corridor to prevent escape, there are bursts of fighting and kicking as some attempt to get past, yet realizing almost at once that there is nowhere to run to. The doors to the outside world are locked. You can only be followed and dragged back and if Matron Glass catches you she will speak angrily, "It's for your own good. Pull yourself together. You've been difficult long enough."

The matron herself does not offer to undergo shock treatment in the way that suspected persons to prove their innocence are sometimes willing to take the first slice of the cake that may contain arsenic.

Floral screens are drawn to conceal the end of the dormitory where the treatment beds have been prepared, the sheets rolled back and the pillows placed at an angle, ready to receive the unconscious patient. And now everybody wants to go again to the lavatory, and again, as the panic grows, and the nurse locks the door for the last time, and the lavatory is inaccessible. We yearn to go there, and sit on the cold china bowls and in the simplest way try to relieve ourselves of the mounting distress in our minds, as if a process of the body could change the distress and flush it away as burning drops of water.

And now there is the sound of an early morning catarrhal cough, the springing squeak of rubber-soled shoes on the polished corridor outside, syncopated with the hasty ping-pong steps of cuban-heeled duty shoes, and Dr. Howell and Matron Glass arrive, she unlocking the dormitory door and standing aside while he enters, and both passing in royal procession to join Sister Honey already waiting in the treatment room. At the last minute, because there are not enough nurses, the newly appointed Social Worker who has been asked to help with treatment comes leaping in (we call her Pavlova).

"Nurses, will you send up the first patient."

Many times I have offered to go first because I like to remind myself that by the time I am awake, so brief is the period of unconsciousness, most of the group will still be waiting in a daze of anxiety which sometimes confuses them into thinking that perhaps they have had treatment, perhaps it has been sneaked upon them without their being aware of it.

The people behind the screen begin to moan and cry.

We are taken strictly according to "volts."

We wait while the Ward Two people are "done."

We know the rumors attached to E.S.T.—it is training for Sing Sing when we are at last convicted of murder and sentenced to death and sit strapped in the electric chair with the electrodes touching our skin through slits in our clothing;

our hair is singed as we die and the last smell in our nostrils is the smell of ourselves burning. And the fear leads in some patients to more madness. And they
say it is a session to get you to talk, that your secrets are filed and kept in the
treatment room, and I have had proof of this, for I have passed through the
treatment room with a basket of dirty linen, and seen my card. Impulsive and
dangerous, it reads. Why? And how? How? What does it all mean?

It is nearly my turn. I walk down to the treatment room door to wait, for so
many treatments have to be performed that the doctor becomes impatient at
any delay. Production, as it were, is speeded up (like laundry economics—one
set of clothes on, one set clean, one in the wash) if there is a patient waiting at
the door, one on the treatment table, and another being given a final "rub-up"
ready to take her place at the door.

Suddenly the inevitable cry or scream sounds from behind the closed doors
which after a few minutes swing open and Molly or Goldie or Mrs. Gregg,
convulsed and snorting, is wheeled out. I close my eyes tight as the bed passes
me, yet I cannot escape seeing it, or the other beds where people are lying,
perhaps heavily asleep, or whimperingly awake, their faces flushed, their eyes
bloodshot. I can hear someone moaning and weeping; it is someone who has
woken up in the wrong time and place, for I know that the treatment snatches
these things from you leaves you alone and blind in a nothingness of being and
you try to fumble your way like a newborn animal to the flowing of first com-
forts; then you wake, small and frightened, and the tears keep falling in a grief
that you cannot name.

Beside me is the bed, sheets turned back pillow arranged where I will lie
after treatment. They will lift me into it and I shall not know. I look at the bed
as if I must establish contact with it. Few people have advance glimpses of their
coffin; if they did they might be tempted to charm it into preserving in the
satin lining a few trinkets of their identity. In my mind, I slip under the pillow
of my treatment bed a docket of time and place so that when and if I ever wake
I shall not be wholly confused in a panic of scrabbling through the darkness of
not knowing and of being nothing. I go into the room then. How brave I am!
Everybody remarks on my bravery! I climb on to the treatment table. I try to
breathe deeply and evenly as I have heard it is wise in moments of fear. I try not
to mind when the matron whispers to one of the nurses, in a hoarse voice like
an assassin, "Have you got the gag?"

And over and over inside myself I am saying a poem which I learned at
school when I was eight. I say the poem, as I wear the gray woolen socks, to ward
off Death. They are not relevant lines because very often the law of extremity
demands an attention to irrelevancies; the dying man wonders what they will
think when they cut his toenails; the man in grief counts the cups in a flower. I

see the face of Miss Swap who taught us the poem. I see the mole on the side of her nose, its two mounds like a miniature cottage loaf and the sprout of ginger hair growing out the top. I see myself standing in the classroom reciting and feeling the worn varnished desk top jutting against my body against my belly-button that has specks of grit in it when I put my finger in; I see from the corner of my left eye my neighbor's pencil case which I coveted because it was a triple decker with a rose design on the lid and a wonderful dent thumb-size for sliding the lid along the groove.

"Moonlit Apples," I say. "By John Drinkwater."

> At the top of the house the apples are laid in rows
> And the skylight lets the moonlight in and those
> Apples are deep-sea apples of green.

I get no further than three lines. The doctor busily attending the knobs and switches of the machine which he respects because it is his ally in the struggle against overwork and the difficulties depressions obsessions manias of a thousand women, has time to smile a harassed Good Morning before he gives the signal to Matron Glass.

"Close your eyes," Matron says.

But I keep them open, observing the secretive signal and engulfed with helplessness while the matron and four nurses and Pavlova press upon my shoulders and my knees and I feel myself dropping as if a trap door had opened into darkness. I imagine as I fall my eyes turning inward to face and confound each other with a separate truth which they prove without my help. Then I rise disembodied from the dark to grasp and attach myself like a homeless parasite to the shape of my identity and its position in space and time. At first I cannot find my way, I cannot find myself where I left myself, someone has removed all trace of me. I am crying.

A cup of sweet tea is being poured down my throat. I grasp the nurse's arm.

"Have I had it? Have I had it?"

"You have had treatment," she answers. "Now go to sleep. You are awake too early."

But I am wide awake and the anxiety begins again to accumulate.

Will I be for treatment tomorrow?

V

The approach of night provided a signal for the release of even more screaming and shouting than had been heard during the day in the park or the yard.

No sedatives were given, and from the time the people from the dirty dayroom went to bed at four o'clock, the Brick Building was a riot of noise. And always, among the others, one could distinguish Brenda's pedantic protesting voice.

I remembered Brenda from Ward four. I remembered her as one of the first to have the "new" operation to change the personality, and how, with much talk of retraining her to adjust to what were called the ways of the world, Pavlova used to take her and the three or four other lobotomy cases, for special walks in the gardens, naming the flowers and the clouds and the incidental people and interesting her patients once more in the affairs of the world, assuming, for something must be assumed to start with, even after a lobotomy, that the affairs of the world were worthy of interest. Brenda, I learned, had been a talented girl, a pianist who was shortly to have taken a scholarship overseas. And now, five years later, she was in Ward Two, having had another operation—performed it seemed in a desperate attempt to remedy the too-soon evident and frightful effects of the first. She remembered me. I tried not to weep when I saw her condition.

When she walked she moved her hands, trying to make elaborate sculptures of the intractable air, taking careful chicken steps and at times supporting herself by sliding her hand along the wall. Forced to move from one side of a room to the other she panicked and clung to the wall until she was propelled by the scruff of her neck. Sometimes suddenly alone in the center of the room, she would overbalance and then laugh delightedly yet nervously, saying in rush of breath, Oh dear, oh dear; and then she would turn to her brother who always followed her and whom she addressed formally as Mr. Frederick Barnes. She would curse him and add, "Get out of here, Mr. Frederick Barnes."

She called me Miss Istina Mavet. She would heave a great sigh, "Oh I envy you Miss Istina Mavet!" Then she would put her hand up the leg of her striped pants and drawing forth, after a little manipulation, a lump of feces would exclaim, "Look Miss Istina Mavet. Just look. I'm terrible aren't I? I blame Mr. Frederick Barnes for this." Her voice would deepen then and become tremendous and, her face would flush purple. She would scream. Since her first operation she suffered from convulsions; often we saw her fall in a fit.

Although Brenda was more often confined in the dirty dayroom, as a special treat Sister Bridge would let her come to the clean dayroom to play the piano. She would sneak in, moving her hand along the wall, and approach the piano and, after lifting the lid of the stool the correct number of times in accord with her secret personal rhythm, she would sit down, shrugging her shoulders with pleasure, and begin to giggle in a deprecating way, blushing and staring at the piano as if it had begun to pay her compliments. It shone ebony; she could see her face in it, even the shadowy hint of her dark mustache. She would continue to giggle, clasping and unclasping her hands and adopting now postures of delight as if the piano were communicating good news to her; and then, in a flash, she would remember Mr. Frederick Barnes.

"Get out of here, Mr. Frederick Barnes," she would rage, dropping her hands quickly to her lap as if she had been putting them to immodest use without knowing that she had been observed. "Get out, Mr. Frederick Barnes."

And turning to the patients who were now interested and waiting for her to play, for we liked her playing, she would excuse herself. "It's Mr. Frederick Barnes. I hate him. I hate him. Ho Ho, Mr. Frederick Barnes. And I, of course, am Miss Brenda Barnes of Cliffhaven Mental Hospital."

Then she would smile wistfully and break into a giggle and begin to play, gently and carefully, a few bars of what the patients called "classical."

Carol would interrupt. "That's classical. Play *Moonlight Sonata*."

Carol, a dwarf, and Big Betty, over six feet tall, were in self-appointed command of the clean dayroom.

So Brenda tempered the music to the demands of pale freckle-faced Carol who, in talking of her own origins used to say, "I'm jitimate. My mother had me before she married. She didn't want me to grow."

"Play Butterfly Grieg Brenda. Play *I'm Always Chasing Rainbows*."

(*I'm Always Chasing Rainbows* was a Chopin melody made popular when Cornel Wilde as Chopin, in the film *A Song to Remember*, found time between gazing tenderly into Mlle. Dupin's eyes, to flick his fingers over the piano keys and be ghosted into playing brief catchy versions of his own alleged compositions.)

At first Brenda played lovingly, remembering every note, although her sense of time seemed to have suffered. She played on and on after a while ignoring Carol's pleas "not to play classical." Listening to her, one experienced a deep uneasiness as of having avoided an urgent responsibility, like someone who, walking at night along the banks of a stream, catches a glimpse in the water of a white face or a moving limb and turns quickly away, refusing to help or to search for help. We all see the faces in the water. We smother our memory of them, even our belief in their reality, and become calm people of the world; or we can neither forget or help them. Sometimes by a trick of circumstances or dream or a hostile neighborhood of light we see our own face.

In the midst of her playing Brenda would suddenly stop, clearly struck by the irrevocability of her situation, and begin to rage and scream and thump violently and abusively, upon the keys, banishing the music which retreated like an animal that, awakened from hibernation by the warmth and light of a false spring, is forsaken by the sun and faced with the continuing desolation of winter.

A restlessness would invade the dayroom. One or two patients would wander up to the piano and tinker with the treble notes or plong the bass and shout to Brenda to go to hell.

Carol would take command again. "We've had enough of you, Brenda. We want the radio on anyway. Let Minnie Cleave play something."

In disgrace Brenda would be led back to the dirty dayroom while Sister Bridge could be heard threatening, "Never again, Brenda. It always ends up like this with your shouting and rampaging."

So we sat around in the clean dayroom, frustrated and uneasy. The spectacle of Brenda at the piano gave the feeling that one had witnessed the kind of earth tremor that in two instants uncovers and reburies the lost kingdom.

But, "Minnie Cleave play for us," Carol would be shouting, and Minnie would look up from her handkerchief which she studied like a plan all day. "No no," she quavered, at the same time deciding that she would enjoy playing, and then her small bowed figure, bag in hand, would creep up to the piano, and Minnie, a former Mother Superior in a convent, would tinkle monotonously over and over until she was forced to stop,

> *The Campbells are coming, hurrah, hurrah,*
> *The Campbells are coming, hurrah.*

VII

There is an aspect of madness which is seldom mentioned in fiction because it would damage the romantic popular idea of the insane as a person whose speech appeals as immediately poetic; but it is seldom the easy Opheliana recited like the pages of a seed catalog or the outpourings of Crazy Janes who provide, in fiction, an outlet for poetic abandon. Few of the people who roamed the dayroom would have qualified as acceptable heroines, in popular taste; few were charmingly uninhibited eccentrics. The mass provoked mostly irritation hostility and impatience. Their behavior affronted, caused uneasiness; they wept and moaned; they quarreled and complained. They were a nuisance and were treated as such. It was forgotten that they too possessed a prized humanity which needed care and love, that a tiny poetic essence could be distilled from their overflowing squalid truth.

Springtime came, as far as spring happens in northern New Zealand where summer is impatient to striptease the sky and reveal brilliant days with the veils of warmth shimmering, like memory mists on the films; where winter too is importunate and will not tolerate the preceding slow melancholy of changing colors and autumn dews that are part of the southern year. The quick spring brought swelling tides of softness and warmth in the dry cold air and the smell of blossoms, the heavy honey-smell of the bush flowers, the fiery blossom of the rata tree and the fuchsia with its purple flowers like intimate folds of bruised flesh. The tuis and bell-birds returned from the deep bush and sang side by side with the migrant English thrush and blackbird; and wax-eyes, drunk with honey, teetered around by the yard fence and the fuchsia tree beyond it. Down in the yard we sniffed the air and stamped in the old puddles and watched the wet corners and the shaded places becoming dry again; and we looked over at the slate-cold sea with its scratches and patterns of depth.

The sun shone. The flies arrived, fat, and expecting to grow fatter. We had our typhoid injections. We sat on an old chair in the middle of the yard while our hair had its weekly combing with kerosene, to keep the lice at bay.

Bickerings and fist fights increased, and more people were put in seclusion; and people danced with good reason which is without reason; and the quiet people gave no sign except a twitching of their lips over their toothless gums, and their eyes stared dully from their wrinkled leaf-brown faces—the brown color that most of us had and that I had thought to be sunburn and windburn but that I realized was a stain of something else, a color of stagnancy spreading from inside and rising to the surface of the skin.

I had been allowed to keep my pink cretonne bag. I took it with me wherever I went, and it was soiled now with crumbs of old cake stuck under the cardboard base and stickings of honey on the inside. I had a copy of Shakespeare its pages thin like tissue paper and the print packed small and black and seeming wet like perpetually new footprints on the beach preserved against the obsessive shiftings of the tide. I seldom read my book yet it became more and more dilapidated physically, with pictures falling out and pages unleaving as if an unknown person were devoting time to studying it. This evidence of secret reading gave me a feeling of gratitude. It seemed as if the book understood how things were and agreed to be company for me and to breathe, even without my opening it, an overwhelming dignity of riches; but because, after all, the first passion of books is to be read, it had decided to read itself; which explained the gradual falling out of the pages. Yet at night, in the shuttered and locked room where I now slept and there was no light to read by, I would remember and say to myself, thinking of the people of Lawn Lodge, and the desperate season of their lives,

> Poor naked wretches wheresoe'er you are
> That bide the pelting of this pitiless storm,
> How shall your houseless heads and unfed sides,
> Your looped and windowed raggedness defend you
> From seasons such as these.

And I thought of the confusion of people, like Gloucester, being led near the cliffs,

> *Methinks the ground is even.*
> *Horrible steep. . . .*
> *Hark, do you hear the sea?*

And over and over in my mind I saw King Lear wandering on the moor and I remembered the old men at Cliffhaven sitting outside their dreary ward, and nobody at home, not in themselves or anywhere.

The Yellow Wallpaper

CHARLOTTE PERKINS GILMAN

IT IS VERY seldom that mere ordinary people like John and myself secure ancestral halls for the summer.

A colonial mansion, a hereditary estate, I would say a haunted house, and reach the height of romantic felicity—but that would be asking too much of fate!

Still I will proudly declare that there is something queer about it.

Else, why should it be let so cheaply? And why have stood so long untenanted?

John laughs at me, of course, but one expects that in marriage.

John is practical in the extreme. He has no patience with faith, an intense horror of superstition, and he scoffs openly at any talk of things not to be felt and seen and put down in figures.

John is a physician, and *perhaps*—(I would not say it to a living soul, of course, but this is dead paper and a great relief to my mind)—*perhaps* that is one reason I do not get well faster.

You see he does not believe I am sick!

And what can one do?

If a physician of high standing, and one's own husband, assures friends and relatives that there is really nothing the matter with one but temporary nervous depression—a slight hysterical tendency—what is one to do?

My brother is also a physician, and also of high standing, and he says the same thing.

So I take phosphates or phosphites—whichever it is, and tonics, and journeys, and air, and exercise, and am absolutely forbidden to "work" until I am well again.

Personally, I disagree with their ideas.

Personally, I believe that congenial work, with excitement and change, would do me good.

But what is one to do?

I did write for a while in spite of them; but it *does* exhaust me a good deal—having to be so sly about it, or else meet with heavy opposition.

I sometimes fancy that in my condition if I had less opposition and more society and stimulus—but John says the very worst thing I can do is to think about my condition, and I confess it always makes me feel bad.

So I will let it alone and talk about the house.

The most beautiful place! It is quite alone, standing well back from the road, quite three miles from the village. It makes me think of English places that you read about, for there are hedges and walls and gates that lock, and lots of separate little houses for the gardeners and people.

There is a *delicious* garden! I never saw such a garden—large and shady, full of box-bordered paths, and lined with long grape-covered arbors with seats under them.

There were greenhouses, too, but they are all broken now.

There was some legal trouble, I believe, something about the heirs and co-heirs; anyhow, the place has been empty for years.

That spoils my ghostliness, I am afraid, but I don't care—there is something strange about the house—I can feel it.

I even said so to John one moonlight evening, but he said what I felt was a *draught,* and shut the window.

I get unreasonably angry with John sometimes. I'm sure I never used to be so sensitive. I think it is due to this nervous condition.

But John says if I feel so, I shall neglect proper self-control; so I take pains to control myself—before him, at least, and that makes me very tired.

I don't like our room a bit. I wanted one downstairs that opened on the piazza and had roses all over the window, and such pretty old-fashioned chintz hangings! but John would not hear of it.

He said there was only one window and not room for two beds, and no near room for him if he took another.

He is very careful and loving, and hardly lets me stir without special direction.

I have a scheduled prescription for each hour in the day; he takes all care from me, and so I feel basely ungrateful not to value it more.

He said we came here solely on my account, that I was to have perfect rest and all the air I could get. "Your exercise depends on your strength, my dear," said he, "and your food somewhat on your appetite; but air you can absorb all the time." So we took the nursery at the top of the house.

It is a big, airy room, the whole floor nearly, with windows that look all ways, and air and sunshine galore. It was nursery first and then playroom and gymnasium, I should judge; for the windows are barred for little children, and there are rings and things in the wall.

The paint and paper look as if a boys' school had used it. It is stripped off—the paper—in great patches all around the head of my bed, about as far as I can reach, and in a great place on the other side of the room low down. I never saw a worse paper in my life.

One of those sprawling flamboyant patterns committing every artistic sin.

It is dull enough to confuse the eye in following, pronounced enough to constantly irritate and provoke study, and when you follow the lame uncertain curves for a little distance they suddenly commit suicide—plunge off at outrageous angles, destroy themselves in unheard of contradictions.

The color is repellent, almost revolting; a smouldering unclean yellow, strangely faded by the slow-turning sunlight.

It is a dull yet lurid orange in some places, a sickly sulphur tint in others.

No wonder the children hated it! I should hate it myself if I had to live in this room long.

There comes John, and I must put this away,—he hates to have me write a word.

We have been here two weeks, and I haven't felt like writing before, since that first day.

I am sitting by the window now, up in this atrocious nursery, and there is nothing to hinder my writing as much as I please, save lack of strength.

John is away all day, and even some nights when his cases are serious.

I am glad my case is not serious!

But these nervous troubles are dreadfully depressing.

John does not know how much I really suffer. He knows there is no *reason* to suffer, and that satisfies him.

Of course it is only nervousness. It does weigh on me so not to do my duty in any way!

I meant to be such a help to John, such a real rest and comfort, and here I am a comparative burden already!

Nobody would believe what an effort it is to do what little I am able,—to dress and entertain, and order things.

It is fortunate Mary is so good with the baby. Such a dear baby!

And yet I *cannot* be with him, it makes me so nervous.

I suppose John never was nervous in his life. He laughs at me so about this wall-paper!

At first he meant to repaper the room, but afterwards he said that I was letting it get the better of me, and that nothing was worse for a nervous patient than to give way to such fancies.

He said that after the wall-paper was changed it would be the heavy bed-stead, and then the barred windows, and then that gate at the head of the stairs, and so on.

"You know the place is doing you good," he said, "and really, dear, I don't care to renovate the house just for a three months' rental."

"Then do let us go downstairs," I said, "there are such pretty rooms there."

Then he took me in his arms and called me a blessed little goose, and said he would go down to the cellar, if I wished, and have it whitewashed into the bargain.

But he is right enough about the beds and windows and things.

It is an airy and comfortable room as any one need wish, and, of course, I would not be so silly as to make him uncomfortable just for a whim.

I'm really getting quite fond of the big room, all but that horrid paper.

Out of one window I can see the garden, those mysterious deep-shaded arbors, the riotous old-fashioned flowers, and bushes and gnarly trees.

Out of another I get a lovely view of the bay and a little private wharf belonging to the estate. There is a beautiful shaded lane that runs down there from the house. I always fancy I see people walking in these numerous paths and arbors, but John has cautioned me not to give way to fancy in the least. He says that with my imaginative power and habit of story-making, a nervous weakness like mine is sure to lead to all manner of excited fancies, and that I ought to use my will and good sense to check the tendency. So I try.

I think sometimes that if I were only well enough to write a little it would relieve the press of ideas and rest me.

But I find I get pretty tired when I try.

It is so discouraging not to have any advice and companionship about my work. When I get really well, John says we will ask Cousin Henry and Julia down for a long visit; but he says he would as soon put fireworks in my pillow-case as to let me have those stimulating people about now.

I wish I could get well faster.

But I must not think about that. This paper looks to me as if it *knew* what a vicious influence it had!

There is a recurrent spot where the pattern lolls like a broken neck and two bulbous eyes stare at you upside down.

I get positively angry with the impertinence of it and the everlastingness. Up and down and sideways they crawl, and those absurd, unblinking eyes are everywhere. There is one place where two breadths didn't match, and the eyes go all up and down the line, one a little higher than the other.

I never saw so much expression in an inanimate thing before, and we all know how much expression they have! I used to lie awake as a child and get more entertainment and terror out of blank walls and plain furniture than most children could find in a toy-store.

I remember what a kindly wink the knobs of our big, old bureau used to have, and there was one chair that always seemed like a strong friend.

I used to feel that if any of the other things looked too fierce I could always hop into that chair and be safe.

The furniture in this room is no worse than inharmonious, however, for we had to bring it all from downstairs. I suppose when this was used as a play-room they had to take the nursery things out, and no wonder! I never saw such ravages as the children have made here.

The wall-paper, as I said before, is torn off in spots, and it sticketh closer than a brother—they must have had perseverance as well as hatred.

Then the floor is scratched and gouged and splintered, the plaster itself is dug out here and there, and this great heavy bed which is all we found in the room, looks as if it had been through the wars.

But I don't mind it a bit—only the paper.

There comes John's sister. Such a dear girl as she is, and so careful of me! I must not let her find me writing.

She is a perfect and enthusiastic housekeeper, and hopes for no better pro-fession. I verily believe she thinks it is the writing which made me sick!

But I can write when she is out, and see her a long way off from these windows.

There is one that commands the road, a lovely shaded winding road, and one that just looks off over the country. A lovely country, too, full of great elms and velvet meadows.

This wall-paper has a kind of sub-pattern in a different shade, a particularly irritating one, for you can only see it in certain lights, and not clearly then.

But in the places where it isn't faded and where the sun is just so—I can see a strange, provoking, formless sort of figure, that seems to skulk about behind that silly and conspicuous front design.

There's sister on the stairs!

Well, the Fourth of July is over! The people are all gone and I am tired out. John thought it might do me good to see a little company, so we just had mother and Nellie and the children down for a week.

Of course I didn't do a thing. Jennie sees to everything now.

But it tired me all the same.

John says if I don't pick up faster he shall send me to Weir Mitchell in the fall.

But I don't want to go there at all. I had a friend who was in his hands once, and she says he is just like John and my brother, only more so!

Besides, it is such an undertaking to go so far.

I don't feel as if it was worth while to turn my hand over for anything, and I'm getting dreadfully fretful and querulous.

I cry at nothing, and cry most of the time.

Of course I don't when John is here, or anybody else, but when I am alone.

And I am alone a good deal just now. John is kept in town very often by serious cases, and Jennie is good and lets me alone when I want her to.

So I walk a little in the garden or down that lovely lane, sit on the porch under the roses, and lie down up here a good deal.

I'm getting really fond of the room in spite of the wall-paper. Perhaps *because* of the wall-paper.

It dwells in my mind so!

I lie here on this great immovable bed—it is nailed down, I believe—and follow that pattern about by the hour. It is as good as gymnastics, I assure you. I start, we'll say, at the bottom, down in the corner over there where it has not been touched, and I determine for the thousandth time that I *will* follow that pointless pattern to some sort of a conclusion.

I know a little of the principle of design, and I know this thing was not arranged on any laws of radiation, or alternation, or repetition, or symmetry, or anything else that I ever heard of.

It is repeated, of course, by the breadths, but not otherwise.

Looked at in one way each breadth stands alone, the bloated curves and flourishes—a kind of "debased Romanesque" with *delirium tremens*—go waddling up and down in isolated columns of fatuity.

But, on the other hand, they connect diagonally, and the sprawling outlines run off in great slanting waves of optic horror, like a lot of wallowing seaweeds in full chase.

The whole thing goes horizontally, too, at least it seems so, and I exhaust myself in trying to distinguish the order of its going in that direction.

They have used a horizontal breadth for a frieze, and that adds wonderfully to the confusion.

There is one end of the room where it is almost intact, and there, when the crosslights fade and the low sun shines directly upon it, I can almost fancy radiation after all,—the interminable grotesques seem to form around a common centre and rush off in headlong plunges of equal distraction.

It makes me tired to follow it. I will take a nap I guess.

I don't know why I should write this.

I don't want to.

I don't feel able.

And I know John would think it absurd. But I *must* say what I feel and think in some way—it is such a relief!

But the effort is getting to be greater than the relief.

Half the time now I am awfully lazy, and lie down ever so much.

John says I mustn't lose my strength, and has me take cod liver oil and lots of tonics and things, to say nothing of ale and wine and rare meat.

Dear John! He loves me very dearly, and hates to have me sick. I tried to have a real earnest reasonable talk with him the other day, and tell him how I wish he would let me go and make a visit to Cousin Henry and Julia.

But he said I wasn't able to go, nor able to stand it after I got there; and I did not make out a very good case for myself, for I was crying before I had finished.

It is getting to be a great effort for me to think straight. Just this nervous weakness I suppose.

And dear John gathered me up in his arms, and just carried me upstairs and laid me on the bed, and sat by me and read to me till it tired my head.

He said I was his darling and his comfort and all he had, and that I must take care of myself for his sake, and keep well.

He says no one but myself can help me out of it, that I must use my will and self-control and not let any silly fancies run away with me.

There's one comfort, the baby is well and happy, and does not have to occupy this nursery with the horrid wall-paper.

If we had not used it, that blessed child would have! What a fortunate escape! Why, I wouldn't have a child of mine, an impressionable little thing, live in such a room for worlds.

I never thought of it before, but it is lucky that John kept me here after all, I can stand it so much easier than a baby, you see.

Of course I never mention it to them any more—I am too wise,—but I keep watch of it all the same.

There are things in that paper that nobody knows but me, or ever will.

Behind that outside pattern the dim shapes get clearer every day.

It is always the same shape, only very numerous.

And it is like a woman stooping down and creeping about behind that pattern. I don't like it a bit. I wonder—I begin to think—I wish John would take me away from here!

It is so hard to talk with John about my case, because he is so wise, and because he loves me so.

But I tried it last night.

It was moonlight. The moon shines in all around just as the sun does.

I hate to see it sometimes, it creeps so slowly, and always comes in by one window or another.

John was asleep and I hated to waken him, so I kept still and watched the moonlight on that undulating wall-paper till I felt creepy.

The faint figure behind seemed to shake the pattern, just as if she wanted to get out.

I got up softly and went to feel and see if the paper *did* move, and when I came back John was awake.

"What is it, little girl?" he said. "Don't go walking about like that—you'll get cold."

I thought it was a good time to talk, so I told him that I really was not gaining here, and that I wished he would take me away.

"Why darling!" said he, "our lease will be up in three weeks, and I can't see how to leave before."

"The repairs are not done at home, and I cannot possibly leave town just now. Of course if you were in any danger, I could and would, but you really are better, dear, whether you can see it or not. I am a doctor, dear, and I know. You are gaining flesh and color, your appetite is better, I feel really much easier about you."

"I don't weigh a bit more," said I, "nor as much; and my appetite may be better in the evening when you are here, but it is worse in the morning when you are away!"

"Bless her little heart!" said he with a big hug, "she shall be as sick as she pleases! But now let's improve the shining hours by going to sleep, and talk about it in the morning!"

"And you won't go away?" I asked gloomily.

"Why, how can I, dear? It is only three weeks more and then we will take a nice little trip of a few days while Jennie is getting the house ready. Really dear you are better!"

"Better in body perhaps—" I began, and stopped short, for he sat up straight and looked at me with such a stern, reproachful look that I could not say another word.

"My darling," said he, "I beg of you, for my sake and for our child's sake, as well as for your own, that you will never for one instant let that idea enter your mind! There is nothing so dangerous, so fascinating, to a temperament like yours. It is a false and foolish fancy. Can you not trust me as a physician when I tell you so?"

So of course I said no more on that score, and we went to sleep before long. He thought I was asleep first, but I wasn't, and lay there for hours trying to decide whether that front pattern and the back pattern really did move together or separately.

On a pattern like this, by daylight, there is a lack of sequence, a defiance of law, that is a constant irritant to a normal mind.

The color is hideous enough, and unreliable enough, and infuriating enough, but the pattern is torturing.

You think you have mastered it, but just as you get well underway in following, it turns a back-somersault and there you are. It slaps you in the face, knocks you down, and tramples upon you. It is like a bad dream.

The outside pattern is a florid arabesque, reminding one of a fungus. If you can imagine a toadstool in joints, an interminable string of toadstools, budding and sprouting in endless convolutions—why, that is something like it.

That is, sometimes!

There is one marked peculiarity about this paper, a thing nobody seems to notice but myself, and that is that it changes as the light changes.

When the sun shoots in through the east window—I always watch for that first long, straight ray—it changes so quickly that I never can quite believe it.

That is why I watch it always.

By moonlight—the moon shines in all night when there is a moon—I wouldn't know it was the same paper.

At night in any kind of light, in twilight, candle light, lamplight, and worst of all by moonlight, it becomes bars! The outside pattern I mean, and the woman behind it is as plain as can be.

I didn't realize for a long time what the thing was that showed behind, that dim sub-pattern, but now I am quite sure it is a woman.

By daylight she is subdued, quiet. I fancy it is the pattern that keeps her so still. It is so puzzling. It keeps me quiet by the hour.

I lie down ever so much now. John says it is good for me, and to sleep all I can.

Indeed he started the habit by making me lie down for an hour after each meal.

It is a very bad habit I am convinced, for you see I don't sleep.

And that cultivates deceit, for I don't tell them I'm awake—O no!

The fact is I am getting a little afraid of John.

He seems very queer sometimes, and even Jennie has an inexplicable look.

It strikes me occasionally, just as a scientific hypothesis,—that perhaps it is the paper!

I have watched John when he did not know I was looking, and come into the room suddenly on the most innocent excuses, and I've caught him several times *looking at the paper!* And Jennie too. I caught Jennie with her hand on it once.

She didn't know I was in the room, and when I asked her in a quiet, a very quiet voice, with the most restrained manner possible, what she was doing with the paper—she turned around as if she had been caught stealing, and looked quite angry—asked me why I should frighten her so!

Then she said that the paper stained everything it touched, that she had found yellow smooches on all my clothes and John's, and she wished we would be more careful!

Did not that sound innocent? But I know she was studying that pattern, and I am determined that nobody shall find it out but myself!

Life is very much more exciting now than it used to be. You see I have something more to expect, to look forward to, to watch. I really do eat better, and am more quiet than I was.

John is so pleased to see me improve! He laughed a little the other day, and said I seemed to be flourishing in spite of my wall-paper.

I turned it off with a laugh. I had no intention of telling him it was *because* of the wall-paper—he would make fun of me. He might even want to take me away.

I don't want to leave now until I have found it out. There is a week more, and I think that will be enough.

I'm feeling ever so much better! I don't sleep much at night, for it is so interesting to watch developments; but I sleep a good deal in the daytime.

In the daytime it is tiresome and perplexing.

There are always new shoots on the fungus, and new shades of yellow all over it. I cannot keep count of them, though I have tried conscientiously.

It is the strangest yellow, that wall-paper! It makes me think of all the yellow things I ever saw—not beautiful ones like buttercups, but old foul, bad yellow things.

But there is something else about that paper—the smell! I noticed it the moment we came into the room, but with so much air and sun it was not bad. Now we have had a week of fog and rain, and whether the windows are open or not, the smell is here.

It creeps all over the house.

I find it hovering in the dining-room, skulking in the parlor, hiding in the hall, lying in wait for me on the stairs.

It gets into my hair.

Even when I go to ride, if I turn my head suddenly and surprise it—there is that smell!

Such a peculiar odor, too! I have spent hours in trying to analyze it, to find what it smelled like.

It is not bad—at first, and very gentle, but quite the subtlest, most enduring odor I ever met.

In this damp weather it is awful, I wake up in the night and find it hanging over me.

It used to disturb me at first. I thought seriously of burning the house—to reach the smell.

But now I am used to it. The only thing I can think of that it is like is the *color* of the paper! A yellow smell.

There is a very funny mark on this wall, low down, near the mopboard. A streak that runs round the room. It goes behind every piece of furniture, except the bed, a long, straight, even *smooch*, as if it had been rubbed over and over.

I wonder how it was done and who did it, and what they did it for. Round and round and round—round and round and round—it makes me dizzy!

I really have discovered something at last.

Through watching so much at night, when it changes so, I have finally found out.

The front pattern *does* move—and no wonder! The woman behind shakes it!

Sometimes I think there are a great many women behind, and sometimes only one, and she crawls around fast, and her crawling shakes it all over.

Then in the very bright spots she keeps still, and in the very shady spots she just takes hold of the bars and shakes them hard.

And she is all the time trying to climb through. But nobody could climb through that pattern—it strangles so; I think that is why it has so many heads.

They get through, and then the pattern strangles them off and turns them upside down, and makes their eyes white!

If those heads were covered or taken off it would not be half so bad.

I think that woman gets out in the daytime!

And I'll tell you why—privately—I've seen her!

I can see her out of every one of my windows!

It is the same woman, I know, for she is always creeping, and most women do not creep by daylight.

I see her on that long road under the trees, creeping along, and when a carriage comes she hides under the blackberry vines.

I don't blame her a bit. It must be very humiliating to be caught creeping by daylight!

I always lock the door when I creep by daylight. I can't do it at night, for I know John would suspect something at once.

And John is so queer now, that I don't want to irritate him. I wish he would take another room! Besides, I don't want anybody to get that woman out at night but myself.

I often wonder if I could see her out of all the windows at once.

But, turn as fast as I can, I can only see out of one at one time.

And though I always see her, she *may* be able to creep faster than I can turn!

I have watched her sometimes away off in the open country, creeping as fast as a cloud shadow in a high wind.

If only that top pattern could be gotten off from the under one! I mean to try it, little by little.

I have found out another funny thing, but I shan't tell it this time! It does not do to trust people too much.

There are only two more days to get this paper off, and I believe John is beginning to notice. I don't like the look in his eyes.

And I heard him ask Jennie a lot of professional questions about me. She had a very good report to give.

She said I slept a good deal in the daytime.

John knows I don't sleep very well at night, for all I'm so quiet!

He asked me all sorts of questions, too, and pretended to be very loving and kind.

As if I couldn't see through him!

Still, I don't wonder he acts so, sleeping under this paper for three months.

It only interests me, but I feel sure John and Jennie are secretly affected by it.

Hurrah! This is the last day, but it is enough. John to stay in town over night, and won't be out until this evening.

Jennie wanted to sleep with me—the sly thing! but I told her I should undoubtedly rest better for a night all alone.

That was clever, for really I wasn't alone a bit! As soon as it was moonlight and that poor thing began to crawl and shake the pattern, I got up and ran to help her.

I pulled and she shook, I shook and she pulled, and before morning we had peeled off yards of that paper.

A strip about as high as my head and half around the room.

And then when the sun came and that awful pattern began to laugh at me, I declared I would finish it to-day!

We go away to-morrow, and they are moving all my furniture down again to leave things as they were before.

Jennie looked at the wall in amazement, but I told her merrily that I did it out of pure spite at the vicious thing.

She laughed and said she wouldn't mind doing it herself, but I must not get tired.

How she betrayed herself that time!

But I am here, and no person touches this paper but me,—not *alive!*

She tried to get me out of the room—it was too patent! But I said it was so quiet and empty and clean now that I believed I would lie down again and sleep all I could; and not to wake me even for dinner—I would call when I woke.

So now she is gone, and the servants are gone, and the things are gone, and there is nothing left but that great bedstead nailed down, with the canvas mattress we found on it.

We shall sleep downstairs to-night, and take the boat home tomorrow.

I quite enjoy the room, now it is bare again.

How those children did tear about here!

This bedstead is fairly gnawed!

But I must get to work.

I have locked the door and thrown the key down into the front path.

I don't want to go out, and I don't want to have anybody come in, till John comes.

I want to astonish him.

I've got a rope up here that even Jennie did not find. If that woman does get out, and tries to get away, I can tie her!

But I forgot I could not reach far without anything to stand on!

This bed will *not* move!

I tried to lift and push it until I was lame, and then I got so angry I bit off a little piece at one corner—but it hurt my teeth.

Then I peeled off all the paper I could reach standing on the floor. It sticks horribly and the pattern just enjoys it! All those strangled heads and bulbous eyes and waddling fungus growths just shriek with derision!

I am getting angry enough to do something desperate. To jump out of the window would be admirable exercise, but the bars are too strong even to try.

Besides I wouldn't do it. Of course not. I know well enough that a step like that is improper and might be misconstrued.

I don't like to *look* out of the windows even—there are so many of those creeping women, and they creep so fast.

I wonder if they all come out of that wall-paper as I did?

But I am securely fastened now by my well-hidden rope—you don't get *me* out in the road there!

I suppose I shall have to get back behind the pattern when it comes night, and that is hard!

It is so pleasant to be out in this great room and creep around as I please!

I don't want to go outside. I won't, even if Jennie asks me to.

For outside you have to creep on the ground, and everything is green instead of yellow.

But here I can creep smoothly on the floor, and my shoulder just fits in that long smooch around the wall, so I cannot lose my way.

Why there's John at the door!

It is no use, young man, you can't open it!

How he does call and pound!

Now he's crying for an axe.

It would be a shame to break down that beautiful door!

"John dear!" said I in the gentlest voice, "the key is down by the front steps, under a plantain leaf!"

That silenced him for a few moments.

Then he said—very quietly indeed, "Open the door, my darling!"

"I can't," said I. "The key is down by the front door under a plantain leaf!"

And then I said it again, several times, very gently and slowly, and said it so often that he had to go and see, and he got it of course, and came in. He stopped short by the door.

"What is the matter?" he cried. "For God's sake, what are you doing!"

I kept on creeping just the same, but I looked at him over my shoulder.

"I've got out at last," said I, "in spite of you and Jennie. And I've pulled off most of the paper, so you can't put me back!"

Now why should that man have fainted? But he did, and right across my path by the wall, so that I had to creep over him every time!

The Woman Hanging
from the Thirteenth Floor Window

JOY HARJO

She is the woman hanging from the 13th floor
window. Her hands are pressed white against the
concrete moulding of the tenement building. She
hangs from the 13th floor window in east Chicago,
with a swirl of birds over her head. They could
be a halo, or a storm of glass waiting to crush her.

She thinks she will be set free.

The woman hanging from the 13th floor window
on the east side of Chicago is not alone.

She is a woman of children, of the baby, Carlos,
and of Margaret, and of Jimmy who is the oldest.
She is her mother's daughter and her father's son.
She is several pieces between the two husbands
she has had. She is all the women of the apartment
building who stand watching her, watching themselves.

When she was young she ate wild rice on scraped down
plates in warm wood rooms. It was in the farther
north and she was the baby then. They rocked her.

She sees Lake Michigan lapping at the shores of
herself. It is a dizzy hole of water and the rich
live in tall glass houses at the edge of it. In some
places Lake Michigan speaks softly, here, it just sputters
and butts itself against the asphalt. She sees
other buildings just like hers. She sees other

women hanging from many-floored windows
counting their lives in the palms of their hands
and in the palms of their children's hands.

She is the woman hanging from the 13th floor window
on the Indian side of town. Her belly is soft from
her children's births, her worn levis swing down below
her waist, and then her feet, and then her heart.
She is dangling.

The woman hanging from the 13th floor hears voices.
They come to her in the night when the lights have gone
dim. Sometimes they are little cats mewing and scratching
at the door, sometimes they are her grandmother's voice,
and sometimes they are gigantic men of light whispering
to her to get up, to get up, to get up. That's when she wants
to have another child to hold onto in the night, to be able
to fall back into dreams.

And the woman hanging from the 13th floor window
hears other voices. Some of them scream out from below
for her to jump, they would push her over. Others cry softly
from the sidewalks, pull their children up like flowers and gather
them into their arms. They would help her, like themselves.

But she is the woman hanging from the 13th floor window,
and she knows she is hanging by her own fingers, her
own skin, her own thread of indecision.

She thinks of Carlos, of Margaret, of Jimmy.
She thinks of her father, and of her mother.
She thinks of all the women she has been, of all
the men. She thinks of the color of her skin, and
of Chicago streets, and of waterfalls and pines.
She thinks of moonlight nights, and of cool spring storms.
Her mind chatters like neon and northside bars.
She thinks of the 4 A.M. lonelinesses that have folded
her up like death, discordant, without logical and
beautiful conclusion. Her teeth break off at the edges.
She would speak.

The woman hangs from the 13th floor window crying for
the lost beauty of her own life. She sees the
sun falling west over the grey plane of Chicago.
She thinks she remembers listening to her own life
break loose, as she falls from the 13th floor
window on the east side of Chicago, or as she
climbs back up to claim herself again.

The Avalanche

LINDA HOGAN

Just last month
the avalanches like good women
were headed for a downfall. I saw one
throw back her head
and let go of the world.

No more free soup bones for that one.
No more faces of friends at the door
with doilies and lace,
with ivory charms
carved of the elephant's great collapse.

Once an avalanche makes up her mind
not to cling,
there's no more covering up the cliff face
and hiding the truth,
and in her breakdown
she knows everything

and knows what she knows
about the turning wheel of earth,
love, markets, and even the spring
coming soon with its wildflowers.

"No Name Woman," from The Woman Warrior

MAXINE HONG KINGSTON

"YOU MUST NOT tell anyone," my mother said, "what I am about to tell you. In China your father had a sister who killed herself. She jumped into the family well. We say that your father has all brothers because it is as if she had never been born.

"In 1924 just a few days after our village celebrated seventeen hurry-up weddings—to make sure that every young man who went 'out on the road' would responsibly come home—your father and his brothers and your grand-father and his brothers and your aunt's new husband sailed for America, the Gold Mountain. It was your grandfather's last trip. Those lucky enough to get contracts waved good-bye from the decks. They fed and guarded the stow-aways and helped them off in Cuba, New York, Bali, Hawaii. 'We'll meet in California next year,' they said. All of them sent money home.

"I remember looking at your aunt one day when she and I were dressing; I had not noticed before that she had such a protruding melon of a stomach. But I did not think, 'She's pregnant,' until she began to look like other pregnant women, her shirt pulling and the white tops of her black pants showing. She could not have been pregnant, you see, because her husband had been gone for years. No one said anything. We did not discuss it. In early summer she was ready to have the child, long after the time when it could have been possible.

"The village had also been counting. On the night the baby was to be born the villagers raided our house. Some were crying. Like a great saw, teeth strung with lights, files of people walked zigzag across our land, tearing the rice. Their lanterns doubled in the disturbed black water, which drained away through the broken bunds. As the villagers closed in, we could see that some of them, probably men and women we knew well, wore white masks. The people with long hair hung it over their faces. Women with short hair made it stand up on end. Some had tied white bands around their foreheads, arms, and legs.

"At first they threw mud and rocks at the house. Then they threw eggs and began slaughtering our stock. We could hear the animals scream their deaths—the roosters, the pigs, a last great roar from the ox. Familiar wild heads flared in our night windows; the villagers encircled us. Some of the faces stopped to peer at us, their eyes rushing like searchlights. The hands flattened against the panes, framed heads, and left red prints.

"The villagers broke in the front and the back doors at the same time, even though we had not locked the doors against them. Their knives dripped with the blood of our animals. They smeared blood on the doors and walls. One woman swung a chicken, whose throat she had slit, splattering blood in red arcs about her. We stood together in the middle of our house, in the family hall with the pictures and tables of the ancestors around us, and looked straight ahead.

"At that time the house had only two wings. When the men came back, we would build two more to enclose our courtyard and a third one to begin a second courtyard. The villagers pushed through both wings, even your grandparents' rooms, to find your aunt's, which was also mine until the men returned. From this room a new wing for one of the younger families would grow. They ripped up her clothes and shoes and broke her combs, grinding them underfoot. They tore her work from the loom. They scattered the cooking fire and rolled the new weaving in it. We could hear them in the kitchen breaking our bowls and banging the pots. They overturned the great waist-high earthenware jugs; duck eggs, pickled fruits, vegetables burst out and mixed in acrid torrents. The old woman from the next field swept a broom through the air and loosed the spirits-of-the-broom over our heads. 'Pig.' 'Ghost.' 'Pig,' they sobbed and scolded while they ruined our house.

"When they left, they took sugar and oranges to bless themselves. They cut pieces from the dead animals. Some of them took bowls that were not broken and the clothes that were not torn. Afterward we swept up the rice and sewed it back up into sacks. But the smells from the spilled preserves lasted. Your aunt gave birth in the pigsty that night. The next morning when I went for the water, I found her and the baby plugging up the family well.

"Don't let your father know that I told you. He denies her. Now that you have started to menstruate, what happened to her could happen to you. Don't humiliate us. You wouldn't like to be forgotten as if you had never been born. The villagers are watchful."

Whenever she had to warn us about life, my mother told stories that ran like this one, a story to grow up on. She tested our strength to establish realities. Those in the emigrant generations who could not reassert brute survival died young and far from home. Those of us in the first American generations have had to figure out how the invisible world the emigrants built around our childhoods fit in solid America.

The emigrants confused the gods by diverting their curses, misleading them with crooked streets and false names. They must try to confuse their offspring as well, who, I suppose, threaten them in similar ways—always trying to get things straight, always trying to name the unspeakable. The Chinese I know hide their names; sojourners take new names when their lives change and guard their real names with silence.

Chinese-Americans, when you try to understand what things in you are Chinese, how do you separate what is peculiar to childhood, to poverty, insanities, one family, your mother who marked your growing with stories, from what is Chinese? What is Chinese tradition and what is the movies?

If I want to learn what clothes my aunt wore, whether flashy or ordinary, I would have to begin, "Remember Father's drowned-in-the-well sister?" I cannot ask that. My mother has told me once and for all the useful parts. She will add nothing unless powered by Necessity, a riverbank that guides her life. She plants vegetable gardens rather than lawns; she carries the odd-shaped tomatoes home from the fields and eats food left for the gods.

Whenever we did frivolous things, we used up energy; we flew high kites. We children came up off the ground over the melting cones our parents brought home from work and the American movie on New Years' Day—*Oh, You Beautiful Doll* with Betty Grable one year, and *She Wore a Yellow Ribbon* with John Wayne another year. After the one carnival ride each, we paid in guilt; our tired father counted his change on the dark walk home.

Adultery is extravagance. Could people who hatch their own chicks and eat the embryos and the heads for delicacies and boil the feet in vinegar for party food, leaving only the gravel, eating even the gizzard lining—could such people engender a prodigal aunt? To be a woman, to have a daughter in starvation time was a waste enough. My aunt could not have been the lone romantic who gave up everything for sex. Women in the old China did not choose. Some man had commanded her to lie with him and be his secret evil. I wonder whether he masked himself when he joined the raid on her family.

Perhaps she encountered him in the fields or on the mountain where the daughters-in-law collected fuel. Or perhaps he first noticed her in the marketplace. He was not a stranger because the village housed no strangers. She had to have dealings with him other than sex. Perhaps he worked an adjoining field, or he sold her the cloth for the dress she sewed and wore. His demand must have surprised, then terrified her. She obeyed him; she always did as she was told.

When the family found a young man in the next village to be her husband, she stood tractably beside the best rooster, his proxy, and promised before they met that she would be his forever. She was lucky that he was her age and she would be the first wife, an advantage secure now. The night she first saw him, he had sex with her. Then he left for America. She had almost forgotten what he looked like. When she tried to envision him, she only saw the black and white face in the group photograph the men had taken before leaving.

The other man was not, after all, much different from her husband. They both gave orders: she followed. "If you tell your family, I'll beat you. I'll kill you. Be here again next week." No one talked sex, ever. And she might have separated the rapes from the rest of living if only she did not have to buy her oil from him or gather wood in the same forest. I want her fear to have lasted just as long as rape lasted so that the fear could have been contained. No drawn-out fear. But women at sex hazarded birth and hence lifetimes. The fear did not stop but permeated everywhere. She told the man, "I think I'm pregnant." He organized the raid against her.

On nights when my mother and father talked about their life back home, sometimes they mentioned an "outcast table" whose business they still seemed to be settling, their voices tight. In a commensal tradition, where food is precious, the powerful older people made wrongdoers eat alone. Instead of letting them start separate new lives like the Japanese, who could become samurais and geishas, the Chinese family, faces averted but eyes glowering sideways, hung on to the offenders and fed them leftovers. My aunt must have lived in the same house as my parents and eaten at an outcast table. My mother spoke about the raid as if she had seen it, when she and my aunt, a daughter-in-law to a different household, should not have been living together at all. Daughters-in-law lived with their husbands' parents, not their own; a synonym for marriage in Chinese is "taking a daughter-in-law." Her husband's parents could have sold her, mortgaged her, stoned her. But they had sent her back to her own mother and father, a mysterious act hinting at disgraces not told me. Perhaps they had thrown her out to deflect the avengers.

She was the only daughter; her four brothers went with her father, husband, and uncles "out on the road" and for some years became western men. When the goods were divided among the family, three of the brothers took land, and the youngest, my father, chose an education. After my grandparents gave their daughter away to her husband's family, they had dispensed all the adventure and all the property. They expected her alone to keep traditional ways, which her brothers, now among the barbarians, could fumble without detection. The heavy, deep-rooted women were to maintain the past against the flood, safe for returning. But the rare urge west had fixed upon our family, and so my aunt crossed boundaries not delineated in space.

The work of preservation demands that the feelings playing about in one's guts not be turned into action. Just watch their passing like cherry blossoms. But perhaps my aunt, my forerunner, caught in a slow life, let dreams grow and fade and after some months or years went toward what persisted. Fear at the enormities of the forbidden kept her desires delicate, wire and bone. She looked at a man because she liked the way the hair was tucked behind his ears, or she liked the question-mark line of a long torso curving at the shoulder and straight at the hip. For warm eyes or a soft voice or a slow walk—that's all—a few hairs, a line, a brightness, a sound, a pace, she gave up family. She offered us up for charm that vanished with tiredness, a pigtail that didn't toss when the wind died. Why, the wrong lighting could erase the dearest thing about him.

It could very well have been, however, that my aunt did not take the subtle enjoyment of her friend, but, a wild woman, kept rollicking company. Imagining her free with sex doesn't fit, though. I don't know any women like that, or men either. Unless I see her life branching into mine, she gives me no ancestral help.

To sustain her being in love, she often worked at herself in the mirror, guessing at the colors and shapes that would interest him, changing them frequently in order to hit on the right combination. She wanted him to look back.

On a farm near the sea, a woman who tended her appearance reaped a reputation for eccentricity. All the married women blunt-cut their hair in flaps about their ears or pulled it back in tight buns. No nonsense. Neither style blew easily into heart-catching tangles. And at their weddings they displayed themselves in their long hair for the last time. "It brushed the backs of my knees," my mother tells me. "It was braided, and even so, it brushed the backs of my knees."

At the mirror my aunt combed individuality into her bob. A bun could have been contrived to escape into black streamers blowing in the wind or in quiet wisps about her face, but only the older women in our picture album wear buns. She brushed her hair back from her forehead, tucking the flaps behind her ears. She looped a piece of thread, knotted into a circle between her index finger and thumbs, and ran the double strand across her forehead. When she closed her fingers as if she were making a pair of shadow geese bite, the string twisted together catching the little hairs. Then she pulled the thread away from her skin, ripping the hairs out neatly, her eyes watering from the needles of pain. Opening her fingers, she cleaned the thread, then rolled it along her hairline and the tops of her eyebrows. My mother did the same to me and my sisters and herself. I used to believe that the expression "caught by the short hairs" meant a captive held with a depilatory string. It especially hurt at the temples, but my mother said we were lucky we didn't have to have our feet bound when we were seven. Sisters used to sit on their beds and cry together, she said, as their mothers or their slave removed the bandages for a few minutes each night and let the blood gush back into their veins. I hope that the man my aunt loved appreciated a smooth brow, that he wasn't just a tits-and-ass man.

Once my aunt found a freckle on her chin, at a spot that the almanac said predestined her for unhappiness. She dug it out with a hot needle and washed the wound with peroxide.

More attention to her looks than these pullings of hairs and pickings at spots would have caused gossip among the villagers. They owned work clothes and good clothes, and they wore good clothes for feasting the new seasons. But since a woman combing her hair hexes beginnings, my aunt rarely found an occasion to look her best. Women looked like great sea snails—the corded wood, babies, and laundry they carried were the whorls on their backs. The Chinese did not admire a bent back; goddesses and warriors stood straight. Still there must have been a marvelous freeing of beauty when a worker laid down her burden and stretched and arched.

Such commonplace loveliness, however, was not enough for my aunt. She dreamed of a lover for the fifteen days of New Year's, the time for families to exchange visits, money, and food. She plied her secret comb. And sure enough she cursed the year, the family, the village, and herself.

Even as her hair lured her imminent lover, many other men looked at her. Uncles, cousins, nephews, brothers would have looked, too, had they been home between journeys. Perhaps they had already been restraining their curiosity, and they left, fearful that their glances, like a field of nesting birds, might be startled and caught. Poverty hurt, and that was their first reason for leaving. But another, final reason for leaving the crowded house was the never-said.

She may have been unusually beloved, the precious only daughter, spoiled and mirror gazing because of the affection the family lavished on her. When her husband left, they welcomed the chance to take her back from the in-laws; she could live like the little daughter for just a while longer. There are stories that my grandfather was different from other people, "crazy ever since the little Jap bayoneted him in the head." He used to put his naked penis on the dinner table, laughing. And one day he brought home a baby girl, wrapped up inside his brown western-style greatcoat. He had traded one of his sons, probably my father, the youngest, for her. My grandmother made him trade back. When he finally got a daughter of his own, he doted on her. They must have all loved her, except perhaps my father, the only brother who never went back to China, having once been traded for a girl.

Brothers and sisters, newly men and women, had to efface their sexual color and present plain miens. Disturbing hair and eyes, a smile like no other, threatened the ideal of five generations living under one roof. To focus blurs, people shouted face to face and yelled from room to room. The immigrants I know have loud voices, unmodulated to American tones even after years away from the villages where they called their friendships out across the fields. I have not been able to stop my mother's screams in public libraries or over telephones. Walking erect (knees straight, toes pointed forward, not pigeon-toed, which is Chinese-feminine) and speaking in an inaudible voice, I have tried to turn myself American-feminine. Chinese communication was loud, public. Only sick people had to whisper. But at the dinner table, where the family members came nearest one another, no one could talk, not the outcast nor any eaters. Every word that falls from the mouth is a coin lost. Silently they gave and accepted food with both hands. A preoccupied child who took his bowl with one hand got a sideways glare. A complete moment of total attention is due everyone alike. Children and lovers have no singularity here, but my aunt used a secret voice, a separate attentiveness.

She kept the man's name to herself throughout her labor and dying; she did not accuse him that he be punished with her. To save her inseminator's name she gave silent birth.

He may have been somebody in her own household, but intercourse with a man outside the family would have been no less abhorrent. All the village were kinsmen, and the titles shouted in loud country voices never let kinship be forgotten. Any man within visiting distance would have been neutralized as a lover— "brother," "younger brother," "older brother"—one hundred and fifteen relationship titles. Parents researched birth charts probably not so much to assure good fortune as to circumvent incest in a population that has but one hundred surnames. Everybody has eight million relatives. How useless then sexual mannerisms, how dangerous.

As if it came from an atavism deeper than fear, I used to add "brother" silently to boys' names. It hexed the boys, who would or would not ask me to dance, and made them less scary and as familiar and deserving of benevolence as girls.

But, of course, I hexed myself also—no dates. I should have stood up, both arms waving, and shouted across libraries, "Hey, you! Love me back." I had no idea, though, how to make attraction selective, how to control its direction and magnitude. If I made myself American-pretty so that the five or six Chinese boys in the class fell in love with me, everyone else—the Caucasian, Negro, and Japanese boys—would too. Sisterliness, dignified and honorable, made much more sense.

Attraction eludes control so stubbornly that whole societies designed to organize relationships among people cannot keep order, not even when they bind people to one another from childhood and raise them together. Among the very poor and the wealthy brothers married their adopted sisters, like doves. Our family allowed some romance, paying adult brides prices and providing dowries so that their sons and daughters could marry strangers. Marriage promises to turn strangers into friendly relatives—a nation of siblings.

In the village structure, spirits shimmered among the live creatures, balanced and held in equilibrium by time and land. But one human being flaring up into violence could open up a black hole, a maelstrom that pulled in the sky. The frightened villagers, who depended on one another to maintain the real, went to my aunt to show her a personal, physical representation of the break she had made in the "roundness." Misallying couples snapped off the future, which was to be embodied in true offspring. The villagers punished her for acting as if she could have a private life, secret and apart from them.

If my aunt had betrayed the family at a time of large grain yields and peace, when many boys were born, and wings were being built on many houses, perhaps she might have escaped such severe punishment. But the men—hungry, greedy, tired of planting in dry soil, cuckolded—and had to leave the village in order to send food-money home. There were ghost plagues, bandit plagues, wars with the Japanese, floods. My Chinese brother and sister had died of an unknown sickness. Adultery, perhaps only a mistake during good times, became a crime when the village needed food.

The round moon cakes and round doorways, the round tables of graduated size that fit one roundness inside another, round windows and rice bowls—these talismans had lost their power to warn this family of the law: a family must be whole, faithfully keeping the descent line by having sons to feed the old and the dead, who in turn look after the family. The villagers came to show my aunt and her lover-in-hiding a broken house. The villagers were speeding up the circling of events because she was too shortsighted to see that her infidelity had already harmed the village, that waves of consequences would return unpredictably, sometimes in disguise, as now, to hurt her. This roundness had to be made coin-sized so that she would see its circumference: punish her at the birth of her baby. Awaken her to the inexorable. People who refused fatalism because they could invent small resources insisted on culpability. Deny accidents and wrest fault from the stars.

After the villagers left, their lanterns now scattering in various directions toward home, the family broke their silence and cursed her. "Aiaa, we're going to die. Death is coming. Death is coming. Look what you've done. You've killed us. Ghost! Dead ghost! Ghost! You've never been born." She ran out into the fields, far enough from the house so that she could no longer hear their voices, and pressed herself against the earth, her own land no more. When she felt the birth coming, she thought that she had been hurt. Her body seized together. "They've hurt me too much." she thought. "This is gall, and it will kill me." With forehead and knees against the earth, her body convulsed and then relaxed. She turned on her back, lay on the ground. The black well of sky and stars went out and out and out forever; her body and her complexity seemed to disappear. She was one of the stars, a bright dot in blackness, without home, without a companion, in eternal cold and silence. An agoraphobia rose in her, speeding higher and higher, bigger and bigger, she would not be able to contain it; there would be no end to fear.

Flayed, unprotected against space, she felt pain return, focusing her body. This pain chilled her—a cold steady kind of surface pain. Inside, spasmodically, the other pain, the pain of the child, heated her. For hours she lay on the ground, alternately body and space. Sometimes a vision of normal comfort obliterated reality: she saw the family in the evening gambling at the dinner table, the young people massaging their elders' backs. She saw them congratulating one another, high joy on the mornings the rice shoots came up. When these pictures burst, the stars drew yet further apart. Black space opened.

She got to her feet to fight better and remembered that old-fashioned women gave birth in their pigsties to fool the jealous, pain-dealing gods, who do not snatch piglets. Before the next spasms could stop her, she ran to the pigsty, each step a rushing out into emptiness. She climbed over the fence and knelt in the dirt. It was good to have a fence enclosing her, a tribal person alone.

Laboring, this woman who had carried her child as a foreign growth that sickened her every day, expelled it at last. She reached down to touch the hot, wet, moving mass, surely smaller than anything human, and could feel that it was human after all—fingers, toes, nails, nose. She pulled it up on to her belly, and it lay curled there, butt in the air, feet precisely tucked one under the other. She opened her loose shirt and buttoned the child inside. After resting, it squirmed and thrashed and she pushed it up to her breast. It turned its head this way and that until it found her nipple. There, it made little snuffling noises. She clenched her teeth at its preciousness, lovely as a young calf, a piglet, a little dog.

She may have gone to the pigsty as a last act of responsibility: she would protect this child as she had protected its father. It would look after her soul, leaving supplies on her grave. But how would this tiny child without family find her grave when there would be no marker for her anywhere, neither in the earth nor the family hall? No one would give her a family hall name. She had taken the child with her into the wastes. At its birth the two of them had felt the raw pain of separation, a wound that only the family pressing tight could close. A child with no descent line would not soften her life but only trail after her, ghostlike, begging her to give it purpose. At dawn the villagers on their way to the fields would stand around the fence and look.

Full of milk, the little ghost slept. When it awoke, she hardened her breasts against the milk that crying loosens. Toward morning she picked up the baby and walked to the well.

Carrying the baby to the well shows loving. Otherwise abandon it. Turn its face into the mud. Mothers who love their children take them along. It was probably a girl; there is some hope of forgiveness for boys.

"Don't tell anyone you had an aunt. Your father does not want to hear her name. She has never been born." I have believed that sex was unspeakable and words so strong and fathers so frail that "aunt" would do my father mysterious harm. I have thought that my family, having settled among immigrants who had also been neighbors in ancestral land, needed to clean their name, and a wrong word would incite the kinspeople even here. But there is more to the silence: they want me to participate in her punishment. And I have.

In the twenty years since I heard this story I have not asked for details nor said my aunt's name; I do not know it. People who can comfort the dead can also chase after them to hurt them further—a reverse ancestor worship. The real punishment was not the raid swiftly inflicted by the villagers, but the family's deliberately forgetting her. Her betrayal so maddened them, they saw to it that she would suffer forever, even after death. Always hungry, always needing, she would have to beg food from other ghosts, snatch and steal it from those whose living descendants give them gifts. She would have to fight the ghosts massed at crossroads for the buns a few thoughtful citizens leave to decoy her away from the village and home so that the ancestral spirits could feast unharassed. At peace, they could act like gods, not ghosts, their descent lines providing them with paper suits and dresses, spirit money, paper houses, paper automobiles, chicken, meat, and rice into eternity—essences delivered up in smoke and flames, steam and incense rising from each rice bowl. In an attempt to make the Chinese care for people outside the family, Chairman Mao encourages us now to give our paper replicas to the spirits of outstanding soldiers and workers, no matter whose ancestors they may be. My aunt remains forever hungry. Goods are not distributed evenly among the dead.

My aunt haunts me—her ghost drawn to me because now, after fifty years of neglect, I alone devote pages of paper to her, though not origamied into houses and clothes. I do not think she always means me well. I am telling on her, and she was a spite suicide, drowning herself in the drinking water. The Chinese are always very frightened of the drowned one, whose weeping ghost, wet hair hanging and skin bloated, waits silently by the water to pull down a substitute.

Three Poems

Anne Sexton

You, Doctor Martin

You, Doctor Martin, walk
from breakfast to madness. Late August,
I speed through the antiseptic tunnel
where the moving dead still talk
of pushing their bones against the thrust
of cure. And I am queen of this summer hotel
or the laughing bee on a stalk

of death. We stand in broken
lines and wait while they unlock
the door and count us at the frozen gates
of dinner. The shibboleth is spoken
and we move to gravy in our smock
of smiles. We chew in rows, our plates
scratch and whine like chalk

in school. There are no knives
for cutting your throat. I make
moccasins all morning. At first my hands
kept empty, unraveled for the lives
they used to work. Now I learn to take
them back, each angry finger that demands
I mend what another will break

tomorrow. Of course, I love you;
you lean above the plastic sky,
god of our block, prince of all the foxes.
The breaking crowns are new

that Jack wore. Your third eye
moves among us and lights the separate boxes
where we sleep or cry.

What large children we are
here. All over I grow most tall
in the best ward. Your business is people,
you call at the madhouse, an oracular
eye in our nest. Out in the hall
the intercom pages you. You twist in the pull
of the foxy children who fall

like floods of life in frost.
And we are magic talking to itself,
noisy and alone. I am queen of all my sins
forgotten. Am I still lost?
Once I was beautiful. Now I am myself,
counting this row and that row of moccasins
waiting on the silent shelf.

SAID THE POET TO THE ANALYST

My business is words. Words are like labels,
or coins, or better, like swarming bees.
I confess I am only broken by the sources of things;
as if words were counted like dead bees in the attic,
unbuckled from their yellow eyes and their dry wings.
I must always forget how one word is able to pick
out another, to manner another, until I have got
something I might have said . . .
but did not.

Your business is watching my words. But I
admit nothing. I work with my best, for instance,
when I can write my praise for a nickel machine,
that one night in Nevada: telling how the magic jackpot
came clacking three bells out, over the lucky screen.
But if you should say this is something it is not,

then I grow weak, remembering how my hands felt funny
and ridiculous and crowded with all
the believing money.

NOON WALK ON THE ASYLUM LAWN

The summer sun ray
shifts through a suspicious tree.
though I walk through the valley of the shadow
It sucks the air
and looks around for me.

The grass speaks.
I hear green chanting all day.
I will fear no evil, fear no evil
The blades extend
and reach my way.

The sky breaks.
It sags and breathes upon my face.
in the presence of mine enemies, mine enemies
The world is full of enemies.
There is no safe place.

SECTION FOUR

Men's Experiences with War Trauma, Including
Post-Traumatic Stress Disorder
§

"1919," *from* Sula

TONI MORRISON

EXCEPT FOR World War II, nothing ever interfered with the celebration of National Suicide Day. It had taken place every January third since 1920, although Shadrack, its founder, was for many years the only celebrant. Blasted and permanently astonished by the events of 1917, he had returned to Medallion handsome but ravaged, and even the most fastidious people in the town sometimes caught themselves dreaming of what he must have been like a few years back before he went off to war. A young man of hardly twenty, his head full of nothing and his mouth recalling the taste of lipstick, Shadrack had found himself in December, 1917, running with his comrades across a field in France. It was his first encounter with the enemy and he didn't know whether his company was running toward them or away. For several days they had been marching, keeping close to a stream that was frozen at its edges. At one point they crossed it, and no sooner had he stepped foot on the other side than the day was adangle with shouts and explosions. Shellfire was all around him, and though he knew that this was something called *it,* he could not muster up the proper feeling—the feeling that would accommodate *it.* He expected to be terrified or exhilarated—to feel *something* very strong. In fact, he felt only the bite of a nail in his boot, which pierced the ball of his foot whenever he came down on it. The day was cold enough to make his breath visible, and he wondered for a moment at the purity and whiteness of his own breath among the dirty, gray explosions surrounding him. He ran, bayonet fixed, deep in the great sweep of men flying across this field. Wincing at the pain in his foot, he turned his head a little to the right and saw the face of a soldier near him fly off. Before he could register shock, the rest of the soldier's head disappeared under the inverted soup bowl of his helmet. But stubbornly, taking no direction from the brain, the body of the headless soldier ran on, with energy and grace, ignoring altogether the drip and slide of brain tissue down its back.

When Shadrack opened his eyes he was propped up in a small bed. Before him on a tray was a large tin plate divided into three triangles. In one triangle was rice, in another meat, and in the third stewed tomatoes. A small round depression held a cup of whitish liquid. Shadrack stared at the soft colors that filled these triangles: the lumpy whiteness of the rice, the quivering blood tomatoes, the grayish-brown meat. All their repugnance was contained in the neat balance of the triangles—a balance that soothed him, transferred some of its equilibrium to him. Thus reassured that the white, the red and the brown would stay where they were—would not explode or burst forth from their restricted zones—he suddenly felt hungry and looked around for his hands. His glance was cautious at first, for he had to be very careful—anything could be anywhere. Then he noticed two lumps beneath the beige blanket on either side of his hips. With extreme care he lifted one arm and was relieved to find his hand attached to his wrist. He tried the other and found it also. Slowly he directed one hand toward the cup and, just as he was about to spread his fingers, they began to grow in higgledy-piggledy fashion like Jack's beanstalk all over the tray and the bed. With a shriek he closed his eyes and thrust his huge growing hands under the covers. Once out of sight they seemed to shrink back to their normal size. But the yell had brought a male nurse.

"Private? We're not going to have any trouble today, are we? Are we, Private?"

Shadrack looked up at a balding man dressed in a green-cotton jacket and trousers. His hair was parted low on the right side so that some twenty or thirty yellow hairs could discreetly cover the nakedness of his head.

"Come on. Pick up that spoon. Pick it up, Private. Nobody is going to feed you forever."

Sweat slid from Shadrack's armpits down his sides. He could not bear to see his hands grow again and he was frightened of the voice in the apple-green suit.

"Pick it up, I said. There's no point to this . . ." The nurse reached under the cover for Shadrack's wrist to pull out the monstrous hand. Shadrack jerked it back and overturned the tray. In panic he raised himself to his knees and tried to fling off and away his terrible fingers, but succeeded only in knocking the nurse into the next bed.

When they bound Shadrack into a straitjacket, he was both relieved and grateful, for his hands were at last hidden and confined to whatever size they had attained.

Laced and silent in his small bed, he tried to tie the loose cords in his mind. He wanted desperately to see his own face and connect it with the word "private"—the word the nurse (and the others who helped bind him) had called him. "Private" he thought was something secret, and he wondered why they looked at him and called him a secret. Still, if his hands behaved as they had done, what might he expect from his face? The fear and longing were too much for him, so he began to think of other things. That is, he let his mind slip into whatever cave mouths of memory it chose.

He saw a window that looked out on a river which he knew was full of fish. Someone was speaking softly just outside the door...

Shadrack's earlier violence had coincided with a memorandum from the hospital executive staff in reference to the distribution of patients in high-risk areas. There was clearly a demand for space. The priority or the violence earned Shadrack his release, $217 in cash, a full suit of clothes and copies of very official-looking papers.

When he stepped out of the hospital door the grounds overwhelmed him: the cropped shrubbery, the edged lawns, the undeviating walks. Shadrack looked at the cement stretches: each one leading clearheadedly to some presumably desirable destination. There were no fences, no warnings, no obstacles at all between concrete and green grass, so one could easily ignore the tidy sweep of stone and cut out in another direction—a direction of one's own.

Shadrack stood in front of the hospital steps watching the heads of trees tossing ruefully but harmlessly, since their trunks were rooted too deeply in the earth to threaten him. Only the walks made him uneasy. He shifted his weight, wondering how he could get to the gate without stepping on the concrete. While plotting his course—where he would have to leap, where to skirt a clump of bushes—a loud guffaw startled him. Two men were going up the steps. Then he noticed that there were many people about, and that he was now just seeing them, or else they had just materialized. They were thin slips, like paper dolls floating down the walks. Some were seated in chairs with wheels, propelled by other paper figures from behind. All seemed to be smoking, and their arms and legs curved in the breeze. A good high wind would pull them up and away and they would land perhaps among the tops of the trees.

Shadrack took the plunge. Four steps and he was on the grass heading for the gate. He kept his head down to avoid seeing the paper people swerving and bending here and there, and he lost his way. When he looked up, he was standing by a low red building separated from the main building by a covered walkway. From somewhere came a sweetish smell which reminded him of something painful. He looked around for the gate and saw that he had gone directly away from it in his complicated journey over the grass. Just to the left of the low building was a graveled driveway that appeared to lead outside the grounds. He trotted quickly to it and left, at last, a haven of more than a year, only eight days of which he fully recollected.

Once on the road, he headed west. The long stay in the hospital had left him weak—too weak to walk steadily on the gravel shoulders of the road. He shuffled, grew dizzy, stopped for breath, started again, stumbling and sweating but refusing to wipe his temples, still afraid to look at his hands. Passengers in dark, square cars shuttered their eyes at what they took to be a drunken man.

The sun was already directly over his head when he came to a town. A few blocks of shaded streets and he was already at its heart—a pretty, quietly regulated downtown.

Exhausted, his feet clotted with pain, he sat down at the curbside to take off his shoes. He closed his eyes to avoid seeing his hands and fumbled with the laces of the heavy high-topped shoes. The nurse had tied them into a double knot, the way one does for children, and Shadrack, long unaccustomed to the manipulation of intricate things, could not get them loose. Uncoordinated, his fingernails tore away at the knots. He fought a rising hysteria that was not merely anxiety to free his aching feet; his very life depended on the release of the knots. Suddenly without raising his eyelids, he began to cry. Twenty-two years old, weak, hot, frightened, not daring to acknowledge the fact that he didn't even know who or what he was . . . with no past, no language, no tribe, no source, no address book, no comb, no pencil, no clock, no pocket handkerchief, no rug, no bed, no can opener, no faded postcard, no soap, no key, no tobacco pouch, no soiled underwear and nothing nothing nothing to do . . . he was sure of one thing only: the unchecked monstrosity of his hands. He cried soundlessly at the curbside of a small Midwestern town wondering where the window was, and the river, and the soft voices just outside the door . . .

Through his tears he saw the fingers joining the laces, tentatively at first, then rapidly. The four fingers of each hand fused into the fabric, knotted themselves and zigzagged in and out of the tiny eyeholes.

By the time the police drove up, Shadrack was suffering from a blinding headache, which was not abated by the comfort he felt when the policemen pulled his hands away from what he thought was a permanent entanglement with his shoelaces. They took him to jail, booked him for vagrancy and intoxication, and locked him in a cell. Lying on a cot, Shadrack could only stare helplessly at the wall, so paralyzing was the pain in his head. He lay in this agony for a long while and then realized he was staring at the painted-over letters of a command to fuck himself. He studied the phrase as the pain in his head subsided.

Like moonlight stealing under a window shade an idea insinuated itself: his earlier desire to see his own face. He looked for a mirror; there was none. Finally, keeping his hands carefully behind his back he made his way to the toilet bowl and peeped in. The water was unevenly lit by the sun so he could make nothing out. Returning to his cot he took the blanket and covered his head, rendering the water dark enough to see his reflection. There in the toilet water he saw a grave black face. A black so definite, so unequivocal, it astonished him. He had been harboring a skittish apprehension that he was not real—that he didn't exist at all. But when the blackness greeted him with its indisputable presence, he wanted nothing more. In his joy he took the risk of letting one edge of the blanket drop and glanced at his hands. They were still. Courteously still.

Shadrack rose and returned to the cot, where he fell into the first sleep of his new life. A sleep deeper than the hospital drugs; deeper than the pits of plums, steadier than the condor's wing; more tranquil than the curve of eggs.

The sheriff looked through the bars at the young man with the matted hair. He had read through his prisoner's papers and hailed a farmer. When Shadrack awoke, the sheriff handed him back his papers and escorted him to the back of a wagon. Shadrack got in and in less than three hours he was back in Medallion, for he had been only twenty-two miles from his window, his river, and his soft voices just outside the door.

In the back of the wagon, supported by sacks of squash and hills of pumpkins, Shadrack began a struggle that was to last for twelve days, a struggle to order and focus experience. It had to do with making a place for fear as a way of controlling it. He knew the smell of death and was terrified of it, for he could not anticipate it. It was not death or dying that frightened him, but the unexpectedness of both. In sorting it all out, he hit on the notion that if one day a year were devoted to it, everybody could get it out of the way and the rest of the year would be safe and free. In this manner he instituted National Suicide Day.

On the third day of the new year, he walked through the Bottom down Carpenter's Road with a cowbell and a hangman's rope calling the people together. Telling them that this was their only chance to kill themselves or each other.

At first the people in the town were frightened; they knew Shadrack was crazy but that did not mean that he didn't have any sense or, even more important, that he had no power. His eyes were so wild, his hair so long and matted, his voice was so full of authority and thunder that he caused panic on the first, or Charter, National Suicide Day in 1920. The next one, in 1921, was less frightening but still worrisome. The people had seen him a year now in between. He lived in a shack on the riverbank that once belonged to his grandfather long time dead. On Tuesday and Friday he sold the fish he had caught that morning, the rest of the week he was drunk, loud, obscene, funny and outrageous. But he never touched anybody, never fought, never caressed. Once the people understood the boundaries and nature of his madness, they could fit him, so to speak, into the scheme of things.

Then, on subsequent National Suicide Days, the grown people looked out from behind curtains as he rang his bell: a few stragglers increased their speed, and little children screamed and ran. The tetter heads tried goading him (although he was only four or five years older then they) but not for long, for his curses were stingingly personal.

As time went along, the people took less notice of these January thirds, or rather they thought they did, thought they had no attitudes or feelings one way or another about Shadrack's annual solitary parade. In fact they had simply stopped remarking on the holiday because they had absorbed it into their thoughts, into their language, into their lives.

Someone said to a friend, "You sure was a long time delivering that baby. How long was you in labor?"

And the friend answered, "'Bout three days. The pains started on Suicide Day and kept up till the following Sunday. Was borned on Sunday. All my boys is Sunday boys."

Some lover said to his bride-to-be, "Let's do it after New Years, 'stead of before. I get paid New Year's Eve."

And his sweetheart answered, "OK, but make sure it ain't on Suicide Day. I ain't 'bout to be listening to no cowbells whilst the weddin's going on."

Somebody's grandmother said her hens always started a laying of double yolks right after Suicide Day.

Then Reverend Deal took it up, saying the same folks who had sense enough to avoid Shadrack's call were the ones who insisted on drinking themselves to death or womanizing themselves to death. "May's well go on with Shad and save the Lamb the trouble of redemption."

Easily, quietly Suicide Day became a part of the fabric of life up in the Bottom of Medallion, Ohio.

Night March

Tim O' Brien

THE PLATOON of thirty-two soldiers moved slowly in the dark, single file, not talking. One by one, like sheep in a dream, they passed through the hedgerow, crossed quietly over a meadow and came down to the paddy. There they stopped. Lieutenant Sidney Martin knelt down, motioning with his hand, and one by one the others squatted or knelt or sat in the shadows. For a long time they did not move. Except for the sounds of their breathing, and, once, a soft fluid trickle as one of them urinated, the thirty-two men were silent: some of them excited by the adventure, some afraid, some exhausted by the long march, some of them looking forward to reaching the sea where they would be safe. There was no talking now. No more jokes. At the rear of the column, Private First Class Paul Berlin lay quietly with his forehead resting on the black plastic stock of his rifle. His eyes were closed. He was pretending that he was not in the war. Pretending he had not watched Billy Boy Watkins die of fright on the field of battle. He was pretending he was a boy again, camping with his father in the midnight summer along the Des Moines River. "Be calm," his father said. "Ignore the bad stuff, look for the good." In the dark, eyes closed, he pretended. He pretended that when he opened his eyes his father would be there by the campfire and, father and son, they would begin to talk softly about whatever came to mind, minor things, trivial things, and then roll into their sleeping bags. And later, he pretended, it would be morning and there would not be a war.

In the morning, when they reached the sea, it would be better. He would bathe in the sea. He would shave. Clean his nails, work out the scum. In the morning he would wash himself and brush his teeth. He would forget the first day, and the second day would not be so bad. He would learn.

There was a sound beside him, a movement, then, "Hey," then louder, "Hey!"

He opened his eyes.

"Hey, we're movin'. Get up."

"Okay."

"You sleeping?"

"No, I was resting. Thinking." He could see only part of the soldier's face. It was a plump, round, child's face. The child was smiling.

"No problem," the soldier whispered. "Up an' at 'em."

And he followed the boy's shadow into the paddy, stumbling once, almost dropping his rifle, cutting his knee, but he followed the shadow and did not stop. The night was clear. Before him, strung out across the paddy, he could make out the black forms of the other soldiers, their silhouettes hard against the sky. Already the Southern Cross was out. And other stars he could not yet name. Soon, he thought, he would learn the names. And puffy night clouds. And a peculiar glow to the west. There was not yet a moon.

Wading through the paddy, listening to the lullaby sounds of his boots, and many other boots, he tried hard not to think. Dead of a heart attack, that was what Doc Peret had said. Only he did not know Doc Peret's name. All he knew was what Doc Peret had said, dead of a heart attack, but he tried hard not to think of this, and instead he thought about not thinking. The fear wasn't so bad now. Now, as he stepped out of the paddy and onto a narrow dirt path, now the fear was mostly the fear of being so dumbly afraid ever again.

So he tried not to think.

There were tricks to keep from thinking. Counting. He counted his steps along the dirt path, concentrating on the numbers, pretending that the steps were dollar bills and that each step through the night made him richer and richer, so that soon he would become a wealthy man, and he kept counting, considering the ways he might spend the wealth, what he would buy and do and acquire and own. He would look his father in the eye and shrug and say, "It was pretty bad at first, sure, but I learned a lot and I got used to it. I never joined them—not them—but I learned their names and I got along, I got used to it." Then he would tell his father the story of Billy Boy Watkins, only a story, just a story, and he would never let on about the fear. "Not so bad," he would say instead, making his father proud.

And songs, another trick to stop the thinking—*Where have you gone, Billy Boy, Billy Boy, oh, where have you gone, charming Billy?* and other songs, *I got a girl, her name is Jill, she won't do it but her sister will,* and *Sound Off!* and other songs that he sang in his head as he marched toward the sea. And when he reached the sea he would dig a hole in the sand and he would sleep like the high clouds, he would swim and dive into the breakers and hunt crayfish and smell the salt, and he would laugh when the others made jokes about Billy Boy, and he would not be afraid ever again.

He walked, and counted, and later the moon came out. Pale, shrunken to the size of a dime.

The helmet was heavy on his head. In the morning he would adjust the leather binding. In the morning, at the end of the long march, his boots would have lost their shiny black stiffness, turning red and clay-colored like all the other boots, and he would have a start on a beard, his clothes would begin to smell of the country, the mud and algae and cow manure and chlorophyll, decay, mosquitoes like mice, all this: He could begin to smell like the others, even look like them, but, by God, he would not join them. He would adjust. He would play the part. But he would not join them. He would shave, he would clean himself, he would clean his weapon and keep it clean. He would clean the breech and trigger assembly and muzzle and magazines, and later, next time, he would not be afraid to use it. In the morning, when he reached the sea, he would learn the soldiers' names and maybe laugh at their jokes. When they joked about Billy Boy he would laugh, pretending it was funny, and he would not let on.

Walking, counting in his walking, and pretending, he felt better. He watched the moon come higher.

The trick was not to take it personally. Stay aloof. Follow the herd but don't join it. That would be the real trick. The trick would be to keep himself separate. To watch things. "Keep an eye out for the good stuff," his father had said by the river. "Keep your eyes open and your ass low, that's my only advice." And he would do it. A low profile. Look for the beauties: the moon sliding higher now, the feeling of the march, all the ironies and truths, and don't take any of it seriously. That would be the trick.

Once, very late in the night, they skirted a sleeping village. The smells again—straw, cattle, mildew. The men were quiet. On the far side of the village, coming like light from the dark, a dog barked. The barking was fierce. Then, nearby, another dog took up the bark. The column stopped. They waited there until the barking died out, then, fast, they marched away from the village, through a graveyard with conical burial mounds and miniature stone altars. The place had a perfumy smell. His mother's dresser, rows of expensive lotions and colognes, eau de bain: She used to hide booze in the larger bottles, but his father found out and carried the whole load out back, started a fire, and, one by one, threw the bottles into the incinerator, where they made sharp exploding sounds like gunfire; a perfumy smell, yes; a nice spot to spend the night, to sleep in the perfumery, the burial mounds making fine strong battlements, the great quiet of the place.

But they went on, passing through a hedgerow and across another paddy and east toward the sea.

He walked carefully. He remembered what he'd been taught. Billy Boy hadn't remembered. And so Billy died of fright, his face going pale and the veins in his arms and neck popping out, the crazy look in his eyes.

He walked carefully.

Stretching ahead of him in the night was the string of shadow-soldiers whose names he did not yet know. He knew some of the faces. And he knew their shapes, their heights and weights and builds, the way they carried themselves on the march. But he could not tell them apart. All alike in the night, a piece, all of them moving with the same sturdy silence and calm and steadiness.

So he walked carefully, counting his steps. And when he had counted to eight thousand and sixty, the column suddenly stopped. One by one the soldiers knelt or squatted down.

The grass along the path was wet. Private First Class Paul Berlin lay back and turned his head so he could lick at the dew with his eyes closed, another trick, closing his eyes. He might have slept. Eyes closed, pretending came easy . . . When he opened his eyes, the same child-faced soldier was sitting beside him, quietly chewing gum. The smell of Doublemint was clean in the night.

"Sleepin' again?" the boy said.

"No. Hell, no."

The boy laughed a little, very quietly, chewing on his gum. Then he twisted the cap off a canteen and took a swallow and handed it through the dark.

"Take some," he said. He didn't whisper. The voice was high, a child's voice, and there was no fear in it. A big blue baby. A genie's voice.

Paul Berlin drank and handed back the canteen. The boy pressed a stick of gum into his fingers.

"Chew it quiet, okay? Don't blow no bubbles or nothing."

It was impossible to make out the soldier's face. It was a huge face, almost perfectly round.

They sat still. Private First Class Paul Berlin chewed the gum until all the sugars were gone. Then in the dark beside him the boy began to whistle. There was no melody.

"You have to do that?"

"Do what?"

"Whistle like that."

"Geez, was I whistling?"

"Sort of."

The boy laughed. His teeth were big and even and white. "Sometimes I forget. Kinda dumb, isn't it?"

"Forget it."

"Whistling! Sometimes I just forget where I'm at. The guys, they get pissed at me, but I just forget. You're new here, right?"

"I guess I am."

"Weird."

"What's weird?"

"Weird," the boy said, "that's all. The way I forget. Whistling! Was I whistling?"

"If you call it that."

"Geez!"

They were quiet awhile. And the night was quiet, no crickets or birds, and it was hard to imagine it was truly a war. He searched again for the soldier's face, but there was just a soft fullness under the helmet. The white teeth: chewing, smiling. But it did not matter. Even if he saw the kid's face, he would not know the name; and if he knew the name, it would still not matter.

"Haven't got the time?"

"No."

"Rats." The boy popped the gum on his teeth, a sharp smacking sound. "Don't matter."

"How about—"

"Time goes faster when you don't know the time. That's why I never bought no watch. Oscar's got one, an' Billy . . . Billy, he's got *two* of 'em. Two watches, you believe that? I never bought none, though. Goes fast when you don't know the time."

And again they were quiet. They lay side by side in the grass. The moon was very high now, and very bright, and they were waiting for cloud cover. After a time there was the crinkling of tinfoil, then the sound of heavy chewing. A moist, loud sound.

"I hate it when the sugar's gone," the boy said. "You want more?"

"I'm okay."

"Just ask. I got about a zillion packs. Pretty weird, wasn't it?"

"What?"

"Today . . . it was pretty weird what Doc said. About Billy Boy."

"Yes, pretty weird."

The boy smiled his big smile. "You like that gum? I got other kinds if you don't like it. I got—"

"I like it."

"I got Black Jack here. You like Black Jack? Geez, I love it! Juicy Fruit's second, but Black Jack's first. I save it up for rainy days, so to speak. Know what I mean? What you got there is Doublemint."

"I like it."

"Sure," the round soldier said, the child, "except for Black Jack and Juicy Fruit it's my favorite. You like Black Jack gum?"

Paul Berlin said he'd never tried it. It scared him, the way the boy kept talking, too loud. He sat up and looked behind him. Everything was dark.

"Weird," the boy said.

"I guess so. Why don't we be a little quiet?"

"Weird. You never even *tried* it?"

"What?"

"Black Jack. You never even chewed it once?"

Someone up the trail hissed at them to shut up. The boy shook his head, put a finger to his lips, smiled, and lay back. Then a long blank silence. It lasted for perhaps an hour, maybe more, and then the boy was whistling again, softly at first but then louder, and Paul Berlin nudged him.

"Really weird," the solider whispered. "About Billy Boy. What Doc said, wasn't that the weirdest thing you ever heard? You ever hear of such a thing?"

"What?"

"What Doc said."

"No, I never did."

"Me neither." The boy was chewing again, and the smell now was licorice. The moon was a bit lower. "Me neither. I never heard once of no such thing. But Doc, he's a pretty smart cookie. Pretty darned smart."

"Is he?"

"You bet he is. When he says something, man, you know he's tellin' the truth. You *know* it." The soldier turned, rolling onto his stomach, and began to whistle, drumming with his fingers. Then he caught himself. "Dang it!" He gave his cheek a sharp whack. "Whistling again! I got to stop that dang whistling." He smiled and thumped his mouth. "But, sure enough, Doc's a smart one. He knows stuff. You wouldn't believe the stuff Doc knows. A lot. He knows a lot."

Paul Berlin nodded. The boy was talking too loud again.

"Well, you'll find out yourself. Doc knows his stuff." Sitting up, the boy shook his head. "A heart attack!" He made a funny face, filling his cheeks like balloons, then letting them deflate. "A heart attack! You hear Doc say that? A heart attack on the field of battle, isn't that what Doc said?"

"Yes," Paul Berlin whispered. He couldn't help giggling.

"Can you believe it? Billy Boy getting heart attacked? Scared to death?"

Paul Berlin giggled, he couldn't help it.

"Can you imagine it?"

"Yes," Paul Berlin whispered, and he imagined it clearly. He couldn't stop giggling.

"Geez!"

He giggled. He couldn't stop it, so he giggled, and he imagined it clearly. He imagined the medic's report. He imagined Billy's surprise. He giggled, imagining Billy's father opening the telegram: SORRY TO INFORM YOU THAT YOUR SON BILLY BOY WAS YESTERDAY SCARED TO DEATH IN ACTION IN THE REPUBLIC OF VIETNAM. Yes, he could imagine it clearly.

He giggled. He rolled onto his belly and pressed his face in the wet grass and giggled, he couldn't help it.

"Not so loud," the boy said. But Paul Berlin was shaking with the giggles: scared to death on the field of battle, and he couldn't help it.

"Not so loud."

But he was coughing with the giggles, he couldn't stop. Giggling and re-membering the hot afternoon, and poor Billy, how they'd been drinking Coke from bright aluminum cans, and how the men lined the cans up in a row and shot them full of practice holes, how funny it was and how dumb and how hot the day, and how they'd started on the march and how the war hadn't seemed so bad, and how a little while later Billy tripped the mine, and how it made a tinny little sound, unimportant, *poof*, that was all, just *poof*, and how Billy Boy stood there with his mouth open and grinning, sort of embarrassed and dumb-looking, how he just stood and stood there, looking down at where his foot had been, and then how he finally sat down, still grinning, not saying a word, his boot lying there with his foot still in it, just *poof*, nothing big or dramatic, and how hot and fine and clear the day had been.

"Hey," he heard the boy saying in the dark, "not so loud, okay?" But he kept giggling. He put his nose in the wet grass and he giggled, then he bit his arm, trying to stifle it, but remembering—"War's over, Billy," Doc Peret said, "that's a million-dollar wound."

"Hey, not so *loud*."

But Billy was holding the boot now. Unlacing it, trying to force it back on, except it was already on, and he kept trying to tie the boot and foot on, working with the laces, but it wouldn't go, and how everyone kept saying, "The war's over, man, be cool." And Billy couldn't get the boot on, because it was already on: He kept trying but it wouldn't go. Then he got scared. "Fuckin boot won't go on," he said. And he got scared. His face went pale and the veins in his arms and neck popped out, and he was yanking at the boot to get it on, and then he was crying. "Bullshit," the medic said, Doc Peret, but Billy boy kept bawling, tightening up, saying he was going to die, but the medic said, "Bullshit, that's a million-dollar wound you got there," but Billy went crazy, pulling at the boot with his foot still in it, crying, saying he was going to die. And even when Doc Peret stuck him with morphine, even then Billy kept crying and working at the boot.

"Shut up!" the soldier hissed, or seemed to, and the smell of licorice was all over him, and the smell made Paul Berlin giggle harder. His eyes stung. Giggling in the wet grass in the dark, he couldn't help it.

"Come on, man, be quiet."

But he couldn't stop. He heard the giggles in his stomach and tried to keep them there, but they were hard and hurting and he couldn't stop them, and he couldn't stop remembering how it was when Billy Boy Watkins died of fright on the field of battle.

Billy tugging away at the boot, rocking, and Doc Peret and two others hold-ing him. "You're okay, man," Doc Peret said, but Billy wasn't hearing it, and he kept getting tighter, making fists, squeezing his eyes shut and teeth scraping, everything tight and squeezing.

Afterward Doc Peret explained that Billy Boy really died of a heart attack, scared to death. "No lie," Doc said, " I seen it before. The wound wasn't what killed him, it was the heart attack. No lie." So they wrapped Billy in a plastic poncho, his eyes still squeezed shut to make wrinkles in his cheeks, and they carried him over the meadow to a dried-up paddy, and they threw out yellow smoke for the chopper, and they put him aboard, and then Doc wrapped the boot in a towel and placed it next to Billy, and that was how it happened. The chopper took Billy away. Later, Eddie Lazzutti, who loved to sing, remembered the song, and the jokes started, and Eddie sang *where have you gone, Billy Boy, Billy Boy, oh, where have you gone, charming Billy?* They sang until dark, marching to the sea.

Giggling, lying now on his back, Paul Berlin saw the moon move. He could not stop. Was it the moon? Or the clouds moving, making the moon seem to move? Or the boy's round face, pressing him, forcing out the giggles. "It wasn't so bad," he would tell his father. "I was a man. I saw it the first day, the very first day at the war, I saw all of it from the start, I learned it, and it wasn't so bad, and later on, later on it got better, later on, once I learned the tricks, later on it wasn't so bad." He couldn't stop.

The soldier was on top of him.

"Okay, man, *okay.*"

He saw the face then, clearly, for the first time.

"It's okay."

The face of the moon, and later the moon went under clouds, and the column was moving.

The boy helped him up.

"Okay?"

"Sure, okay."

The boy gave him a stick of gum. It was Black Jack, the precious stuff. "You'll do fine," Cacciato said. "You will. You got a terrific sense of humor."

Mental Cases

WILFRED OWEN

Who are these? Why sit they here in twilight?
Wherefore rock they, purgatorial shadows,
Drooping tongues from jaws that slob their relish,
Baring teeth that leer like skulls' teeth wicked?
Stroke on stroke of pain,—but what slow panic,
Gouged these chasms round their fretted sockets?
Ever from their hair and through their hands' palms
Misery swelters. Surely we have perished
Sleeping, and walk hell; but who these hellish?

—These are men whose minds the Dead have ravished.
Memory fingers in their hair of murders,
Multitudinous murders they once witnessed.
Wading sloughs of flesh these helpless wander,
Treading blood from lungs that had loved laughter.
Always they must see these things and hear them,
Batter of guns and shatter of flying muscles,
Carnage incomparable, and human squander
Rucked too thick for these men's extrication.

Therefore still their eyeballs shrink tormented
Back into their brains, because on their sense
Sunlight seems a bloodsmear; night comes blood-black;
Dawn breaks open like a wound that bleeds afresh.
—Thus their heads wear this hilarious, hideous,
Awful falseness of set-smiling corpses.
—Thus their hands are plucking at each other;
Picking at the rope-knots of their scourging;
Snatching after us who smote them, brother,
Pawing us who dealt them war and madness.

From Ceremony

LESLIE MARMON SILKO

TAYO DIDN'T SLEEP WELL that night. He tossed in the old iron bed, and the coiled springs kept squeaking even after he lay still again, calling up humid dreams of black night and loud voices rolling him over and over again like debris caught in a flood. Tonight the singing had come first, squeaking out of the iron bed, a man singing in Spanish, the melody of a familiar love song, two words again and again, "*Y volveré.*" Sometimes the Japanese voices came first, angry and loud, pushing the song far away, and then he could hear the shift in his dreaming, like a slight afternoon wind changing its direction, coming less and less from the south, moving into the west, and the voices would become Laguna voices, and he could hear Uncle Josiah calling to him, Josiah bringing him the fever medicine when he had been sick a long time ago. But before Josiah could come, the fever voices would drift and whirl and emerge again— Japanese soldiers shouting orders to him, suffocating damp voices that drifted out in the jungle steam, and he heard the women's voices then; they faded in and out until he was frantic because he thought the Laguna words were his mother's, but when he was about to make out the meaning of the words, the voice suddenly broke into a language he could not understand; and it was then that all the voices were drowned by the music—loud, loud music from a big juke box, its flashing red and blue lights pulling the darkness closer.

He lay there early in the morning and watched the high small window above the bed; dark gray gradually became lighter until it cast a white square on the opposite wall at dawn. He watched the room grow brighter then, as the square of light grew steadily warmer, more yellow with the climbing sun. He had not been able to sleep for a long time—for as long as all things had become tied together like colts in single file when he and Josiah had taken them to the mountain, with the halter rope of one colt tied to the tail of the colt ahead of it, and the lead colt's rope tied to the wide horn on Josiah's Mexican saddle. He could still see them now—the creamy sorrel, the bright red bay, and the gray roan— their slick summer coats reflecting the sunlight as it came up from behind the yellow mesas, shining on them, strung out behind Josiah's horse like an old-time pack train. He could get no rest as long as the memories were tangled with the present, tangled up like colored threads from old Grandma's wicker sewing basket when he was a child, and he had carried them outside to play and they had spilled out of his arms into the summer weeds and rolled away in all directions, and then he had hurried to pick them up before Auntie found him. He could feel it inside his skull—the tension of little threads being pulled and how it was with tangled things, things tied together, and as he tried to pull them apart and rewind them into their places, they snagged and tangled even more. So Tayo had to sweat through those nights when thoughts became entangled; he had to sweat to think of something that wasn't unraveled or tied in knots to the past—something that existed by itself, standing alone like a deer. And if he could hold that image of the deer in his mind long enough, his stomach might shiver less and let him sleep for a while. It worked as long as the deer was alone, as long as he could keep it a gray buck on an unrecognized hill; but if he did not hold it tight, it would spin away from him and become the deer he and Rocky had hunted. That memory would unwind into the last day when they had sat together, oiling their rifles in the jungle of some nameless Pacific island. While they used up the last of the oil in Rocky's pack, they talked about the deer that Rocky had hunted, and the corporal next to them shook his head, and kept saying he had dreamed the Japs would get them that day.

The humid air turned into sweat that had run down the corporal's face while he repeated his dream to them. That was the first time Tayo had realized that the man's skin was not much different from his own. The skin. He saw the skin of the corpses again and again, in ditches on either side of the long muddy road—skin that was stretched shiny and dark over bloated hands; even white men were darker after death. There was no difference when they were swollen and covered with flies. That had become the worst thing for Tayo: they looked too familiar even when they were alive. When the sergeant told them to kill all the Japanese soldiers lined up in front of the cave with their hands on their heads, Tayo could not pull the trigger. The fever made him shiver, and the sweat was stinging his eyes and he couldn't see clearly; in that instant he saw Josiah standing there; the face was dark from the sun, and the eyes were squinting as though he were about to smile at Tayo. So Tayo stood there, stiff with nausea, while they fired at the soldiers, and he watched his uncle fall, and he *knew* it was Josiah; and even after Rocky started shaking him by the shoulders and telling him to stop crying, it was *still* Josiah lying there. They forced medicine into Tayo's mouth, and Rocky pushed him toward the corpses and told him to look, look past the blood that was already dark like the jungle mud, with only flecks of bright red shimmering in it. Rocky made him look at the corpse and said, "Tayo, this is a *Jap!* This is a *Jap* uniform!" And then he rolled the body over with his boot and said, "Look, Tayo, look at the face," and that was when Tayo started screaming because it wasn't a Jap, it was Josiah, eyes shrinking back into the skull and all their shining black light glazed over by death.

The sergeant had called for a medic and somebody rolled up Tayo's sleeve; they told him to sleep, and the next day they all acted as though nothing had happened. They called it battle fatigue, and they said hallucinations were common with malarial fever.

Rocky had reasoned it out with him; it was impossible for the dead man to be Josiah, because Josiah was an old Laguna man, thousands of miles from the Philippine jungles and Japanese armies. "He's probably up on some mesa right now, chopping wood," Rocky said. He smiled and shook Tayo's shoulders. "Hey, I know you're homesick. But, Tayo, we're *supposed* to be here. This is what we're supposed to do."

Tayo nodded, slapped at the insects mechanically and staring straight ahead, past the smothering dampness of the green jungle leaves. He examined the facts and logic again and again, the way Rocky had explained it to him; the facts made what he had seen an impossibility. He felt the shivering then; it began at the tips of his fingers and pulsed into his arms. He shivered because all the facts, all the reasons made no difference any more; he could hear Rocky's words, and he could follow the logic of what Rocky said, but he could not feel anything except a swelling in his belly, a great swollen grief that was pushing into his throat.

He had to keep busy; he had to keep moving so that the sinews connected behind his eyes did not slip loose and spin his eyes to the interior of his skull where the scenes waited for him. He got out of the bed quickly while he could still see the square of yellow sunshine on the wall opposite the bed, and he pulled on his jeans and the scuffed brown boots he had worn before the war, and the red plaid western shirt old Grandma gave him the day he had come home after the war.

The air outside was still cool; it smelled like night dampness, faintly of rain. He washed his face in the steel-cold water of the iron trough by the windmill. The yellow striped cat purred and wrapped herself around his legs while he combed his hair. She ran ahead of him to the goat pen and shoved her head under his left arm when he knelt down to milk the black goat. He poured milk for her in the lid of an old enamel coffeepot, and then he opened the pen and let them run, greedy for the tender green shoots of tumbleweeds pushing through the sand. The kid was almost too big to nurse any more, and it knelt by the doe and hunched down to reach the tits, butting her to make the milk come faster, wiggling its tail violently until the nanny jumped away and turned on the kid, butting it away from her. The process of weaning had gone on like this for weeks, but the nanny was more intent on weeds than the lesson, and when Tayo left them, the kid goat was back at the tits, a little more careful this time.

The sun was climbing then, and it looked small in that empty morning sky. He knew he should eat, but he wasn't hungry any more. He sat down in the kitchen, at the small square table with the remains of a white candle melted to a nub on the lid of a coffee can; he wondered how long the candle had been there, he wondered if Josiah had been the one to light it last. He thought he would cry then, thinking of Josiah and how he had been here and touched all these things, sat in this chair. So he jerked his head away from the candle, and looked at the soot around the base of the coffeepot. He wouldn't waste firewood to heat up yesterday's coffee or maybe it was day-before-yesterday's coffee. He had lost track of the days there.

The drought years had returned again, as they had after the First World War and in the twenties, when he was a child and they had to haul water to the sheep in big wooden barrels in the old wagon. The windmill near the sheep camp had gone dry, so the gray mules pulled the wagon from the springs, moving slowly so that the water would not splash over the rims. He sat close to his uncle then, on the wagon seat, above the bony gray rumps of the mules. After they had dumped water for the sheep, they went to burn the spines from the cholla and prickly pear. They stood back by the wagon and watched the cows walk up to the cactus cautiously, sneezing at the smoldering ashes. The cows were patient while the scorched green pulp cooled, and then they brought out their wide spotted tongues and ate those strange remains because the hills were barren those years and only the cactus could grow.

Now there was no wagon or wooden barrels. One of the gray mules had eaten a poison weed near Acoma, and the other one was blind; it stayed close to the windmill at the ranch, grazing on the yellow rice grass that grew in the blow sand. It walked a skinny trail, winding in blind circles from the grass to the water trough, where it dipped its mouth in the water and let the water dribble out again, rinsing its mouth four or five times a day to make sure the water was still there. The dry air shrank the wooden staves of the barrels; they pulled loose, and now the rusty steel hoops were scattered on the ground behind the corral in the crazy patterns of some flashy Kiowa hoop dancer at the Gallup Ceremonials, throwing his hoops along the ground where he would hook and flip them into the air again and they would skim over his head and shoulders down to his dancing feet, like magic. Tayo stepped in one that was half buried in the reddish blow sand; he hooked an edge with the toe of his boot, and then he let it slip into the sand again.

The wind had blown since late February and it did not stop after April. They said it had been that way for the past six years while he was gone. And all this time they had watched the sky expectantly for the rainclouds to come. Now it was late May, and when Tayo went to the outhouse he left the door open wide, facing the dry empty hills and the light blue sky. He watched the sky over the distant Black Mountains the way Josiah had many years before, because sometimes when the rain finally came, it was from the southwest.

Jungle rain had no beginning or end; it grew like foliage from the sky, branching and arching to the earth, sometimes in solid thickets entangling the islands, and, other times, in tendrils of blue mist curling out of coastal clouds. The jungle breathed an eternal green that fevered men until they dripped sweat the way rubbery jungle leaves dripped the monsoon rain. It was there that Tayo began to understand what Josiah had said. Nothing was all good or all bad either; it all depended. Jungle rain lay suspended in the air, choking their lungs as they marched; it soaked into their boots until the skin on their toes peeled away dead and wounds turned green. This was not the rain he and Josiah had prayed for, this was not the green foliage they sought out in sandy canyons as a sign of a spring. When Tayo prayed on the long muddy road to the prison camp, it was for dry air, dry as a hundred years squeezed out of yellow sand, air to dry out the oozing wounds of Rocky's leg, to let the torn flesh and broken bones breathe, to clear the sweat that filled Rocky's eyes. It was that rain which filled the tire ruts and made the mud so deep that the corporal began to slip and fall with his end of the muddy blanket that held Rocky. Tayo hated this unending rain as if it were the jungle green rain and not the miles of marching or the Japanese grenade that was killing Rocky. He would blame the rain if the Japs saw how the corporal staggered; if they saw how weak Rocky had become, and came to crush his head with the butt of a rifle, then it would be the rain and the green all around that killed him.

Tayo talked to the corporal almost incessantly, walking behind him with his end of the blanket stretcher, telling him that it wasn't much farther now, and all down hill from there. He made a story for all of them, a story to give them strength. The words of the story poured out of his mouth as if they had substance, pebbles and stone extending to hold the corporal up, to keep his knees from buckling, to keep his hands from letting go of the blanket.

The sound of the rain got louder, pounding on the leaves, splashing into the ruts; it splattered on his head, and the sound echoed inside his skull. It streamed down his face and neck like jungle flies with crawling feet. He wanted to turn loose the blanket to wipe the rain away; he wanted to let go for only a moment. But as long as the corporal was still standing, still moving, they had to keep going. Then from somewhere, within the sound of the rain falling, he could hear it approaching like a summer flash flood, the rumble still faint and distant, floodwater boiling down a narrow canyon. He could smell the foaming flood water, stagnant and ripe with the rotting debris it carried past each village, sucking up their sewage, their waste, the dead animals. He tried to hold it back, but the wind swept down from the green coastal mountains, whipping the rain into gray waves that blinded him. The corporal fell, jerking the ends of the blanket from his hands, and he felt Rocky's foot brush past his own leg. He slid to his knees, trying to find the ends of the blanket again, and he started repeating "Goddamn, goddamn!"; it flooded out of the last warm core in his chest and echoed inside his head. He damned the rain until the words were a chant, and he sang it while he crawled through the mud to find the corporal and get him up before the Japanese saw them. He wanted the words to make a cloudless blue sky, pale with a summer sun pressing across wide and empty horizons. The words gathered inside him and gave him strength. He pulled on the corporal's arm; he lifted him to his knees and all the time he could hear his own voice praying against the rain.

It was summertime
and Iktoa'ak'o'ya-Reed Woman
was always taking a bath.
She spent all day long
sitting in the river
splashing down
the summer rain.

But her sister
Corn Woman
worked hard all day
sweating in the sun
getting sore hands
in the corn field.
Corn Woman got tired of that
she got angry
she scolded
her sister
for bathing all day long.

Iktoa'ak'o'ya-Reed Woman
went away then
she went back
to the original place
down below.

And there was no more rain then.
Everything dried up
all the plants
the corn
the beans
they all dried up
and started blowing away
in the wind.

The people and the animals
were thirsty.
They were starving.

So he had prayed the rain away, and for the sixth year it was dry; the grass turned yellow and it did not grow. Wherever he looked, Tayo could see the consequences of his praying; the gray mule grew gaunt, and the goat and kid had to wander farther and farther each day to find weeds or dry shrubs to eat. In the evenings they waited for him, chewing their cuds by the shed door, and the mule stood by the gate with blind marble eyes. He threw them a little dusty hay and sprinkled some cracked corn over it. The nanny crowded the kid away from the corn. The mule whinnied and leaned against the sagging gate; Tayo reached into the coffee can and he held some corn under the quivering lips. When the corn was gone, the mule licked for the salt taste on his hand; the tongue was rough and wet, but it was also warm and precise across his fingers. Tayo looked at the long white hairs growing out of the lips like antennas, and he got the choking in his throat again, and he cried for all of them, and for what he had done.

From Mrs. Dalloway

VIRGINIA WOOLF

SEPTIMUS WAS ONE of the first to volunteer. He went to France to save an England which consisted almost entirely of Shakespeare's plays and Miss Isabel Pole in a green dress walking in a square. There in the trenches the change which Mr. Brewer desired when he advised football was produced instantly; he developed manliness; he was promoted; he drew the attention, indeed the affection of his officer, Evans by name. It was a case of two dogs playing on a hearth-rug; one worrying a paper screw, snarling, snapping, giving a pinch, now and then, at the old dog's ear; the other lying somnolent, blinking at the fire, raising a paw, turning and growling good-temperedly. They had to be together, share with each other, fight with each other, quarrel with each other. But when Evans (Rezia who had only seen him once called him "a quiet man," a sturdy red-haired man, undemonstrative in the company of women), when Evans was killed, just before the Armistice, in Italy, Septimus, far from showing any emotion or recognizing that here was the end of a friendship, congratulated himself upon feeling very little and very reasonably. The War had taught him. It was sublime. He had gone through the whole show, friendship, European War, death, had won promotion, was still under thirty and was bound to survive. He was right there. The last shells missed him. He watched them explode with indifference. When peace came he was in Milan, billeted in the house of an innkeeper with a courtyard, flowers in tubs, little tables in the open, daughters making hats, and to Lucrezia, the younger daughter, he became engaged one evening when the panic was on him—that he could not feel.

For now that it was all over, truce signed, and the dead buried, he had, especially in the evening, these sudden thunder-claps of fear. He could not feel. As he opened the door of the room where the Italian girls sat making hats, he could see them; could hear them; they were rubbing wires among coloured beads in saucers; they were turning buckram shapes this way and that; the table was all strewn with feathers, spangles, silks, ribbons; scissors were rapping on the table; but something failed him; he could not feel. Still, scissors rapping, girls laughing, hats being made protected him; he was assured of safety; he had a refuge. But he could not sit there all night. There were moments of waking in the early morning. The bed was falling; he was falling. Oh for the scissors and the lamplight and the buckram shapes! He asked Lucrezia to marry him, the younger of the two, the gay, the frivolous, with those little artist's fingers that she would hold up and say "It is all in them." Silk, feathers, what not were alive to them.

"It is the hat that matters most," she would say, when they walked out together. Every hat that passed, she would examine; and the cloak and the dress and the way the woman held herself. Ill-dressing, over-dressing she stigmatized, not savagely, rather with impatient movements of the hands, like those of a painter who puts from him some obvious well-meant glaring imposture; and then, generously, but always critically, she would welcome a shopgirl who had turned her little bit of stuff gallantly, or praise, wholly, with enthusiastic and professional understanding, a French lady descending from her carriage, in chinchilla, robes, pearls.

"Beautiful!" she would murmur, nudging Septimus, that he might see. But beauty was behind a pane of glass. Even taste (Rezia liked ices, chocolates, sweet things) had no relish to him. He put down his cup on the little marble table. He looked at people outside; happy they seemed, collecting in the middle of the street, shouting, laughing, squabbling over nothing. But he could not taste, he could not feel. In the teashop among the tables and the chattering waiters the appalling fear came over him—he could not feel. He could reason; he could read, Dante for example, quite easily ("Septimus, do put down your book," said Rezia, gently shutting the *Inferno*), he could add up his bill; his brain was perfect; it must be the fault of the world then—that he could not feel.

"The English are so silent," Rezia said. She liked it, she said. She respected these Englishmen, and wanted to see London, and the English horses, and the tailormade suits, and could remember hearing how wonderful the shops were, from an Aunt who had married and lived in Soho.

It might be possible, Septimus thought, looking at England from the train window, as they left Newhaven; it might be possible that the world itself is without meaning.

At the office they advanced him to a post of considerable responsibility. They were proud of him; he had won crosses. "You have done your duty; it is up to us—" began Mr. Brewer; and could not finish, so pleasurable was his emotion. They took admirable lodgings off the Tottenham Court Road.

Here he opened Shakespeare once more. That boy's business of the intoxication of language—*Antony and Cleopatra*—had shriveled utterly. How Shakespeare loathed humanity—the putting on of clothes, the getting of children, the sordidity of the mouth and the belly! This was now revealed to Septimus; the message hidden in the beauty of words. The secret signal which one generation passes, under disguise, to the next is loathing, hatred, despair. Dante the same. Aeschylus (translated) the same. There Rezia sat at the table trimming hats. She trimmed hats for Mrs. Filmer's friends; she trimmed hats by the hour. She looked pale, mysterious, like a lily, drowned, under water, he thought.

"The English are so serious," she would say, putting her arms round Septimus, her cheek against his.

Love between man and woman was repulsive to Shakespeare. The business of copulation was filth to him before the end. But, Rezia said, she must have children. They had been married five years.

They went to the Tower together; to the Victoria and Albert museum; stood in the crowd to see the King open Parliament. And there were the shops—hat shops, dress shops, shops with leather bags in the window, where she would stand staring. But she must have a boy.

She must have a son like Septimus, she said. But nobody could be like Septimus; so gentle; so serious; so clever. Could she not read Shakespeare too? Was Shakespeare a difficult author? she asked.

One cannot bring children into a world like this. One cannot perpetuate suffering, or increase the breed of these lustful animals, who have no lasting emotions, but only whims and vanities, eddying them now this way, now that.

He watched her snip, shape, as one watches a bird hop, flit in the grass, without daring to move a finger. For the truth is (let her ignore it) that human beings have neither kindness, nor faith, nor charity beyond what serves to increase the pleasure of the moment. They hunt in packs. Their packs scour the desert and vanish screaming into the wilderness. They desert the fallen. They are plastered over with grimaces. There was Brewer at the office, with his waxed moustache, coral tie-pin, white slip, and pleasurable emotions—all coldness and clamminess within,—his geraniums ruined in the War—his cook's nerves destroyed; or Amelia What's-her-name, handing round cups of tea punctually at five—a leering, sneering obscene little harpy; and the Toms and Berties in their starched shirt fronts oozing thick drops of vice. They never saw him drawing pictures of them naked at their antics in his notebook. In the street, vans roared past him; brutality blared out on placards; men were trapped in mines; women burnt alive; and once a maimed file of lunatics being exercised or displayed for the diversion of the populace (who laughed aloud), ambled and nodded and grinned past him, in the Tottenham Court Road, each half apologetically, yet triumphantly, inflicting his hopeless woe. And would *he* go mad?

At tea Rezia told him that Mrs. Filmer's daughter was expecting a baby. *She* could not grow old and have no children! She was very lonely, she was very unhappy! She cried for the first time since they were married. Far away he heard her sobbing; he heard it accurately, he noticed it distinctly; he compared it to a piston thumping. But he felt nothing.

His wife was crying, and he felt nothing; only each time she sobbed in this profound, this silent, this hopeless way, he descended another step into the pit.

At last, with a melodramatic gesture which he assumed mechanically and with complete consciousness of its insincerity, he dropped his head on his hands. Now he had surrendered; now other people must help him. People must be sent for. He gave in.

Nothing could rouse him. Rezia put him to bed. She sent for a doctor—Mrs. Filmer's Dr. Holmes. Dr. Holmes examined him. There was nothing whatever the matter, said Dr. Holmes. Oh, what a relief! What a kind man, what a good man! thought Rezia. When he felt like that he went to the Music Hall, said Dr. Holmes. He took a day off with his wife and played golf. Why not try two tabloids of bromide dissolved in a glass of water at bedtime? These old Bloomsbury houses, said Dr. Holmes, tapping the wall, are often full of very fine paneling, which the landlords have the folly to paper over. Only the other day, visiting a patient, Sir Somebody Something in Bedford Square—

So there was no excuse; nothing whatever the matter, except the sin for which human nature had condemned him to death; that he did not feel. He had not cared when Evans was killed; that was worst; but all the other crimes raised their heads and shook their fingers and jeered and sneered over the rail of the bed in the early hours of the morning at the prostrate body which lay realizing its degradation; how he had married his wife without loving her; had lied to her; seduced her; outraged Miss Isabel Pole, and was so pocked and marked with vice that women shuddered when they saw him in the street. The verdict of human nature on such a wretch was death.

Dr. Holmes came again. Large, fresh coloured, handsome, flicking his boots, looking in the glass, he brushed it all aside—headaches, sleeplessness, fears, dreams—nerve symptoms and nothing more, he said. If Dr. Holmes found himself even half a pound below eleven stone six, he asked his wife for another plate of porridge at breakfast. (Rezia would learn to cook porridge.) But, he continued, health is largely a matter in our own control. Throw yourself into outside interests; take up some hobby. He opened Shakespeare—*Antony and Cleopatra*; pushed Shakespeare aside. Some hobby, said Dr. Holmes, for did he not owe his own excellent health (and he worked as hard as any man in London) to the fact that he could always switch off from his patients on to old furniture? And what a very pretty comb, if he might say so, Mrs. Warren Smith was wearing!

When the damned fool came again, Septimus refused to see him. Did he indeed? said Dr. Holmes, smiling agreeably. Really he had to give that charming little lady, Mrs. Smith, a friendly push before he could get past her into her husband's bedroom.

"So you're in a funk," he said agreeably, sitting down by his patient's side. He had actually talked of killing himself to his wife, quite a girl, a foreigner, wasn't she? Didn't that give her a very odd idea of English husbands? Didn't one owe perhaps a duty to one's wife? Wouldn't it be better to do something instead of lying in bed? For he had had forty years' experience behind him; and Septimus could take Dr. Holmes's word for it—there was nothing whatever the matter with him. And next time Dr. Holmes came he hoped to find Smith out of bed and not making that charming little lady his wife anxious about him.

Human nature, in short, was on him—the repulsive brute, with the blood-red nostrils. Holmes was on him. Dr. Holmes came quite regularly every day. Once you stumble, Septimus wrote on the back of a postcard, human nature is on you. Holmes is on you. Their only chance was to escape, without letting Holmes know; to Italy—anywhere, anywhere, away from Dr. Holmes.

But Rezia could not understand him. Dr. Holmes was such a kind man. He was so interested in Septimus. He only wanted to help them, he said. He had four little children and he had asked her to tea, she told Septimus.

So he was deserted. The whole world was clamouring: Kill yourself, kill yourself, for our sakes. But why should he kill himself for their sakes? Food was pleasant; the sun hot; and this killing oneself, how does one set about it, with a table knife, uglily, with floods of blood,—by sucking a gaspipe? He was too weak; he could scarcely raise his hand. Besides, now that he was quite alone, condemned, deserted as those who are about to die are alone, there was a luxury in it, an isolation full of sublimity; a freedom which the attached can never know. Holmes had won of course; the brute with the red nostrils had won. But even Holmes himself could not touch this last relic straying on the edge of the world, this outcast, who gazed back at the inhabited regions, who lay, like a drowned sailor, on the shore of the world.

It was at that moment (Rezia gone shopping) that the great revelation took place. A voice spoke from behind the screen. Evans was speaking. The dead were with him.

"Evans, Evans!" he cried.

Mr. Smith was talking aloud to himself, Agnes the servant girl cried to Mrs. Filmer in the kitchen. "Evans, Evans," he had said as she brought in the tray. She jumped, she did. She scuttled downstairs.

And Rezia came in, with her flowers, and walked across the room, and put the roses in a vase, upon which the sun struck directly, and it went laughing, leaping round the room.

She had had to buy the roses, Rezia said, from a poor man in the street. But they were almost dead already, she said, arranging the roses.

So there was a man outside; Evans presumably; and the roses, which Rezia said were half dead, had been picked by him in the fields of Greece. "Communication is health; communication is happiness, communication—" he muttered.

"What are you saying, Septimus?" Rezia asked, wild with terror, for he was talking to himself.

She sent Agnes running for Dr. Holmes. Her husband, she said, was mad. He scarcely knew her.

"You brute! You brute!" cried Septimus, seeing human nature, that is Dr. Holmes, enter the room.

"Now what's all this about?" said Dr. Holmes in the most amiable way in the world. "Talking nonsense to frighten your wife?" But he would give him something to make him sleep. And if they were rich people, said Dr. Holmes, looking ironically round the room, by all means let them go to Harley Street; if they had no confidence in him, said Dr. Holmes, looking not quite so kind.

It was precisely twelve o'clock; twelve by Big Ben; whose stroke was wafted over the northern part of London; blent with that of other clocks, mixed in a thin ethereal way with the clouds and wisps of smoke, and died up there among the seagulls—twelve o'clock struck as Clarissa Dalloway laid her green dress on her bed, and the Warren Smiths walked down Harley Street. Twelve was the hour of their appointment. Probably, Rezia thought, that was Sir William Bradshaw's house with the grey motor car in front of it. The leaden circles dissolved in the air.

Indeed it was—Sir William Bradshaw's motor car; low, powerful, grey with plain initials interlocked on the panel, as if the pomps of heraldry were incongruous, this man being the ghostly helper, the priest of science; and, as the motor car was grey, so to match its sober suavity, grey furs, silver grey rugs were heaped in it, to keep her ladyship warm while she waited. For often Sir William would travel sixty miles or more down into the country to visit the rich, the afflicted, who could afford the very large fee which Sir William very properly charged for his advice. Her ladyship waited with the rugs about her knees an hour or more, leaning back, thinking sometimes of the patient, sometimes, excusably, of the wall of gold, mounting minute by minute while she waited; the wall of gold that was mounting between them and all shifts and anxieties (she had borne them bravely; they had had their struggles) until she felt wedged on a calm ocean, where only spice winds blow; respected, admired, envied, with scarcely anything left to wish for, though she regretted her stoutness; large dinner-parties every Thursday night to the profession; an occasional bazaar to be opened; Royalty greeted; too little time, alas, with her husband, whose work grew and grew; a boy doing well at Eton; she would have liked a daughter too; interests she had, however, in plenty; child welfare; the aftercare of the epileptic, and photography, so that if there was a church build- ing, or a church decaying, she bribed the sexton, got the key and took photo- graphs, which were scarcely to be distinguished from the work of profes- sionals, while she waited.

Sir William himself was no longer young. He had worked very hard; he had won his position by sheer ability (being the son of a shopkeeper); loved his profession; made a fine figurehead at ceremonies and spoke well—all of which had by the time he was knighted given him a heavy look, a weary look (the stream of patients being so incessant, the responsibilities and privileges of his profession so onerous), which weariness, together with his grey hairs, in- creased the extraordinary distinction of his presence and gave him the repu- tation (of the utmost importance in dealing with nerve cases) not merely of lightning skill, and almost infallible accuracy in diagnosis but of sympathy; tact; understanding of the human soul. He could see the first moment they came into the room (the Warren Smiths they were called); he was certain di- rectly he saw the man; it was a case of extreme gravity. It was a case of complete breakdown—complete physical and nervous breakdown, with every symptom in an advanced stage, he ascertained in two or three minutes (writing answers to questions, murmured discreetly, on a pink card).

How long had Dr. Holmes been attending him?

Six weeks.

Prescribed a little bromide? Said there was nothing the matter? Ah yes (those general practitioners! thought Sir William. It took half his time to undo their blunders. Some were irreparable).

"You served with great distinction in the War?"

The patient repeated the word "war" interrogatively.

He was attaching meanings to words of a symbolical kind. A serious symp- tom, to be noted on the card.

"The War?" the patient asked. The European War—that little shindy of schoolboys with gunpowder? Had he served with distinction? He really forgot. In the War itself he had failed.

"Yes, he served with the greatest distinction," Rezia assured the doctor; "he was promoted."

"And they have the very highest opinion of you at your office?" Sir William murmured, glancing at Mr. Brewer's very generously worded letter. "So that you have nothing to worry you, no financial anxiety, nothing?"

He had committed an appalling crime and been condemned to death by human nature.

"I have—I have," he began, "committed a crime—"

"He has done nothing wrong whatever," Rezia assured the doctor. If Mr. Smith would wait, said Sir William, he would speak to Mrs. Smith in the next room. Her husband was very seriously ill, Sir William said. Did he threaten to kill himself?

Oh, he did, she cried. But he did not mean it, she said. Of course not. It was merely a question of rest, said Sir William; of rest, rest, rest; a long rest in bed. There was a delightful home down in the country where her husband would be perfectly looked after. Away from her? she asked. Unfortunately, yes; the people we care for most are not good for us when we are ill. But he was not mad, was he? Sir William said he never spoke of "madness"; he called it not having a sense of proportion. But her husband did not like doctors. He would refuse to go there. Shortly and kindly Sir William explained to her the state of the case. He had threatened to kill himself. There was no alternative. It was a question of law. He would lie in bed in a beautiful house in the country. The nurses were admirable. Sir William would visit him once a week. If Mrs. Warren Smith was quite sure she had no more questions to ask—he never hurried his patients—they would return to her husband. She had nothing more to ask—not of Sir William.

So they returned to the most exalted of mankind; the criminal who faced his judges; the victim exposed on the heights; the fugitive; the drowned sailor; the poet of the immortal ode; the Lord who had gone from life to death; to Septimus Warren Smith, who sat in the arm-chair under the skylight staring at a photograph of Lady Bradshaw in Court dress, muttering messages about beauty.

"We have had our little talk," said Sir William.

"He says you are very, very ill," Rezia cried.

"We have been arranging that you should go into a home," said Sir William.

"One of Holmes's homes?" sneered Septimus.

The fellow made a distasteful impression. For there was in Sir William, whose father had been a tradesman, a natural respect for breeding and clothing, which shabbiness nettled; again, more profoundly, there was in Sir William, who had never had time for reading, a grudge, deeply buried, against cultivated people who came into his room and intimated that doctors, whose profession is a constant strain upon all the highest faculties, are not educated men.

"One of *my* homes, Mr. Warren Smith," he said, "where we will teach you to rest."

And there was just one thing more.

He was quite certain that when Mr. Warren Smith was well he was the last man in the world to frighten his wife. But he had talked of killing himself.

"We all have our moments of depression," said Sir William.

Once you fall, Septimus repeated to himself, human nature is on you. Holmes and Bradshaw are on you. They scour the desert. They fly screaming into the wilderness. The rack and the thumbscrew are applied. Human nature is remorseless.

"Impulses came upon him sometimes?" Sir William asked, with his pencil on a pink card.

That was his own affair, said Septimus.

"Nobody lives for himself alone," said Sir William, glancing at the photograph of his wife in Court dress.

"And you have a brilliant career before you," said Sir William. There was Mr. Brewer's letter on the table. "An exceptionally brilliant career."

But if he confessed? If he communicated? Would they let him off then, his torturers?

"I—I—" he stammered.

But what was his crime? He could not remember it.

"Yes?" Sir William encouraged him. (But it was growing late.)

Love, trees, there is no crime—what was his message?

He could not remember it.

"I—I—" Septimus stammered.

"Try to think as little about yourself as possible," said Sir William kindly. Really, he was not fit to be about.

Was there anything else they wished to ask him? Sir William would make all arrangements (he murmured to Rezia) and he would let her know between five and six that evening he murmured.

"Trust everything to me," he said, and dismissed them.

Never, never had Rezia felt such agony in her life! She had asked for help and been deserted! He had failed them! Sir William Bradshaw was not a nice man.

The upkeep of that motor car alone must cost him quite a lot, said Septimus, when they got out into the street.

She clung to his arm. They had been deserted.

But what more did she want?

To his patients he gave three-quarters of an hour; and if in this exacting science which has to do with what, after all, we know nothing about— the nervous system, the human brain—a doctor loses his sense of proportion, as a doctor he fails. Health we must have; and health is proportion; so that when a man comes into your room and says he is Christ (a common delusion), and has a message, as they mostly have, and threatens, as they often do, to kill himself, you invoke proportion; order rest in bed; rest in solitude; silence and rest; rest without friends, without books, without messages; six months' rest; until a man who went in weighing seven stone six comes out weighing twelve.

Proportion, divine proportion, Sir William's goddess, was acquired by Sir William walking hospitals, catching salmon, begetting one son in Harley Street by Lady Bradshaw, who caught salmon herself and took photographs scarcely to be distinguished from the work of professionals. Worshiping proportion, Sir William not only prospered himself but made England prosper, secluded her lunatics, forbade childbirth, penalized her despair, made it impossible for the unfit to propagate their views until they, too, shared his sense of proportion—his, if they were men, Lady Bradshaw's if they were women (she embroidered, knitted, spent four nights out of seven at home with her son), so that not only did his colleagues respect him, his subordinates fear him, but the friends and relations of his patients felt for him the keenest gratitude for insisting that these prophetic Christs and Christesses, who prophesied the end of the world, or the advent of God, should drink milk in bed, as Sir William ordered; Sir William with his thirty years' experience of these kinds of cases, and his infallible instinct, this is madness, this sense; in fact, his sense of proportion.

But Proportion has a sister, less smiling, more formidable, a Goddess even now engaged—in the heat and sands of India, the mud and swamp of Africa, the purlieus of London, wherever in short the climate or the devil tempts men to fall from the true belief which is her own—is even now engaged in dashing down shrines, smashing idols, and setting up in their place her own stern countenance. Conversion is her name and she feasts on the wills of the weakly, loving to impress, to impose, adoring her own features stamped on the face of the populace. At Hyde Park Corner on a tub she stands preaching; shrouds herself in white and walks penitentially disguised as brotherly love through factories and parliaments; offers help, but desires power; smites out of her way roughly the dissentient, or dissatisfied; bestows her blessing on those who, looking upward, catch submissively from her eyes the light of their own. This lady too (Rezia Warren Smith divined it) had her dwelling in Sir William's heart, though concealed, as she mostly is, under some plausible disguise; some venerable name; love, duty, self sacrifice. How he would work—how toil to raise funds, propagate reforms, initiate institutions! But conversion, fastidious Goddess, loves blood better than brick, and feasts most subtly on the human will. For example, Lady Bradshaw. Fifteen years ago she had gone under. It was nothing you could put your finger on; there had been no scene, no snap; only the slow sinking, water-logged, of her will into his. Sweet was her smile, swift her submission; dinner in Harley Street, numbering eight or nine courses, feeding ten or fifteen guests of the professional classes, was smooth and urbane. Only as the evening wore on a very slight dullness, or uneasiness perhaps, a nervous twitch, fumble, stumble and confusion indicated, what it was really painful to believe—that the poor lady lied. Once, long ago, she had caught salmon freely: now, quick to minister to the craving which lit her husband's eye so oilily for dominion, for power, she cramped, squeezed, pared, pruned, drew back, peeped through; so that without knowing precisely what made the evening disagreeable, and caused this pressure on the top of the head (which might well be imputed to the professional conversation, or the fatigue of a great doctor whose life, Lady Bradshaw said, "is not his own but his patients'") disagreeable it was: so that guests, when the clock struck ten, breathed in the air of Harley Street even with rapture; which relief, however, was denied to his patients.

There in the grey room, with the pictures on the wall, and the valuable furniture, under the ground glass skylight, they learnt the extent of their transgressions; huddled up in arm-chairs, they watched him go through, for their benefit, a curious exercise with the arms, which he shot out, brought sharply back to his hip, to prove (if the patient was obstinate) that Sir William was master of his own actions, which the patient was not. There some weakly broke down; sobbed, submitted; others, inspired by Heaven knows what intemperate madness, called Sir William to his face a damnable humbug; questioned, even more impiously, life itself. Why live? they demanded. Sir William replied that life was good. Certainly Lady Bradshaw in ostrich feathers hung over the mantelpiece, and as for his income it was quite twelve thousand a year. But to us, they protested, life has given no such bounty. He acquiesced. They lacked a sense of proportion. And perhaps, after all, there is no God? He shrugged his shoulders. In short, this living or not living is an affair of our own? But there they were mistaken. Sir William had a friend in Surrey where they taught, what Sir William frankly admitted was a difficult art—a sense of proportion. There were, moreover, family affection; honour; courage; and a brilliant career. All of these had in Sir William a resolute champion. If they failed him, he had to support police and the good of society, which, he remarked very quietly, would take care, down in Surrey, that these unsocial impulses, bred more than anything by the lack of good blood, were held in control. And then stole out from her hiding-place and mounted her throne that Goddess whose lust is to override opposition, to stamp indelibly in the sanctuaries of others the image of herself. Naked, defenseless, the exhausted, the friendless received the impress of Sir William's will. He swooped; he devoured. He shut people up. It was this combination of decision and humanity that endeared Sir William so greatly to the relations of his victims.

But Rezia Warren Smith cried, walking down Harley Street, that she did not like that man.

Shredding and slicing, dividing and subdividing, the clocks of Harley Street nibbled at the June day, counseled submission, upheld authority, and pointed out in chorus the supreme advantages of a sense of proportion, until the mound of time was so far diminished that a commercial clock, suspended above a shop in Oxford Street, announced, genially and fraternally, as if it were a pleasure to Messrs. Rigby and Lowndes to give the information gratis, that it was half-past one.

Men & Mental Disorders

Panic

PHILIP BOOTH

It is to be out
of familiar walls
with no place left
but the Halfway
House far up
the block: it is,
this first after-
noon, to carefully
ask your new self
for a walk beyond
the drugstore around
the block, but then
to have to refuse;
it is to remember
how trees grow out
of the sidewalk, to
figure how this time
to face him: the one
with hair like old vines,
who steps out of
nowhere, trying to
take you over, back
where he always
comes from; it is
having moved here
instead: here to
sleep, to learn
to get up: it is,

at supper the always
first night, to
try to ask for
the salt. And having it
passed, it's to weep.

King of the Bingo Game

RALPH ELLISON

THE WOMAN in front of him was eating roasted peanuts that smelled so good that he could barely contain his hunger. He could not even sleep and wished they'd hurry and begin the bingo game. There, on his right, two fellows were drinking wine out of a bottle wrapped in a paper bag, and he could hear soft gurgling in the dark. His stomach gave a low, gnawing growl. "If this was down South," he thought, "all I'd have to do is lean over and say, 'Lady, gimme a few of those peanuts, please ma'm,' and she'd pass me the bag and never think nothing of it." Or he could ask the fellows for a drink in the same way. Folks down South stuck together that way; they didn't even have to know you. But up here it was different. Ask somebody for something, and they'd think you were crazy. Well, I ain't crazy. I'm just broke, 'cause I got no birth certificate to get a job, and Laura 'bout to die 'cause we got no money for a doctor. But I ain't crazy. And yet a pinpoint of doubt was focused in his mind as he glanced toward the screen and saw the hero stealthily entering a dark room and sending the beam of a flashlight along a wall of bookcases. This is where he finds the trapdoor, he remembered. The man would pass abruptly through the wall and find the girl tied to a bed, her legs and arms spread wide, and her clothing torn to rags. He laughed softly to himself. He had seen the picture three times, and this was one of the best scenes.

On his right the fellow whispered wide-eyed to his companion, "Man, look a-yonder!"

"Damn!"

"Wouldn't I like to have her tied up like that . . ."

"Hey! That fool's letting her loose!"

"Aw, man, he loves her."

"Love or no love!"

The man moved impatiently beside him, and he tried to involve himself in the scene. But Laura was on his mind. Tiring quickly of watching the picture he looked back to where the white beam filtered from the projection room above the balcony. It started small and grew large, specks of dust dancing in its whiteness as it reached the screen. It was strange how the beam always landed right on the screen and didn't mess up and fall somewhere else. But they had it all fixed. Everything was fixed. Now suppose when they showed that girl with her dress torn the girl started taking off the rest of her clothes, and when the guy came in he didn't untie her but kept her there and went to taking off his own clothes? *That* would be something to see. If a picture got out of hand like that those guys up there would go nuts. Yeah, and there'd be so many folks in here you couldn't find a seat for nine months! A strange sensation played over his skin. He shuddered. Yesterday he'd seen a bedbug on a woman's neck as they walked out into the bright street. But exploring his thigh through a hole in his pocket he found only goose pimples and old scars.

The bottle gurgled again. He closed his eyes. Now a dreamy music was accompanying the film and train whistles were sounding in the distance, and he was a boy again walking along a railroad trestle down South, and seeing the train coming, and running back as fast as he could go, and hearing the whistle blowing, and getting off the trestle to solid ground just in time, with the earth trembling beneath his feet, and feeling relieved as he ran down the cinder-strewn embankment onto the highway, and looking back and seeing with terror that the train had left the track and was following him right down the middle of the street, and all the white people laughing as he ran screaming...

"Wake up there, buddy! What the hell do you mean hollering like that? Can't you see we trying to enjoy this here picture?"

He stared at the man with gratitude.

"I'm sorry, old man," he said. "I musta been dreaming."

"Well, here, have a drink. And don't be making no noise like that, damn!"

His hands trembled as he tilted his head. It was not wine, but whiskey. Cold rye whiskey. He took a deep swoller, decided it was better not to take another, and handed the bottle back to its owner.

"Thanks, old man," he said.

Now he felt the cold whiskey breaking a warm path straight through the middle of him, growing hotter and sharper as it moved. He had not eaten all day, and it made him light-headed. The smell of the peanuts stabbed him like a knife, and he got up and found a seat in the middle aisle. But no sooner did he sit than he saw a row of intense-faced young girls, and got up again, thinking, "You chicks musta been Lindy-hopping somewhere." He found a seat several rows ahead as the lights came on, and he saw the screen disappear behind a heavy red and gold curtain; then the curtain rising, and the man with the microphone and a uniformed attendant coming on the stage.

He felt for his bingo cards, smiling. The guy at the door wouldn't like it if he knew about his having *five* cards: Well, not everyone played the bingo game; and even with five cards he didn't have much of a chance. For Laura, though, he had to have faith. He studied the cards, each with its different numerals, punching the free center hole in each and spreading them neatly across his lap; and when the lights faded he sat slouched in his seat so that he could look from his cards to the bingo wheel with but a quick shifting of his eyes.

Ahead, at the end of the darkness, the man with the microphone was pressing a button attached to a long cord and spinning the bingo wheel and calling out the number each time the wheel came to rest. And each time the voice rang out his finger raced over the cards for the number. With five cards he had to move fast. He became nervous; there were too many cards, and the man went too fast with his grating voice. Perhaps he should just select one and throw the others away. But he was afraid. He became warm. Wonder how much Laura's doctor would cost? Damn that, watch the cards! And with despair he heard the man call three in a row which he missed on all five cards. This way he'd never win . . .

When he saw the row of holes punched across the third card, he sat paralyzed and heard the man call three more numbers before he stumbled forward, screaming,

"Bingo! Bingo!"

"Let that fool up there," someone called.

"Get up there, man!"

He stumbled down the aisle and up the steps to the stage into a light so sharp and bright that for a moment it blinded him, and he felt that he had moved into the spell of some strange, mysterious power. Yet it was as familiar as the sun, and he knew it was the perfectly familiar bingo.

The man with the microphone was saying something to the audience as he held out his card. A cold light flashed from the man's finger as the card left his hand. His knees trembled. The man stepped closer, checking the card against the numbers chalked on the board. Suppose he had made a mistake? The pomade on the man's hair made him feel faint, and he backed away. But the man was checking the card over the microphone now, and he had to stay. He stood tense, listening.

"Under the O, forty-four," the man chanted. "Under the I, seven. Under the G, three. Under the B, ninety-six. Under the N, thirteen!"

His breath came easier as the man smiled at the audience.

"Yessir, ladies and gentlemen, he's one of the chosen people!"

The audience rippled with laughter and applause.

"Step right up to the front of the stage."

He moved slowly forward, wishing that the light was not so bright.

"To win tonight's jackpot of $36.90 the wheel must stop between the double zero, understand?"

He nodded, knowing the ritual from the many days and nights he had watched the winners march across the stage to press the button that controlled the spinning wheel and receive the prizes. And now he followed the instructions as though he'd crossed the slippery stage a million prize-winning times.

The man was making some kind of a joke, and he nodded vacantly. So tense had he become that he felt a sudden desire to cry and shook it away. He felt vaguely that his whole life was determined by the bingo wheel; not only that which would happen now that he was at last before it, but all that had gone before, since his birth, and his mother's birth and the birth of his father. It had always been there, even though he had not been aware of it, handing out the unlucky cards and numbers of his days. The feeling persisted, and he started quickly away. I better get down from here before I make a fool of myself, he thought.

"Here, boy," the man called. "You haven't started yet."

Someone laughed as he went hesitantly back.

"Are you all reet?"

He grinned at the man's jive talk, but no words would come, and he knew it was not a convincing grin. For suddenly he knew that he stood on the slippery brink of some terrible embarrassment.

"Where are you from, boy?" the man asked.

"Down South."

"He's from down South, ladies and gentlemen," the man said. "Where from? Speak right into the mike."

"Rocky Mont," he said. "Rock' Mont, North Car'lina."

"So you decided to come down off that mountain to the U.S.," the man laughed. He felt that the man was making a fool of him, but then something cold was placed in his hand, and the lights were no longer behind him.

Standing before the wheel he felt alone, but that was somehow right, and he remembered his plan. He would give the wheel a short quick twirl. Just a touch of the button. He had watched it many times, and always it came close to double zero when it was short and quick. He steeled himself; the fear had left, and he felt a profound sense of promise, as though he were about to be repaid for all the things he'd suffered all his life. Trembling, he pressed the button. There was a whirl of lights, and in a second he realized with finality that though he wanted to, he could not stop. It was as though he held a high-powered line in his naked hand. His nerves tightened. As the wheel increased its speed it seemed to draw him more and more into his power, as though it held his fate; and with it came a deep need to submit, to whirl, to lose himself in its swirl of color. He could not stop it now, he knew. So let it be.

The button rested snuggly in his palm where the man had placed it. And now he became aware of the man beside him, advising him through the microphone, while behind the shadowy audience hummed with noisy voices. He shifted his feet. There was still that feeling of helplessness within him, making part of him desire to turn back, even now that the jackpot was right in his hand. He squeezed the button until his fist ached. Then, like the sudden shriek of a subway whistle, a doubt tore through his head. Suppose he did not spin the wheel long enough? What could he do, and how could he tell? And then he knew, even as he wondered, that as long as he pressed the button, he could control the jackpot. He and only he could determine whether or not it was to be his. Not even the man with the microphone could do anything about it now. He felt drunk. Then, as though he had come down from a high hill into a valley of people, he heard the audience yelling.

"Come down from there, you jerk!"

"Let somebody else have a chance . . ."

"Ole Jack thinks he done found the end of the rainbow . . ."

The last voice was not unfriendly, and he turned and smiled dreamily into the yelling mouths. Then he turned his back squarely on them.

"Don't take too long, boy," a voice said.

He nodded. They were yelling behind him. Those folks did not understand what had happened to him. They had been playing the bingo game day in and night out for years, trying to win rent money or hamburger change. But not one of those wise guys had discovered this wonderful thing. He watched the wheel whirling past the numbers and experienced a burst of exhaltation: This is God! This is the really true God! He said it aloud, "This is God!"

He said it with such absolute conviction that he feared he would fall fainting into the footlights. But the crowd yelled so loud that they could not hear. Those fools, he thought. I'm here trying to tell them the most wonderful secret in the world, and they're yelling like they gone crazy. A hand fell upon his shoulder.

"You'll have to make a choice now, boy. You've taken too long."

He brushed the hand violently away.

"Leave me alone, man. I know what I'm doing!"

The man looked surprised and held on to the microphone for support. And because he did not wish to hurt the man's feelings he smiled, realizing with a sudden pang that there was no way of explaining to the man just why he had to stand there pressing the button forever.

"Come here," he called tiredly.

The man approached, rolling the heavy microphone across the stage.

"Anybody can play this bingo game, right?" he said.

"Sure, but . . ."

He smiled, feeling inclined to be patient with this slick looking white man with his blue sport shirt and his sharp gabardine suit.

"That's what I thought," he said. "Anybody can win the jackpot as long as they get the lucky number, right?"

"That's the rule, but after all . . ."

"That's what I thought," he said. "And the big prize goes to the man who knows how to win it?"

The man nodded speechlessly.

"Well then, go on over there and watch me win like I want to. I ain't going to hurt nobody," he said, "and I'll show you how to win. I mean to show the whole world how it's got to be done."

And because he understood, he smiled again to let the man know that he held nothing against him for being white and impatient. Then he refused to see the man any longer and stood pressing the button, the voices of the crowd reaching him like sounds in distant streets. Let them yell. All the Negroes down there were just ashamed because he was black like them. He smiled inwardly, knowing how it was. Most of the time he was ashamed of what Negroes did himself. Well, let them be ashamed for something this time. Like him. He was like a long thin black wire that was being stretched and wound upon the bingo wheel; wound until he wanted to scream; wound, but this time himself controlling the winding and the sadness and the shame, and because he did, Laura would be all right. Suddenly the lights flickered. He staggered backwards. Had something gone wrong? All this noise. Didn't they know that although he controlled the wheel, it also controlled him, and unless he pressed the button forever and forever and ever it would stop, leaving him high and dry, dry and high on this hard high slippery hill and Laura dead? There was only one chance; he had to do whatever the wheel demanded. And gripping the button in despair, he discovered with surprise that it imparted a nervous energy. His spine tingled. He felt a certain power.

Now he faced the raging crowd with defiance, its screams penetrating his eardrums like trumpets shrieking from a juke-box. The vague faces glowing in the bingo lights gave him a sense of himself that he had never known before. He was running the show, by God! They had to react to him, for he was their luck. This is *me*, he thought. Let the bastards yell. Then someone was laughing inside him, and he realized that somehow he had forgotten his own name. It was a sad, lost feeling to lose your name, and a crazy thing to do. That name had been given him by the white man who had owned his grandfather a long lost time ago down South. But maybe those wise guys knew his name.

"Who am I?" he screamed.

"Hurry up and bingo, you jerk!"

They didn't know either, he thought sadly. They didn't even know their own names, they were all poor nameless bastards. Well, he didn't need that old name; he was reborn. For as long as he pressed the button he was The-man-who-pressed-the-button-who-held-the-prize-who-was-the-King-of-Bingo. That was the way it was, and he'd have to press the button even if nobody understood, even though Laura did not understand.

"Live!" he shouted.

The audience quieted like the dying of a huge fan.

"Live, Laura, baby. I got holt of it now, sugar. Live!"

He screamed it, tears streaming down his face. "I got nobody but YOU!"

The screams tore from his very guts. He felt as though the rush of blood to his head would burst out in baseball seams of small red droplets, like a head beaten by police clubs. Bending over he saw a trickle of blood splashing the toe of his shoe. With his free hand he searched his head. It was his nose. God, suppose something has gone wrong? He felt that the whole audience had somehow entered him and was stamping its feet in his stomach and he was unable to throw them out. They wanted the prize, that was it. They wanted the secret for themselves. But they'd never get it; he would keep the bingo wheel whirling forever, and Laura would be safe in the wheel. But would she? It had to be, because if she were not safe the wheel would cease to turn; it could not go on. He had to get away, *vomit* all, and his mind formed an image of himself running with Laura in his arms down the tracks of the subway just ahead of an A train, running desperately, *vomit* with people screaming for him to come out but knowing no way of leaving the tracks because to stop would bring the train crushing down upon him and to attempt to leave across the other tracks would mean to run into a hot third rail as high as his waist which threw blue sparks that blinded his eyes until he could hardly see.

He heard singing and the audience was clapping its hands.

> Shoot the liquor to him, Jim, boy!
> Clap-clap-clap
> Well a-calla the cop
> He's blowing his top!
> Shoot the liquor to him, Jim, boy!

Bitter anger grew within him at the singing. They think I'm crazy. Well let 'em laugh. I'll do what I got to do.

He was standing in an attitude of intense listening when he saw that they were watching something on the stage behind him. He felt weak. But when he turned he saw no one. If only his thumb did not ache so. Now they were applauding. And for a moment he thought that the wheel had stopped. But that was impossible, his thumb still pressed the button. Then he saw them. Two men in uniform beckoned from the end of the stage. They were coming toward him, walking in step, slowly, like a tap-dance team returning for a third encore. But their shoulders shot forward, and he backed away, looking wildly about. There was nothing to fight them with. He had only the long black cord which led to a plug somewhere back stage, and he couldn't use that because it operated the bingo wheel. He backed slowly, fixing the men with his eyes as his lips stretched over his teeth in a tight, fixed grin; moved toward the end of the stage and realizing that he couldn't go much further, for suddenly the cord became taut and he couldn't afford to break the cord. But he had to do something. The audience was howling. Suddenly he stopped dead, seeing the men halt, their legs lifted as in an interrupted step of a slow-motion dance. There was nothing to do but run in the other direction and he dashed forward, slipping and sliding. The men fell back, surprised. He struck out violently going past.

"Grab him!"

He ran, but all too quickly the cord tightened, resistingly, and he turned and ran back again. This time he slipped them, and discovered by running in a circle before the wheel he could keep the cord from tightening. But this way he had to flail his arms to keep the men away. Why couldn't they leave a man alone? He ran, circling.

"Bring down the curtain," someone yelled. But they couldn't do that. If they did the wheel flashing from the projection room would be cut off. But they had him before he could tell them so, trying to pry open his fist, and he was wrestling and trying to bring his knees into the fight and holding on to the button, for it was his life. And now he was down, seeing a foot coming down, crushing his wrist cruelly, down, as he saw the wheel whirling serenely above.

"I can't give it up," he screamed. Then quietly, in a confidential tone, "Boys, I really can't give it up."

It landed hard against his head. And in the blank moment they had it away from him, completely now. He fought them trying to pull him up from the stage as he watched the wheel spin slowly to a stop. Without surprise he saw it rest at double-zero.

"You see," he pointed bitterly.

"Sure, boy, sure, it's O. K.," one of the men said smiling.

And seeing the man bow his head to someone he could not see, he felt very, very happy; he would receive what all the winners received.

But as he warmed in the justice of the man's tight smile he did not see the man's slow wink, nor see the bow-legged man behind him step clear of the swiftly descending curtain and set himself for a blow. He only felt the dull pain exploding in his skull, and he knew even as it slipped out of him that his luck had run out on the stage.

"Cash," from As I Lay Dying

WILLIAM FAULKNER

IT WASN'T NOTHING else to do. It was either send him to Jackson, or have Gillespie sue us, because he knowed some way that Darl set fire to it. I dont know how he knowed, but he did. Vardaman see him do it, but he swore he never told nobody but Dewey Dell and that she told him not to tell nobody. But Gillespie knowed it. But he would a suspicioned it sooner or later. He could have done it that night just watching the way Darl acted.

And so pa said, "I reckon there aint nothing else to do," and Jewel said, "You want to fix him now?"

"Fix him?" pa said.

"Catch him and tie him up," Jewel said. "Goddam it, do you want to wait until he sets fire to the goddam team and wagon?"

But there wasn't no use in that. "There aint no use in that," I said. "We can wait till she is underground." A fellow that's going to spend the rest of his life locked up, he ought to be let to have what pleasure he can have before he goes.

"I reckon he ought to be there," pa says. "God knows, it's a trial on me. Seems like it aint no end to bad luck when once it starts."

Sometimes I aint so sho who's got ere a right to say when a man is crazy and when he aint. Sometimes I think it aint none of us pure crazy and aint none of us pure sane until the balance of us talks him that-a-way. It's like it aint so much what a fellow does, but it's the way the majority of folks is looking at him when he does it.

Because Jewel is too hard on him. Of course it was Jewel's horse was traded to get her that nigh to town, and in a sense it was the value of his horse Darl tried to burn up. But I thought more than once before we crossed the river and after, how it would be God's blessing if He did take her outen our hands and get shut of her in some clean way, and it seemed to me that when Jewel worked so to get her outen the river, he was going against God in a way, and then when Darl seen that it looked like one of us would have to do something, I can almost believe he done right in a way. But I dont reckon nothing excuses setting fire to a man's barn and endangering his stock and destroying his property. That's how I reckon a man is crazy. That's how he cant see eye to eye with other folks. And I reckon they aint nothing else to do with him but what the most folks says is right.

But it's a shame, in a way. Folks seems to get away from the olden right teaching that says to drive the nails down and trim the edges well always like it was for your own use and comfort you were making it. It's like some folks has the smooth, pretty boards to build a courthouse with and others dont have no more than rough lumber fitten to build a chicken coop. But it's better to build a tight chicken coop than a shoddy courthouse, and when they both build shoddy or build well, neither because it's one or tother is going to make a man feel the better nor the worse.

So we went up the street, toward the square, and he said, "We better take Cash to the doctor first. We can leave him there and come back for him." That's it. It's because me and him was born close together, and it nigh ten years before Jewel and Dewey Dell and Vardaman begun to come along. I feel kin to them, all right, but I dont know. And me being the oldest, and thinking already the very thing that he done: I dont know.

Pa was looking at me, then at him, mumbling his mouth.

"Go on," I said. "We'll get it done first."

"She would want us all there," pa says.

"Let's take Cash to the doctor first," Darl said. "She'll wait. She's already waited nine days."

"You all dont know," pa says. "The somebody you was young with and you growed old in her and she growed old in you, seeing the old coming on and it was the one somebody you could hear say it dont matter and know it was the truth outen the hard world and all a man's grief and trials. You all dont know."

"We got the digging to do, too," I said.

"Armstid and Gillespie both told you to send word ahead," Darl said. "Dont you want to go to Peabody's now, Cash?"

"Go on," I said. "It feels right easy now. It's best to get things done in the right place."

"If it was just dug," pa says. "We forgot our spade, too."

"Yes," Darl said. "I'll go to the hardware store. We'll have to buy one."

"It'll cost money," pa says.

"Do you begrudge her it?" Darl says.

"Go on and get a spade," Jewel said. "Here. Give me the money."

But pa didn't stop. "I reckon we can get a spade," he said. "I reckon there are Christians here." So Darl set still and we went on, with Jewel squatting on the tail-gate, watching the back of Darl's head. He looked like one of these bull dogs, one of these dogs that dont bark none, squatting against the rope, watching the thing he was waiting to jump at.

He set that way all the time we was in front of Mrs Bundren's house, hearing the music, watching the back of Darl's head with them hard white eyes of hisn.

The music was playing in the house. It was one of them graphophones. It was natural as a music-band.

"Do you want to go to Peabody's?" Darl said. "They can wait here and tell pa, and I'll drive you to Peabody's and come back for them."

"No," I said. It was better to get her underground, now we was this close, just waiting until pa borrowed the shovel. He drove along the street until we could hear the music.

"Maybe they got one here," he said. He pulled up at Mrs Bundren's. It was like he knowed. Sometimes I think that if a working man could see work as far ahead as a lazy man can see laziness. So he stopped there like he knowed, before that little new house, where the music was. We waited there, hearing it. I believe I could have dickered Suratt down to five dollars on that one of his. It's a comfortable thing, music is. "Maybe they got one here," pa says.

"You want Jewel to go," Darl says, "or do you reckon I better?"

"I reckon I better," pa says. He got down and went up the path and around the house to the back. The music stopped, then it started again.

"He'll get it, too," Darl said.

"Ay," I said. It was just like he knowed, like he could see through the walls and into the next ten minutes.

Only it was more than ten minutes. The music stopped and never commenced again for a good spell, where her and pa was talking at the back. We waited in the wagon.

"You let me take you back to Peabody's," Darl said.

"No," I said. "We'll get her underground."

"If he ever gets back," Jewel said. He begun to cuss. He started to get down from the wagon. "I'm going," he said.

Then we saw pa coming back. He had two spades, coming around the house. He laid them in the wagon and got in and we went on. The music never started again. Pa was looking back at the house. He kind of lifted his hand a little and I saw the shade pulled back a little at the window and her face in it.

But the curiousest thing was Dewey Dell. It surprised me. I see all the while how folks could say he was queer, but that was the very reason couldn't nobody hold it personal. It was like he was outside of it too, same as you, and getting mad as it would be kind of like getting mad at a mud-puddle that splashed you when you stepped in it. And then I always kind of had a idea that him and

Dewey Dell kind of knowed things betwixt them. If I'd a said it was ere a one of us she liked better than ere a other, I'd a said it was Darl. But when we got it filled and covered and drove out the gate and turned into the lane where them fellows was waiting, when they come out and come on him and he jerked back, it was Dewey Dell that was on him before even Jewel could get at him. And then I believed I knowed how Gillespie knowed about how his barn taken fire.

She hadn't said a word, hadn't even looked at him, but when them fellows told him what they wanted and that they had come to get him and he throwed back, she jumped on him like a wild cat so that one of the fellows had to quit and hold her and her scratching and clawing at him like a wild cat, while the other one and pa and Jewel throwed Darl down and held him lying on his back, looking up at me.

"I thought you would have told me," he said. "I never thought you wouldn't have."

"Darl," I said. But he fought again, him and Jewel and the fellow, and the other one holding Dewey Dell and Vardaman yelling and Jewel saying,

"Kill him. Kill the son of a bitch."

It was bad so. It was bad. A fellow cant get away from a shoddy job. He cant do it. I tried to tell him, but he just said, "I thought you'd a told me. It's not that I," he said, then he begun to laugh. The other fellow pulled Jewel off of him and he sat there on the ground, laughing.

I tried to tell him. If I could have just moved, even set up. But I tried to tell him and he quit laughing, looking up at me.

"Do you want me to go?" he said.

"It'll be better for you," I said. "Down there it'll be quiet, with none of the bothering and such. It'll be better for you, Darl," I said.

"Better," he said. He began to laugh again. "Better," he said. He couldn't hardly say it for laughing. He sat on the ground and us watching him, laughing and laughing. It was bad. It was bad so. I be durn if I could see anything to laugh at. Because there just aint nothing justifies the deliberate destruction of what a man has built with his own sweat and stored the fruit of his sweat into.

But I aint so sho that ere a man has the right to say what is crazy and what aint. It's like there was a fellow in every man that's done a-past the sanity or the insanity, that watches the sane and the insane doings of that man with the same horror and the same astonishment.

Gogol's Wife

TOMMASO LANDOLFI

AT THIS POINT, confronted with the whole complicated affair of Nikolai Vassilevitch's wife, I am overcome by hesitation. Have I any right to disclose something which is unknown to the whole world, which my unforgettable friend himself kept hidden from the world (and he had his reasons), and which I am sure will give rise to all sorts of malicious and stupid misunderstandings? Something, moreover, which will very probably offend the sensibilities of all sorts of base, hypocritical people, and possibly of some honest people too, if there are any left? And finally, have I any right to disclose something before which my own spirit recoils, and even tends toward a more or less open disapproval?

But the fact remains that, as a biographer, I have certain firm obligations. Believing as I do that every bit of information about so lofty a genius will turn out to be of value to us and to future generations, I cannot conceal something which in any case has no hope of being judged fairly and wisely until the end of time. Moreover, what right have we to condemn? Is it given to us to know, not only what intimate needs, but even what higher and wider ends may have been served by those very deeds of a lofty genius which perchance may appear to us vile? No indeed, for we understand so little of these privileged natures. "It is true," a great man once said, "that I also have to pee, but for quite different reasons."

But without more ado I will come to what I know beyond doubt, and can prove beyond question, about this controversial matter, which will now—I dare to hope—no longer be so. I will not trouble to recapitulate what is already known of it, since I do not think this should be necessary at the present stage of development of Gogol studies.

Let me say it at once: Nikolai Vassilevitch's wife was not a woman. Nor was she any sort of human being, nor any sort of living creature at all, whether animal or vegetable (although something of the sort has sometimes been hinted). She was quite simply a balloon. Yes, a balloon; and this will explain the perplexity, or even indignation, of certain biographers who were also the personal friends of the Master, and who complained that, although they often went to his house, they never saw her and "never even heard her voice." From this they deduced all sorts of dark and disgraceful complications—yes, and criminal ones too. No, gentlemen, everything is always simpler than it appears. You did not hear her voice simply because she could not speak, or to be more exact, she could only speak in certain conditions, as we shall see. And it was always, except once, in tête-a-tête with Nikolai Vassilevitch. So let us not waste time with any cheap or empty refutations but come at once to as exact and complete a description as possible of the being or object in question.

Gogol's so-called wife was an ordinary dummy made of thick rubber, naked at all seasons, buff in tint, or as is more commonly said, flesh-colored. But since women's skins are not all of the same color, I should specify that hers was a light-colored, polished skin, like that of certain brunettes. It, or she, was, it is hardly necessary to add, of feminine sex. Perhaps I should say at once that she was capable of very wide alterations of her attributes without, of course, being able to alter her sex itself. She could sometimes appear to be thin, with hardly any breasts and with narrow hips more like a young lad than a woman, and at other times to be excessively well-endowed or—let us not mince matters—fat. And she often changed the color of her hair, both on her head and elsewhere on her body, though not necessarily at the same time. She could also seem to change in all sorts of other tiny particulars, such as the position of moles, the vitality of the mucous membranes and so forth. She could even to a certain extent change the very color of her skin. One is faced with the necessity of asking oneself who she really was, or whether it would be proper to speak of a single "person"—and in fact we shall see that it would be imprudent to press this point.

The cause of these changes, as my readers will already have understood, was nothing else but the will of Nikolai Vassilevitch himself. He would inflate her to a greater or lesser degree, would change her wig and her other tufts of hair, would grease her with ointments and touch her up in various ways so as to obtain more or less the type of woman which suited him at that moment. Following the natural inclinations of his fancy, he even amused himself sometimes by producing grotesque or monstrous forms; as will be readily understood, she became deformed when inflated beyond a certain point or if she remained below a certain pressure.

But Gogol soon tired of these experiments, which he held to be "after all, not very respectful" to his wife, whom he loved in his own way—however inscrutable it may remain to us. He loved her, but which of these incarnations, we may ask ourselves, did he love? Alas, I have already indicated that the end of the present account will furnish some sort of an answer. And how can I have stated above that it was Nikolai Vassilevitch's will which ruled that woman? In a certain sense, yes, it is true; but it is equally certain that she soon became no longer his slave but his tyrant. And here yawns the abyss, or if you prefer it, the Jaws of Tartarus. But let us not anticipate.

I have said that Gogol obtained with his manipulations *more or less* the type of woman which he needed from time to time. I should add that when, in rare cases, the form he obtained perfectly incarnated his desire, Nikolai Vassilevitch fell in love with it "exclusively," as he said in his own words, and that this was enough to render "her" stable for a certain time—until he fell out of love with "her." I counted no more than three or four of these violent passions—or, as I suppose they would be called today, infatuations—in the life (dare I say in the conjugal life?) of the great writer. It will be convenient to add here that a few years after what one may call his marriage, Gogol had even given a name to his wife. It was Caracas, which is, unless I am mistaken, the capital of Venezuela. I have never been able to discover the reason for this choice: great minds are so capricious!

Speaking only of her normal appearance, Caracas was what is called a fine woman—well built and proportioned in every part. She had every smallest attribute of her sex properly disposed in the proper location. Particularly worthy of attention were her genital organs (if the adjective is permissible in such a context). They were formed by means of ingenious folds in the rubber. Nothing was forgotten, and their operation was rendered easy by various devices, as well as by the internal pressure of the air.

Caracas also had a skeleton, even though a rudimentary one. Perhaps it was made of whalebone. Special care had been devoted to the construction of the thoracic cage, of the pelvic basin and of the cranium. The first two systems were more or less visible in accordance with the thickness of the fatty layer, if I may so describe it, which covered them. It is a great pity that Gogol never let me know the name of the creator of such a fine piece of work. There was an obstinacy in his refusal which was never quite clear to me.

Nikolai Vassilevitch blew his wife up through the anal sphincter with a pump of his own invention, rather like those which you hold down with your two feet and which are used today in all sorts of mechanical workshops. Situated in the anus was a little one-way valve, or whatever the correct technical description would be, like the mitral valve of the heart, which, once the body was inflated, allowed more air to come in but none to go out. To deflate, one unscrewed a stopper in the mouth, at the back of the throat.

And that, I think, exhausts the description of the most noteworthy peculiarities of this being. Unless perhaps I should mention the splendid rows of white teeth which adorned her mouth and the dark eyes which, in spite of their immobility, perfectly simulated life. Did I say simulate? Good heavens, simulate is not the word! Nothing seems to be the word, when one is speaking of Caracas! Even these eyes could undergo a change of color, by means of a special process to which, since it was long and tiresome, Gogol seldom had recourse. Finally, I should speak of her voice, which it was only once given to me to hear. But I cannot do that without going more fully into the relationship between husband and wife, and in this I shall no longer be able to answer to the truth of everything with absolute certitude. On my conscience I could not— so confused, both in itself and in my memory, is that which I now have to tell.

Here, then, as they occur to me, are some of my memories.

The first and, as I said, the last time I ever heard Caracas speak to Nikolai Vassilevitch was one evening when we were absolutely alone. We were in the room where the woman, if I may be allowed the expression, lived. Entrance to this room was strictly forbidden to everybody. It was furnished more or less in the Oriental manner, had no windows and was situated in the most inaccessible part of the house. I did know that she could talk, but Gogol had never explained to me the circumstances under which this happened. There were only the two of us, or three, in there. Nikolai Vassilevitch and I were drinking vodka and discussing Butkov's novel. I remember that we left this topic, and he was maintaining the necessity for radical reforms in the laws of inheritance. We had almost forgotten her. It was then that, with a husky and submissive voice, like Venus on the nuptial couch, she said point-blank: "I want to go poo poo."

I jumped, thinking I had misheard, and looked across at her. She was sitting on a pile of cushions against the wall; that evening she was a soft, blonde beauty, rather well-covered. Her expression seemed commingled of shrewdness and slyness, childishness and irresponsibility. As for Gogol, he blushed violently and, leaping on her, stuck two fingers down her throat. She immediately began to shrink and to turn pale; she took on once again that lost and astonished air which was especially hers, and was in the end reduced to no more than a flabby skin on a perfunctory bony armature. Since, for practical reasons which will readily be divined, she had an extraordinarily flexible backbone, she folded up almost in two, and for the rest of the evening she looked up at us from where she had slithered to the floor, in utter abjection.

All Gogol said was: "She only does it for a joke, or to annoy me, because as a matter of fact she does not have such needs." In the presence of other people, that is to say of me, he generally made a point of treating her with a certain disdain.

We went on drinking and talking, but Nikolai Vassilevitch seemed very much disturbed and absent in spirit. Once he suddenly interrupted what he was saying, seized my hand in his and burst into tears. "What can I do now?" he exclaimed. "You understand, Foma Paskalovitch, that I loved her?"

It is necessary to point out that it was impossible, except by a miracle, ever to repeat any of Caracas' forms. She was a fresh creation every time, and it would have been wasted effort to seek to find again the exact proportions, the exact pressure, and so forth, of a former Caracas. Therefore the plumpish blonde of that evening was lost to Gogol from that time forth forever; this was in fact the tragic end of one of those few loves of Nikolai Vassilevitch, which I described above. He gave me no explanation; he sadly rejected my proffered comfort, and that evening we parted early. But his heart had been laid bare to me in that outburst. He was no longer so reticent with me, and soon had hardly any secrets left. And this, I may say in parenthesis, caused me very great pride.

It seems that things had gone well for the "couple" at the beginning of their life together. Nikolai Vassilevitch had been content with Caracas and slept regularly with her in the same bed. He continued to observe this custom till the end, saying with a timid smile that no companion could be quieter or less importunate than she. But I soon began to doubt this, especially judging by the state he was sometimes in when he woke up. Then, after several years, their relationship began strangely to deteriorate.

All this, let it be said once and for all, is no more than a schematic attempt at an explanation. About that time the woman actually began to show signs of independence or, as one might say, of autonomy. Nikolai Vassilevitch had the extraordinary impression that she was acquiring a personality of her own, indecipherable perhaps, but still distinct from his, and one which slipped through his fingers. It is certain that some sort of continuity was established between each of her appearances—between all those brunettes, those blondes, those redheads and auburn-headed girls, between those plump, those slim, those dusky or snowy or golden beauties, there was a certain something in common. At the beginning of this chapter I cast some doubt on the propriety of considering Caracas as a unitary personality; nevertheless I myself could not quite, whenever I saw her, free myself of the impression that, however unheard of it may seem, this was fundamentally the same woman. And it may be that this was why Gogol felt he had to give her a name.

An attempt to establish in what precisely subsisted the common attributes of the different forms would be quite another thing. Perhaps it was no more and no less than the creative afflatus of Nikolai Vassilevitch himself. But no, it would have been too singular and strange if he had been so much divided off from himself, so much averse to himself. Because whoever she was, Caracas was a disturbing presence and even—it is better to be quite clear—a hostile one. Yet neither Gogol nor I ever succeeded in formulating a remotely tenable hypothesis as to her true nature; when I say formulate, I mean in terms which would be at once rational and accessible to all. But I cannot pass over an extraordinary event which took place at this time.

Caracas fell ill of a shameful disease—or rather Gogol did—though he was not then having, nor had he ever had, any contact with other women. I will not even try to describe how this happened, or where the filthy complaint came from; all I know is that it happened. And that my great, unhappy friend would say to me: "So, Foma Paskalovitch, you see what lay at the heart of Caracas; it was the spirit of syphilis."

Sometimes he would even blame himself in a quite absurd manner; he was always prone to self-accusation. This incident was a real catastrophe as far as the already obscure relationship between husband and wife, and the hostile feelings of Nikolai Vassilevitch himself, were concerned. He was compelled to undergo long-drawn-out and painful treatment—the treatment of those days—and the situation was aggravated by the fact that the disease in the woman did not seem to be easily curable. Gogol deluded himself for some time that, by blowing his wife up and down and furnishing her with the most widely divergent aspects, he could obtain a woman immune from the contagion, but he was forced to desist when no results were forthcoming.

I shall be brief, seeking not to tire my readers, and also because what I remember seems to become more and more confused. I shall therefore hasten to the tragic conclusion. As to this last, however, let there be no mistake. I must once again make it clear that I am very sure of my ground. I was an eyewitness. Would that I had not been!

The years went by. Nikolai Vassilevitch's distaste for his wife became stronger, though his love for her did not show any signs of diminishing. Toward the end, aversion and attachment struggled so fiercely with each other in his heart that he became quite stricken, almost broken up. His restless eyes, which habitually assumed so many different expressions and sometimes spoke so sweetly to the heart of his interlocutor, now almost always shone with a fevered light, as if he were under the effect of a drug. The strangest impulses arose in him, accompanied by the most senseless fears. He spoke to me of Caracas more and more often, accusing her of unthinkable and amazing things. In these regions I could not follow him, since I had but a sketchy acquaintance with his wife, and hardly any intimacy—and above all since my sensibility was so limited compared with his. I shall accordingly restrict myself to reporting some of his accusations, without reference to my personal impressions.

"Believe it or not, Foma Paskalovitch," he would, for example, often say to me: "Believe it or not, *she's aging!*" Then, unspeakably moved, he would, as was his way, take my hands in his. He also accused Caracas of giving herself up to solitary pleasures, which he had expressly forbidden. He even went so far as to charge her with betraying him, but the things he said became so extremely obscure that I must excuse myself from any further account of them.

One thing that appears certain is that toward the end Caracas, whether aged or not, had turned into a bitter creature, querulous, hypocritical and subject to religious excess. I do not exclude the possibility that she may have had an influence on Gogol's moral position during the last period of his life, a position which is sufficiently well known. The tragic climax came one night quite unexpectedly when Nikolai Vassilevitch and I were celebrating his silver wedding— one of the last evenings we were to spend together. I neither can nor should attempt to set down what it was that led to his decision, at a time when to all appearances he was resigned to tolerating his consort. I know not what new events had taken place that day. I shall confine myself to the facts; my readers must make what they can of them.

That evening Nikolai Vassilevitch was unusually agitated. His distaste for Caracas seemed to have reached an unprecedented intensity. The famous "pyre of vanities"—the burning of his manuscripts—had already taken place; I should not like to say whether or not at the instigation of his wife. His state of mind had been further inflamed by other causes. As to his physical condition, this was ever more pitiful, and strengthened my impression that he took drugs. All the same, he began to talk in a more or less normal way about Belinsky, who was giving him some trouble with his attacks on the *Selected Correspondence*. Then suddenly, tears rising to his eyes, he interrupted himself and cried out: "No. No. It's too much, too much. I can't go on any longer," as well as other obscure and disconnected phrases which he would not clarify. He seemed to be talking to himself. He wrung his hands, shook his head, got up and sat down again after having taken four or five anxious steps round the room. When Caracas appeared, or rather when we went in to her later in the evening in her Oriental chamber, he controlled himself no longer and began to behave like an old man, if I may so express myself, in his second childhood, quite giving way to his absurd impulses. For instance, he kept nudging me and winking and senselessly repeating: "There she is, Foma Paskalovitch; there she is!" Meanwhile she seemed to look up at us with a disdainful attention. But behind these "mannerisms" one could feel in him a real repugnance, a repugnance which had, I suppose, now reached the limits of the endurable. Indeed . . .

After a certain time Nikolai Vassilevitch seemed to pluck up courage. He burst into tears, but somehow they were more manly tears. He wrung his hands again, seized mine in his, and walked up and down, muttering: "That's enough! We can't have any more of this. This is an unheard of thing. How can such a thing be happening to me? How can a man be expected to put up with *this*?"

He then leapt furiously upon the pump, the existence of which he seemed just to have remembered, and, with it in his hand, dashed like a whirlwind to

Caracas. He inserted the tube in her anus and began to inflate her. . . . Weeping the while, he shouted like one possessed: "Oh, how I love her, how I love her, my poor, poor darling! . . . But she's going to burst! Unhappy Caracas, most pitiable of God's creatures! But die she must!"

Caracas was swelling up. Nikolai Vassilevitch sweated, wept and pumped. I wished to stop him but, I know not why, I had not the courage. She began to become deformed and shortly assumed the most monstrous aspect; and yet she had not given any signs of alarm—she was used to these jokes. But when she began to feel unbearably full, or perhaps when Nikolai Vassilevitch's intentions became plain to her, she took on an expression of bestial amazement, even a little beseeching, but still without losing that disdainful look. She was afraid, she was even committing herself to his mercy, but still she could not believe in the immediate approach of her fate; she could not believe in the frightful audacity of her husband. He could not see her face because he was behind her. But I looked at her with fascination, and did not move a finger.

At last the internal pressure came through the fragile bones at the base of her skull, and printed on her face an indescribable rictus. Her belly, her thighs, her lips, her breasts and what I could see of her buttocks had swollen to incredible proportions. All of a sudden she belched, and gave a long hissing groan; both these phenomena one could explain by the increase in pressure, which had suddenly forced a way out through the valve in her throat. Then her eyes bulged frantically, threatening to jump out of their sockets. Her ribs flared wide apart and were no longer attached to the sternum, and she resembled a python digesting a donkey. A donkey, did I say? An ox! An elephant! At this point I believed her already dead, but Nikolai Vassilevitch, sweating, weeping and repeating: "My dearest! My beloved! My best!" continued to pump.

She went off unexpectedly and, as it were, all of a piece. It was not one part of her skin which gave way and the rest which followed, but her whole surface at the same instant. She scattered in the air. The pieces fell more or less slowly, according to their size, which was in no case above a very restricted one. I distinctly remember a piece of her cheek, with some lip attached, hanging on the corner of the mantelpiece. Nikolai Vassilevitch stared at me like a madman. Then he pulled himself together and, once more with furious determination, he began carefully to collect those poor rags which once had been the shining skin of Caracas, and all of her.

"Good-by, Caracas," I thought I heard him murmur, "Good-by! You were too pitiable!" And then suddenly and quite audibly: "The fire! The fire! She too must end up in the fire." He crossed himself—with his left hand, of course. Then, when he had picked up all those shriveled rags, even climbing on the furniture so as not to miss any, he threw them straight on the fire in the hearth, where they began to burn slowly and with an excessively unpleasant smell. Nikolai Vassilevitch, like all Russians, had a passion for throwing important things in the fire.

Red in the face, with an inexpressible look of despair, and yet of sinister triumph too, he gazed on the pyre of those miserable remains. He had seized my arm and was squeezing it convulsively. But those traces of what had once been a being were hardly well alight when he seemed yet again to pull himself together, as if he were suddenly remembering something or taking a painful decision. In one bound he was out of the room.

A few seconds later I heard him speaking to me through the door in a broken, plaintive voice: "Foma Paskalovitch, I want you to promise not to look. *Golubchik*, promise not to look at me when I come in."

I don't know what I answered, or whether I tried to reassure him in any way. But he insisted, and I had to promise him, as if he were a child, to hide my face against the wall and only turn round when he said I might. The door then opened violently and Nikolai Vassilevitch burst into the room and ran to the fireplace.

And here I must confess my weakness, though I consider it justified by the extraordinary circumstances. I looked round before Nikolai Vassilevitch told me I could; it was stronger than me. I was just in time to see him carrying something in his arms, something which he threw on the fire with all the rest, so that it suddenly flared up. At that, since the desire to *see* had entirely mastered every other thought in me, I dashed to the fireplace. But Nikolai Vassilevitch placed himself between me and it and pushed me back with a strength of which I had not believed him capable. Meanwhile the object was burning and giving off clouds of smoke. And before he showed any sign of calming down there was nothing left but a heap of silent ashes.

The true reason why I wished to see was because I had already glimpsed. But it was only a glimpse, and perhaps I should not allow myself to introduce even the slightest element of uncertainty into this true story. And yet, an eyewitness account is not complete without a mention of that which the witness knows with less than complete certainty. To cut a long story short, that something was a baby. Not a flesh and blood baby, of course, but more something in the line of a rubber doll or a model. Something, which, to judge by its appearance, could have been called *Caracas's son*.

Was I mad too? That I do not know, but I do know that this was what I saw, not clearly, but with my own eyes. And I wonder why it was that when I was writing this just now I didn't mention that when Nikolai Vassilevitch came back into the room he was muttering between his clenched teeth: "Him too! Him too!"

And that is the sum of my knowledge of Nikolai Vassilevitch's wife. In the next chapter I shall tell what happened to him afterwards, and that will be the last chapter of his life. But to give an interpretation of his feelings for his wife, or indeed for anything, is quite another and more difficult matter, though I have attempted it elsewhere in this volume, and refer the reader to that modest effort. I hope I have thrown sufficient light on a most controversial question and that I have unveiled the mystery, if not of Gogol, then at least of his wife. In the course of this I have implicitly given the lie to the insensate accusation that he ill-treated or even beat his wife, as well as other like absurdities. And what else can be the goal of a humble biographer such as the present writer but to serve the memory of that lofty genius who is the object of this study?

The Tell-Tale Heart

Edgar Allen Poe

TRUE! NERVOUS, very, very dreadfully nervous I had been and am; but why *will* you say that I am mad? The disease had sharpened my senses, not destroyed, not dulled them. Above all was the sense of hearing acute. I heard all things in the heaven and in the earth. I heard many things in hell. How then am I mad? Hearken! and observe how healthily, how calmly, I can tell you the whole story.

It is impossible to say how first the idea entered my brain, but, once conceived, it haunted me day and night. Object there was none. Passion there was none. I loved the old man. He had never wronged me. He had never given me insult. For his gold I had no desire. I think it was his eye! Yes, it was this! One of his eyes resembled that of a vulture—a pale blue eye with a film over it. Whenever it fell upon me my blood ran cold, and so by degrees, very gradually, I made up my mind to take the life of the old man, and thus rid myself of the eye for ever.

Now this is the point. You fancy me mad. Madmen know nothing. But you should have seen *me*. You should have seen how wisely I proceeded—with what caution—with what foresight, with what dissimulation, I went to work! I was never kinder to the old man than during the whole week before I killed him. And every night about midnight I turned the latch of his door and opened it—oh, so gently! And then when I had made an opening sufficient for my head I put in a dark lantern all closed, closed so that no light shone out, and then I thrust in my head. Oh, you would have laughed to see how cunningly I thrust it in! I moved it slowly, very, very slowly, so that I might not disturb the old man's sleep. It took me an hour to place my whole head within the opening so far that I could see him as he lay upon his bed. Ha! would a madman have been so wise as this? And then when my head was well in the room I undid the lantern cautiously—oh, so cautiously—cautiously (for the hinges creaked), I undid it just so much that a single thin ray fell upon the vulture eye. And this I did for seven long nights, every night just at midnight, but I found the eye always closed, and so it was impossible to do the work, for it was not the old man who vexed me but his Evil Eye. And every morning, when the day broke,

I went boldly into the chamber and spoke courageously to him, calling him by name in a hearty tone, and inquiring how he had passed the night. So you see he would have been a very profound old man, indeed, to suspect that every night, just at twelve, I looked in upon him while he slept.

Upon the eighth night I was more than usually cautious in opening the door. A watch's minute hand moves more quickly than did mine. Never before that night had I *felt* the extent of my own powers, of my sagacity. I could scarcely contain my feeling of triumph. To think that there I was opening the door little by little, and he not even to dream of my secret deeds or thoughts. I fairly chuckled at the idea, and perhaps he heard me, for he moved on the bed suddenly as if startled. Now you may think that I drew back—but no. His room was as black as pitch with the thick darkness (for the shutters were close fastened through fear of robbers), and so I knew that he could not see the opening of the door, and I kept pushing it on steadily, steadily.

I had my head in, and was about to open the lantern, when my thumb slipped upon the tin fastening, and the old man sprang up in the bed, crying out, "Who's there?"

I kept quite still and said nothing. For a whole hour I did not move a muscle, and in the meantime I did not hear him lie down. He was still sitting up in the bed, listening; just as I have done night after night hearkening to the death watches in the wall.

Presently I heard a slight groan, and I knew it was the groan of mortal terror. It was not a groan of pain or of grief—oh, no! it was the low stifled sound that arises from the bottom of the soul when overcharged with awe. I knew the sound well. Many a night, just at midnight, when all the world slept, it has welled up from my own bosom, deepening with its dreadful echo, the terrors that distracted me. I say I knew it well. I knew what the old man felt, and pitied him although I chuckled at heart. I knew that he had been lying awake ever since the first slight noise when he had turned in the bed. His fears had been ever since growing upon him. He had been trying to fancy them causeless, but could not. He had been saying to himself, "It is nothing but the wind in the chimney, it is only a mouse crossing the floor," or "It is merely a cricket which has made a single chirp." Yes, he has been trying to comfort himself with these suppositions; but he had found all in vain. *All in vain*, because Death in approaching him had stalked with his black shadow before him and enveloped the victim. And it was the mournful influence of the unperceived shadow that caused him to feel, although he neither saw nor heard, to *feel* the presence of my head within the room.

When I had waited a long time very patiently without hearing him lie down, I resolved to open a little—a very, very little, crevice in the lantern. So I opened it—you cannot imagine how stealthily, stealthily—until at length a single dim ray like the thread of the spider shot out from the crevice and fell upon the vulture eye.

It was open, wide, wide open, and I grew furious as I gazed upon it. I saw it with perfect distinctness—all a dull blue with a hideous veil over it that chilled the very marrow in my bones, but I could see nothing else of the old man's face or person, for I had directed the ray as if by instinct precisely upon the damned spot.

And now have I not told you that what you mistake for madness is but over-acuteness of the senses? now, I say, there came to my ears a low, dull, quick sound, such as a watch makes when enveloped in cotton. I knew *that* sound well, too. It was the beating of the old man's heart. It increased my fury, as the beating of a drum stimulates the soldier into courage.

But even yet I refrained and kept still. I scarcely breathed. I held the lantern motionless. I tried how steadily I could maintain the ray upon the eye. Mean-time the hellish tattoo of the heart increased. It grew quicker and quicker, and louder and louder, every instant. The old man's terror *must* have been extreme! It grew louder, I say, louder every moment!—do you mark me well? I have told you that I am nervous; so I am. And now at the dead hour of the night, amid the dreadful silence of that old house, so strange a noise as this excited me to uncontrollable terror. Yet, for some minutes longer I refrained and stood still. But the beating grew louder, louder! I thought the heart must burst. And now a new anxiety seized me—the sound would be heard by a neighbour! The old man's hour had come! With a loud yell, I threw open the lantern and leaped into the room. He shrieked once—once only. In an instant I dragged him to the floor, and pulled the heavy bed over him. I then smiled gaily, to find the deed so far done. But for many minutes the heart beat on with a muffled sound. This, however, did not vex me; it would not be heard through the wall. At length it ceased. The old man was dead. I removed the bed and examined the corpse. Yes, he was stone, stone dead. I placed my hand upon the heart and held it there many minutes. There was no pulsation. He was stone dead, His eye would trouble me no more.

If still you think me mad, you will think so no longer when I describe the wise precautions I took for the concealment of the body. The night waned, and I worked hastily, but in silence.

I took up three planks from the flooring of the chamber, and deposited all between the scantlings. I then replaced the boards so cleverly, so cunningly, that no human eye—not even *his*—could have detected anything wrong. There was nothing to wash out—no stain of any kind—no blood-spot what-ever. I had been too wary for that.

When I had made an end of these labours, it was four o'clock—still dark as midnight. As the bell sounded the hour, there came a knocking at the street door. I went down to open it with a light heart,—for what had I *now* to fear? There entered three men, who introduced themselves, with perfect suavity, as officers of the police. A shriek had been heard by a neighbour during the night; suspicion of foul play had been aroused; information had been lodged at the police office, and they (the officers) had been deputed to search the premises.

I smiled,—for *what* had I to fear? I bade the gentlemen welcome. The shriek, I said, was my own in a dream. The old man, I mentioned, was absent in the country. I took my visitors all over the house. I bade them search—search *well*. I led them, at length, to *his* chamber. I showed them his treasures, secure, undisturbed. In the enthusiasm of my confidence, I brought chairs into the room, and desired them *here* to rest from their fatigues, while I myself, in the wild audacity of my perfect triumph, placed my own seat upon the very spot beneath which reposed the corpse of the victim.

The officers were satisfied. My *manner* had convinced them. I was singularly at ease. They sat, and while I answered cheerily, they chatted of familiar things. But, ere long, I felt myself getting pale and wished them gone. My head ached, and I fancied a ringing in my ears; but still they sat, and still chatted. The ringing became more distinct;—it continued and became more distinct: I talked more freely to get rid of the feeling: but it continued and gained definitiveness—until, at length, I found that the noise was *not* within my ears.

No doubt I now grew *very* pale;—but I talked more fluently, and with a heightened voice. Yet the sound increased—and what could I do? It was a *low, dull, quick sound—much such a sound as a watch makes when enveloped in cotton.* I gasped for breath—and yet the officers heard it not. I talked more quickly—more vehemently; but the noise steadily increased. I arose and argued about trifles, in a high key and with violent gesticulations; but the noise steadily increased. Why *would* they not be gone? I paced the floor to and fro with heavy strides, as if excited to fury by the observations of the men—but the noise steadily increased. O God! what *could* I do? I foamed—I raved—I swore! I swung the chair upon which I had been sitting, and grated it upon the boards, but the noise arose over all and continually increased. It grew louder— louder—*louder!* And still the men chatted pleasantly, and smiled. Was it possible they heard not? Almighty God!—no, no! They heard!—they suspected!— they *knew!*—they were making a mockery of my horror!—this I thought, and this I think. But anything was better than this agony! Anything was more tolerable than this derision! I could bear those hypocritical smiles no longer! I felt that I must scream or die!—and now—again!—hark! louder! louder! louder! *louder!*—

"Villains!" I shrieked, "dissemble no more! I admit the deed!—tear up the planks!—here, here!— it is the beating of his hideous heart!"

From The Notebooks of Malte Laurids Brigge

RAINER MARIA RILKE

AND NOW THIS illness too, which has always affected me so strangely. I am sure it is underestimated. Just as the importance of other diseases is exaggerated. This disease has no particular characteristics; it takes on those of the person it attacks. With a somnambulic certainty it drags out of each his deepest danger, that seemed passed, and sets it before him again, quite near, imminent. Men, who once in their school-days attempted the helpless vice that has for its duped intimate the poor, hard hands of boys, find themselves at it again; or an illness they had conquered in childhood begins in them again; or a lost habit reappears, a certain hesitant turn of the head that had been peculiar to them years before. And with whatever comes there rises a whole tangle of insane memories, which hangs about it like wet seaweed on some sunken thing. Lives of which one would never have known mount to the surface and mingle with what has actually been, and push aside past matters that one had thought to know: for in that which ascends is a rested, new strength, but that which has always been there is wearied by too frequent remembrance.

I am lying in my bed, five flights up, and my day, which nothing interrupts, is like a dial without hands. As a thing long lost lies one morning in its old place, safe and well, fresher almost than at the time of its loss, quite as though someone had cared for it—: so here and there on my coverlet lie lost things out of my childhood and are as new. All forgotten fears are there again.

The fear that a small, woollen thread that sticks out of the hem of my blanket may be hard, hard and sharp like a steel needle; the fear that this little button on my night-shirt may be bigger than my head, big and heavy; the fear that this crumb of bread now falling from my bed may arrive glassy and shattered on the floor, and the burdensome worry lest at that really everything will be broken, everything for ever; the fear that the torn border of an opened letter may be something forbidden that no one ought to see, something indescribably precious for which no place in the room is secure enough; the fear that if I fell asleep I might swallow the piece of coal lying in front of the stove; the fear that some number may begin to grow in my brain until there is no more room for it inside me; the fear that it may be granite I am lying on, grey granite; the fear that I may shout, and that people may come running to my door and finally break it open; the fear that I may betray myself and tell all that I dread; and the fear that I might not be able to say anything, because everything is beyond utterance,—and the other fears . . . the fears.

I asked for my childhood and it has come back, and I feel that it is just as difficult as it was before, and that it has been useless to grow older.

Alzheimer's & Dementia

To You My Mother Lost in Time

HALE CHATFIELD

Anne Webster Chatfield
May 8, 1914–April 15, 1990

This sun day morning I am come to this
another page through our tears' and loves' history
to sing to my source my gratitude my very great joy

to reaffirm the perfect equality of our shared dying,
the beds we share in the leaning over to care and to harbor
and the beds we have shared in my conception and my birth:
how you have kept me warm!
Mother I have come to celebrate

my not losing you as you simply live and die
during these slow days in which your heaven of words
and the margins from which you laugh or smile
who have taught me the languages of my life
and the love of women who love

to sing! for who could not sing who has been loved
and been made ready for love? who could not sing
who has been stricken with beauty, who has been carried
to the arms of God, who could not sing who has been
himself sung into being?

to my mother lost in the paradoxes between love and spirit
I have come to cover those portions of her flesh
which I have both loved and feared, and how innocent
they are and how beloved in their penultimate simplicity
that were mysterious and meaningful and will not endure:

your shoulders and breasts Mother the paradigms of our human
tenderness, to shudder
at the poignancy of the dear
the loss of the precious ordinary

to weep a little for the vulnerable flesh
of my mother, the disposable stuff
of which the very stuff itself made me to be—
to be here to mourn for its passing,

the beloved broken thumb the garage door emphasized,
the crooked upper incisor, the moles,
the arms which could not let me go.

These lines have their place for my tears,
a moment to dissolve myself in for a moment,
a small place to weep in. Once again.

And yet Mother still we are here
both of us breathing
a while longer to contemplate
each other's similar face
to see or not see into each other's eyes

where the light falls over us
which is eternity, to praise God from whom all blessings flow,
to move together in orderly sequence from the warm
to the warm, from the darkness of love
to the darkness of love.

From My Journey into Alzheimer's Disease

ROBERT DAVIS
WITH HELP FROM HIS WIFE, BETTY

CHAPTER FOUR: THE REACHING POWER OF CHRIST

AS WE HEADED WEST, my body gradually began to gain strength. I was able to stay awake several hours a day. Gradually my physical strength returned so that I was able to leave the car and walk to the various roadside points of interest.

My spiritual life was still most miserable. I could not read the Bible. I could not pray as I wanted because my emotions were dead and cut off. There was no feedback from God the Holy Spirit. As I tried to fall asleep only blackness and misery came, misery so terrifying that I could not drop off to sleep. Nighttime was horrible. My mind could not rest and grow calm but instead raced relentlessly, thinking dreadful thoughts of despair. Invariably I lay there, terrified by a darkness that I could not understand.

My mind also raced about, grasping for the comfort of the Savior whom I knew and loved and for the emotional peace that he could give me, but finding nothing. I concluded that the only reason for such darkness must be spiritual. Unnamed guilt filled me. Yet the only guilt I could put a name to was failure to read my Bible. But I could not read, and would God condemn me for this? I could only lie there and cry, "Oh God, why? Why?"

"If I cannot find fellowship and joy again, what will happen to my professional life? I cannot lead Christ's church into light and truth when I am full of darkness." Why would God allow this to happen at the height of my effectiveness in the ministry? I had given my entire life to become the best pastor I could possibly be. The thought of total retirement had never crossed my mind. I felt that if I should leave the pastorate I would teach in seminary and pass on the things that I had learned to those younger men preparing for the ministry. I had also considered leading in church training organizations to show how to make churches grow in unusual situations. For years one of my favorite expressions had been, "God has no retirement plan." Retirement from Christian service had never entered my mind. But now everything that I had given myself for and studied for these past years was gone, lost in the dark recesses of my mind. As I thought of the sheer waste of this, I groaned out "Why, God? Why?"

In addition to all of these things, there was the plain fear of the unknown. At this time I had no idea whether this was a psychological breakdown, a result of some organic disease that could be cured, or some rare unknown thing that would just lead me downward into complete physical and mental devastation. I had no idea what the consequences of my illness would be, and if it would totally destroy me and my family.

Feasting my eyes on the ever-changing scenery caused me to praise God for the wonder of his creation. The trip became more and more enjoyable as my physical strength returned to normal. During the day, I could praise God as I had reminders to lead my thoughts heavenward. But at night when I could no longer look upon God's handiwork, the darkness returned perhaps magnified by contrast to the grandeur of the day. At night I cried out to Christ by the hour. Why had he deserted me in this, my greatest time of need?

One night in Wyoming, as I lay in a motel crying out to my Lord, my long desperate prayers were suddenly answered. As I lay there in the blackness silently shrieking out my often repeated prayer, there was suddenly a light that seemed to fill my very soul. The sweet, holy presence of Christ came to me. He spoke to my spirit and said, "Take my peace. Stop your struggling. It is all right. This is all in keeping with my will for your life. I now release you from the burden of the heavy yoke of pastoring that I placed upon you. Relax and stop struggling in your desperate search for answers. I will hold you. Lie back in your Shepherd's arms, and take my peace."

What a precious moment this was! At last all my prayers that I had cried out to Christ over the past few weeks were answered in the most complete and precious way that I knew possible. My spiritual and emotional needs had been fully and completely met. I lay in bed and cried like a baby. At last I had my inner pain and rage pacified, and I had all those perplexing inner spiritual questions answered. Furthermore, I had a new direction in life and a peace and release that allowed me to face the world with the absolute answer of, "Yes, it is all true. All that I have preached about the supernatural peace of Christ is true. At last this tremendous peace of Christ has transformed the deepest part of me. Now I can again speak about the peace and power of Christ without the slightest trace of hypocrisy."

In my confused and shattered emotional and mental condition, Christ had to meet me in this special way. He adjusted his way of comforting me so that it would immerse me in the radiance of his very presence. I do not believe there was ever before a time in my life when I needed this kind of miracle. Ever since my salvation experience, I could always reach up to Jesus. Now in my helplessness he reached down to me. His love overwhelmed me as he told me to take and enjoy his peace, and that the yoke of the pastoral ministry that had obsessed me and driven me on to deeper and greater service was now lifted from my shoulders. My new and simple service to him was to rest in him and moment by moment take his peace and use his strength to simply live.

When I awoke the next morning, the winds of confusion and frustration about all the "whys" in my life were gone. The very presence and peace of Christ absolutely overflowed me deep inside, and I had been changed. I discovered in a richer way than I ever knew possible the peace that surpasses all understanding Jesus promised. Now, instead of my reaching out to Christ by prayer, intellectual determination, sheer bull-headed faith, or by aggressively claiming the promises of Scripture, Christ reached down and held me close to him. The only way I can describe it is that my Good Shepherd took me, his special lamb, in his arms and cuddled me close. As he cuddled me he assured me that this was all in his will. I could now rest from my struggles, enjoy my daily life as it came, and have his peace. From now on, my lot in life would be to be especially held by the Shepherd, letting him fully care for me.

The frustration, pain, aggravation, or irrational thinking did not leave immediately. The old saying that, "God did not promise us smooth seas but a safe harbor," is especially meaningful to me now. Life is never a simple all good or all bad experience. Pain and pleasure, sorrow and joy, mingle in the rope of life for all people, the whole and handicapped alike.

This experience that finally lifted the dark veil for a brief moment did not make my brain whole again. I am still handicapped and will continue to become more and more dependent as my disease progresses. But in my darkness I am again assured that I am not alone. As Isaiah 43:2 reminds us of God's words, "When you pass through the waters, I will be with you; and when you pass through the rivers, they will not sweep over you."

I still have the aggravations of daily living. For instance, it is annoying to be unable to remember information such as my license tag. It is embarrassing and irritating to go to a service station and have to make two trips back to the car to check the license plate because I forgot the number between the pump and the cash register. How frightening it is to go into a large, familiar shopping center with crowds and blinking lights and become totally lost! How humiliating it is to be unable to make the right change and ask the cashier to pick the correct coins from my hand!

It is still sometimes terrifying at night. When I let my mind go in order to go to sleep, my mind still slips into blankness and moonlight. However, this is all just surface frustration, brought on by the constant process of losing control at the daily living level. I can either struggle angrily and uselessly against the inevitable, or else I can admit my inadequacy and humbly ask for help. I choose to do the latter and keep a calmer and more peaceful mind. Fortunately,

I can still make this choice, but it is possible with the progress of the brain damage that I will lose this ability.

I must learn a new life-style, accommodating to my limitations to reduce the irritation and frustration of constant failure. I must stay in my limited familiar surroundings or go in absolute blind trust with someone who will take care of me. Many of my old activities are gone forever. Emotionally this is difficult. I naturally mourn the loss of old abilities and skills that are now suddenly gone. I try to focus my attention on the things I can still do and enjoy. For instance, the recorded books for the blind supplied by the Library of Congress have filled the tremendous void left by the inability to read. In my personal emotional struggle, I find that a visit to a rest home increases my gratitude immensely and helps me bring the parameters of my present life into proper perspective. The old Indian proverb expresses this well, "I complained because I had no moccasins until I met a man who had no feet."

I am learning to take strength and comfort wherever and whenever it comes to me. Since it is no longer possible to feed my inner man through the usual channels of prayer, meditation, and Bible study, I am learning to be strengthened by words and instructions that suddenly pop into my mind. To recall definite things, particularly under stress, is very difficult. Somehow the more I try to think of something, the more the thoughts disappear. However, at times certain things pop into my mind, much to my surprise and everyone else's. I cannot read the Bible, but suddenly miscellaneous Bible verses come to mind. I take these and think about them for as long as I can, enjoying their truths and praising God for this facet of blessing. As I do this, I also have a reason to thank God for his goodness.

I have a life that can be either frustrating and frightening or peaceful and submissive. The choice is mine. I choose to take things moment by moment, thankful for everything that I have, instead of raging wildly at the things that I have lost. I must thank God for the ability to do this. I know there must be many people who would like to do this, but in their illness they have lost the power to concentrate enough to make this choice.

In accepting this progressive handicap as from the Lord, I am coming to a fuller understanding of that phrase from the Lord's Prayer, "Thy will be done." My unique meeting with Christ assured me that all that has happened to me was in the center of his will, and I am now able to believe with assurance Romans 8:28, "And we know that in all things God works for the good of those who love him, who have been called according to his purpose." I do love him, and I have loved him with all of my heart. Therefore, this stands true, and all the other circumstances that arise must be put in this perspective of love.

In my weakness and in my confusion that night in a motel in Wyoming, Jesus Christ reached down and ushered me into a new dimension of fellowship with him, "the fellowship of his suffering." In his love, Jesus heard my confused prayers and my unsure thoughts, and he understood my unique and desperate needs. I joined a great host of deeply suffering Christians whom Christ has met in their extremity, those people for whom there is no cure or miracle to make them whole again. Those who, like Humpty-Dumpty, cannot be fixed even by "all the King's horses and all the King's men." Those who must learn, with Paul the apostle, of Christ's sufficient grace.

I never really knew how many people are in this special fellowship because I only looked into the lives of the heroic from my wholeness. Now I have walked through that door and find a great crowd of loving, suffering, unsung heroes who are courageously living with Christ through the fellowship of his suffering. Paul went through this door and, though he sought healing, Christ answered, "My grace is sufficient . . . for my strength is made perfect in weakness." And Paul replied, "I will boast all the more gladly about my weaknesses, so that Christ's power may rest on me."

Since my illness, I have discovered a large group of deeply suffering Christians whom Christ has met in the same way he met me that night in the motel. Many Christians have found that when life completely tumbles in, when they are without strength or any hope or help for themselves, or when their minds become too tangled to even hold thoughts, that God overrules the circumstances and that Christ comes to minister to them at the very point of their need.

I will never again be able to preach or to teach. The only service I can do is listen and pray. However, even in my slight ability to do this, I have been so blessed by the calls of those who have experienced the "fellowship of his suffering." I have received calls from quadriplegics, from people in mental hospitals, from loved ones whose partners have lost their minds, from young people who blew their minds away with drugs, and from those who hurt as they have learned they have a terminal illness. We can pray and cry together and wonderfully identify with the person of Jesus our Savior who is reaching down to help us when life tumbles in.

Shortly after this experience of meeting Jesus Christ in such a wonderful and precious way, my health failed again, and we had to fly home to Miami so I could be hospitalized. However, this time it was different. This time I knew that Christ was with me, and I was determined to finish out my ministry with sermons explaining to my people how all of this could possibly be in the center of God's will. I love my congregation, and I love the people of Miami to whom we minister. I thought about my own predicament, and the thousands of people who had been praying for my healing. I was persuaded that, unless I could share my personal peace from Christ, they might think that their prayers were in vain and that perhaps God had failed. As I lay in the hospital, I resolved that I would ask my church officers for the opportunity to preach a series of five farewell sermons. I felt compelled to preach them regardless of my then stuttering speech and impaired vision. I prayed to God, "Please give me strength to conclude my ministry with praise to thee, and with the triumphant spirit that comes from having run the race and finished that one course that was set before me."

Chapter Seven: The Abnormal Changes So Far

Some may ask, "What is it like to have Alzheimer's disease?"

Obviously the noticeable changes will be very individual according to the life-style and occupation of the person and the demands placed upon him. I know that many people were able to continue in their profession much longer than I. People who have a routine job that does not require mathematical skills or new learning may function at their job until they can no longer find their way to the work place.

Because of the particular demands of the pastoral ministry, I was made aware of my losses very early in the course of the disease. For more than a year, many of these losses were attributed to other causes, and I took every possible treatment to alleviate them. The trauma of surgery then brought considerable new demands on my body, and at this time all the measures to compensate no longer took up the slack. I had reached the point of no return. Life would never again be the same.

In my present condition (February 1988, just seven months since diagnosis) there are times when I feel normal. At other times I cannot follow what is going on around me; as the conversation whips too fast from person to person and before I have processed one comment, the thread has moved to another person or another topic, and I am left isolated from the action—alone in a crowd. If I press myself with greatest concentration to try to keep up, I feel as though something short circuits in my brain. At this point I become disoriented, have difficulty with my balance if I am standing, my speech becomes slow, or I cannot find the right words to express myself.

At my own speed and in keeping with my individual body rhythms, I can still act with the skills and knowledge I have acquired over the years. This book is an example of this. It was dictated at all hours of the day and night, whenever I had a clear enough mind to string thoughts together.

In my rational moments I am still me.

Alzheimer's disease is like a reverse aging process. Having drunk from the fountain of youth one is caught in the time tunnel without a stopping place at the height of beauty and strength. Cruelly, it whips us back to the place of infancy. First the memories go, then perceptions, feelings, knowledge, and, in the last stage, our ability to talk and take care of our most basic human needs. Thrusting us headlong into the seventh age of man, "without teeth, without sight, without everything."

At this stage, while I still have some control of thoughts and feelings, I must learn to take on the role of the infant in order to make use of whatever gifts are left to me.

A baby must have its own special environment to be safe and happy. It starts out in a crib, moves on to a playpen, and then goes into its own room and, after five or more years, is trusted outside the house with minimum supervision. The patient with Alzheimer's disease must move in the opposite direction from freedom. Someone must constantly monitor the amount of freedom and self-determination in order to keep the patient safe and able to function at top level.

Patients have to determine the size of their playpen. If they go outside the playpen in their normal life, then, like a baby, they are liable to be hurt, and they are certainly very vulnerable. All the books written on caring for Alzheimer's disease patients stress this point—to maximize the potential for living, the patient must remain in familiar surroundings and follow an established routine.

Ritual

Now that I am developing a ritual with which I can be comfortable, I begin to see the great value of establishing a routine within my limits. It is easy now to understand the seemingly boring routines our parents got into in their later years. At the time we watched our parents do this we tried to bring more variety into their lives only to be met with rejection or scorn. They intuitively had been doing the very thing that science now tells us to establish in order to reduce confusion to a diminished brain capacity.

In the 1950s, my physiology and psychology textbooks taught that the brain does not get tired. They stated that only the physical functions of muscle fatigue, cramps, and eyestrain intrude on our attention span so that we have greater difficulty thinking. I do not know the proper medical description for what occurs, but I do know that the ability to function intellectually rises and falls with the amount of time I have been trying to concentrate and the amount of external stimuli to which I have been exposed. If I do not listen to my body and withdraw from the overstimulation, it takes several days for my intellectual abilities to return. This is very frightening because I can't help wondering each time this happens if I have pushed myself totally over the line of no return.

This past December we took our little family to Disney World. The rides with their blinking and flashing lights, the confusion of the crowds, the long waits in line, and particularly the special effects shows of Epcot totally exhausted my reserves. It became difficult to maintain my balance without something to steady me. I couldn't make a decision as to what I wanted to do. I needed to go to the room and lie down but I couldn't figure out what to do to relieve my discomfort. Finally, my speech became slow and my wife insisted that I be taken to the room. I lay in a dark room, listening to the tapes that keep my mind from falling into the "black hole" that tries to suck me in every time I stop concentrating on something. I spent six days lying in a dark room upon our return from Orlando. For a while I thought that I had lost everything but I began to recoup my ability to function, to leave the house alone, to visit with friends, to dictate portions of this book after more than two weeks of being a couch potato.

Leaving the routine of being around my familiar home, having more people and excitement around than I am accustomed to, varying my ritual for taking care of my grooming and health care, being unable to lie down and nap at my usual times, all brought me to a place of being unable to make even the most basic decisions for myself, of not even being aware of how to relieve my discomfort. This experience taught me that if I want to function at the top of my limited capacity, I must establish a routine and keep to it. I must stay away from crowds, blinking lights, too much emotional or mental stimulation, and must not become physically exhausted. I have to set the bounds of my playpen, even though it is annoying to give up the freedom of "hanging loose." I must seek out social contacts in groups of ten or less. I must avoid shopping centers and large athletic stadiums.

However, I can still go and work in the yard, I can enjoy church worship services and my friends there, and I can still go out in the midst of nature and enjoy places like the Everglades. The most important thing is finding out where I become the most lost and confused, and then staying away from those places so that I can enjoy life in my safe "playpen." Right now, I am very happy in my playpen, yet I realize that it will grow smaller and I will be compelled to adjust to this if I am to function at my highest level.

Two years ago, I was able to handle sudden surprising situations on a routine basis. Now I am completely paralyzed mentally if I am thrown a question that demands an immediate decision on my part. I must protect myself from being thrust into an unexpected situation. My wife answers the phone, or if she is gone I turn on the answering machine. This gives me a moment to assess who is calling and prepare myself to speak with them.

Betty and I have traveled extensively. We have visited more than thirty countries and almost all of the fifty states. Every vacation was a new experience in learning and relationships. I grew by new experiences. I am naturally adventuresome, and we enjoyed every new adventure possible. Those days are over forever. Because of my disease, the new and the strange have to be eliminated. Fear and tension fill me before any new event, even a wonderful event. I have to stay close to home and have less mental and emotional stimulation if I am going to have a more normal and peaceful life.

Along with the need for ritualism, I find that I am now a victim of obsessive behavior. Whatever I start, I want to get finished as soon as possible with no interruptions. An unfinished task preys on my mind until it is completely finished. This is the direct opposite of what I used to be. I used to read four or five books at a time and leave them turned down throughout the house so I could pick one up and read first one and then the other. I had a dozen projects going at the same time and could leave one and be refreshed by picking up the next one and working on it awhile. I was exhilarated by having dozens of balls bouncing in the air so that life did not become stale. Now I can only concentrate on one thing at a time and, much to everyone's distress, this thing occupies my mind and obsesses me until it is completed.

It is an old military maxim that the best generals win because they choose their battlefields carefully. The same thing is true with the early Alzheimer's patient. There are times when we cannot function and we need to withdraw and regroup. There are situations that we know we cannot handle. In spite of all the pushing and urging of friends and family who insist that we will have a wonderful time, the patient senses that it will lead to his mental devastation. There are times when the patient needs to be alone in order to keep everything in proper perspective, and the request to drop out of life or out of a situation at a particular time should be carefully considered.

At this point in my life I can still sense when I need to retreat from some situations, and my guess is that other patients have a better sense of what they should avoid than care givers may be willing to give them credit for knowing.

Paranoia

Paranoia is another of the painful changes that has accompanied my journey into Alzheimer's disease. I was a strong, self-willed, self-disciplined man, and I thought that nothing could ever shake my mind. For years I have claimed Isaiah 26:3–4 as a promise for those who trust God. "You will keep in perfect peace him whose mind is steadfast, because he trusts in you. Trust in the Lord forever, for the Lord, the Lord, is the Rock eternal." I do trust the Lord completely, not just because of blind faith but also because God has proven himself to provide for my every need in every situation. Yet, the devastation wrought by this disease brought me to despair. Gradually, because of not hearing, not remembering, or not comprehending, fear swept over me as I lost more and more control of my circumstances. I was gripped by paranoia. The saddest part is that I became distrustful of those who loved me and had my best interest at heart.

I saw what was happening in me and I could name it at the time as paranoia. However, even though I saw it happening to me, I could do nothing to stop the feelings. I worried particularly about money. There was no reason to worry about money. The church took care of me wonderfully well as they made sure that my salary continued until our very adequate disability plan took effect. I cannot imagine the pain that it caused my friends, but I know that during this time I kept asking silly questions like "Is the insurance paid?" or other questions of this nature. I had such a great fear. I doubted any financial security. It was irrational, but I could do nothing to control the fear. After several months of constant reassurance from my friends and my wife, I am better able to deal with these paranoid feelings. If I start down the worry path about who or what is out to get me, my wife or daughter brings me back with a gentle reminder that, "Your paranoia is talking again."

Having experienced these feelings makes me wonder if this is the reason why people with dementia are found hoarding strange items. The loss of self, which I was experiencing, the helplessness to control this insidious thief who was little by little taking away my most valued possession, my mind, had made me especially wary of the rest of my possessions in an unreasonable way.

This paranoia that accompanies Alzheimer's makes me fearful of so many things and has completely changed my personality. Right now, I am able to recognize many of these things, but later on as the disease progresses I realize that it is going to be a burden to everyone. My goal now is to try to program myself to let Betty worry about the things that I cannot be reasonable about. I must make more conscious effort to trust God for the future. Each time I dignify the paranoia with an action based on the improper feeling, I strengthen the hold the paranoia has on me. Each time I face a paranoid fear and say, "I reject you and your hold on me for my trust is in the Lord and I will not fear what men can do to me," I have won the battle for my mind one more day.

Failures and Mistakes

Certainly one of the very real fears felt by anyone with early Alzheimer's disease is the fear of failure. I live with the imminent dread that one mistake in my daily life will mean another freedom will be taken from me. Each freedom taken places me in a smaller playpen with a tighter ritual to maintain myself.

For example, any housewife can forget a pan on the stove and burn dinner. She and her family just laugh about it and get a can of something else out for supper. If a person with Alzheimer's gets caught burning something, it is a severe tragedy, another marker of the progress of her incompetency for self-sufficiency. In all likelihood, it will take away forever her opportunity to cook unless she has a very understanding, loving family who will allow her to cook but will be willing to keep an eye on the stove without her knowing it. For the healthy person, this oversight will be just an honest mistake, but for the person with Alzheimer's, it may be the end to a whole line of productivity.

What fear this produces! The thought that one moment of inattention will change your life forever! I can still drive my car. So far my physical response time has not been greatly affected. My great problem is that of getting lost. Therefore, I limit my driving to a small radius around my home unless someone is with me to give directions. I also limit myself to driving only when I am well rested and feeling alert. However, I realize that in the old days I could easily have a fender bender in the Miami traffic and it would be no big deal. It happens all the time. Today if I have a fender bender, in all likelihood it will be the end of my driving career. Mistakes are not easily forgiven or forgotten. They often produce great loss of freedom and sense of person. I find myself becoming much more careful and timid, not from paranoia alone but as a result of these very real fears of failure.

Disorganization

It is very painful to go into crowds. When I sit in the middle of a large audience, I find myself becoming more and more panic-stricken, and quite often I will leave the church service, confused and completely drenched with sweat. I do not enjoy large crowds, and I can barely keep up with the people that I meet in the stream of people without becoming confused and having to sit down and regroup my thoughts.

In other places, such as shopping centers with uneven lighting and crowds of people moving in all directions at once, I become confused and completely lost. It is incredible that I can no longer find my way out of the center of a large shopping center, but my mind completely leaves me as I become totally disoriented. Even going into a large supermarket and looking at rows and rows of cans is mentally exhausting. When I do become exhausted, my walk becomes staggering. In a supermarket I can make it very well if I have a grocery cart to push around; or when walking in crowds I cling to the wall in order to give my hands something to touch to keep from going sideways. There is always the tendency in the confusion of a crowd to suddenly step sideways and perhaps to keep on going until I fall.

Headaches are a common occurrence. Whether they are caused by emotional disturbance or organic problems, I do not know. I do know that in times of emotional stress I have tremendous headaches that produce confusion and finally produce physical exhaustion. At the end, my mind blanks out, and I become unresponsive and uncommunicative. During the worst of these times, recovery does not come in an hour or two, but rather in a day or two. It is entirely different than being physically tired. Being mentally overworked takes a great deal of peace and quiet. I usually lie in my darkened bedroom, listening to tapes. Because I can no longer read, due to an organic disability, I am eligible for talking books for the blind, and these are great comfort to me at such times when my mind needs something to occupy it. This helps me in the middle of the night when I become sleepless and restless, and it helps me during the times when I have to withdraw in order to regather my mental abilities.

Waking up from sleep is a real experience. I have no idea where I am at times, and also I am totally lost. I have run into more objects in our bedroom and have more bruises from getting up and wandering around in the middle of the night than I care to state. Therefore, after I sit on the side of the bed to get myself orientated, I have to turn the light on in order to see. I am totally lost and forget the pattern of my own bedroom, even though it has been my bedroom for the last ten years.

At my worst times, I cannot bring myself out of this state of stupor. I need something to shock or stimulate me awake. I had a talk with one of my friends about making a battery-powered shocking device to try to bring me out of this quickly, but we decided against it as we did not know what the effects would be. One of my dear friends, Dr. Joe Davis, a psychologist who has helped me with this crisis, came up with a very simple solution. He said that if I would lay the roughest kind of indoor-outdoor carpet on my bedroom floor as a path between my bed and the bathroom, I could then follow the carpet with my bare feet, and probably the pain on my feet would rouse me from this state. It is an excellent suggestion, and one that should be considered. Again suggestions of this nature are hard to find because so little has been researched and written.

Hearing

My wife had been telling me to have my hearing checked for two years. I thought that I had a little trouble hearing on the phone at church so I had a special hard-of-hearing headset installed. As some close friends began to insinuate that perhaps I wasn't hearing everything, I began to check myself. I listened for the tick of the clock on the wall, and other little obscure sounds. When I concentrated I could hear perfectly well, so I inferred there was nothing wrong with my hearing. Yet my wife continued to speak loudly to me. I told her over and over again that there was no need to yell, as I could hear perfectly well. Strangely, she insisted that she did not raise her voice until the third repetition. I never heard her say anything three times.

Now it is clear why. I was missing many spoken clues. Whole sentences were passing by without my knowing it, and people could speak for my attention without my noticing. There was nothing the matter with my ears. The trouble was in my brain. I could not make the shift in attention until seconds or even moments after the intrusion. And on some occasions the intrusion never came to my conscious level. It was for this reason that I had to give up counseling, which I dearly love. I can still give wise and scriptural advice, but it is altogether possible that I would not hear the problem fully. Thus, I might give wise advice, but on the wrong subject.

Patterns and Pictures

I have lost my ability to fit patterns and pictures together. I find difficulty grouping things like I used to. A jigsaw puzzle is impossible for me. I cannot see how things fit. I cannot pack a car trunk. I can't figure out how to screw a nut on a bolt or how a piece of wood is supposed to fit into a slot. This ability to see spatial relationships is gone. I sometimes find the same difficulty relating verbal things as well. It is as if I hear things and they get into the wrong slots, which make no sense to me at all.

Forgetfulness

Memory loss is usually the first thing people think of when Alzheimer's disease is mentioned. I had always prided myself on my memory. I very seldom used notes during the day, nor even needed to carry a calendar for the day's appointments. About a year before my diagnosis, forgetfulness began to plague me. I found myself forgetting, not just obscure facts, but the most familiar things. When called upon to introduce the officers of my church whom I knew and loved intimately, I suddenly forgot their names or their wives' names. When called upon to remember the most obvious Bible verses, I would have it slip away. After missing one or two appointments, I began to carry a calendar and note my appointments. I even began carrying slips of paper to remind myself of certain things. Sometimes in teaching I would find myself grasping for the most familiar words.

Things learned in the past by rote were difficult to recall. I could explain the meaning of what I wanted to say but could not repeat verbatim. Recently learned material was more likely to be difficult to recall than things from the far past. With long-term memory, it is more like I have lost the access key to certain memories. Recognition is less impaired than recall. If a photo or a story jogs a past memory it will usually come forth intact.

Physical Exercise and Wandering

Wandering around and restlessness is one of the by-products of Alzheimer's disease. Many people have tried to guess why Alzheimer's disease patients are so restless and want to walk around at all hours of the day and night. I believe I may have a clue. When the darkness and emptiness fill my mind, it is totally terrifying. I cannot think my way out of it. It stays there, and sometimes images stay stuck in my mind. Thoughts increasingly haunt me. The only way that I can break this cycle is to move. Vigorous exercise to the point of exhaustion gets my mind out of the black hole. At first, it meant for me to go to a quiet room in our home and ride furiously on an exercise bicycle until I was panting and exhausted and my mind was clear. Now I try to schedule my daily routine with productive, physically demanding activity. Following this I rest quietly, listening to my tapes and sometimes fall asleep. When I wake, I am refreshed and usually more alert mentally. When I have had a particularly difficult night and awaken foggy and disoriented, I find that a stretch of vigorous activity helps me to clear my head.

Adaptation

My psychologist told me one evidence that I had been laboring under diminished capacity for some time before I was aware of the loss was the many compensatory techniques I was employing unknowingly. Some compensatory techniques are helping me maximize my potential. I must learn new ways to get things programmed into my brain, and I must find new ways to get my communication out to others. I must adapt to these handicaps for as long as I still have enough undamaged brain to do it. As noted earlier, tape-recorded books for the blind have filled the gap that my reading loss left.

A keyboard has taken up the slack that the writing loss left. Strangely, when I attempt to communicate in my own handwriting I leave words out, put down incomplete thoughts, and write in a scrawl, legible only to my wife. When I read over what I have done, it looks all right to me. I am unaware of the omitted words. Upon being made aware of the poor quality of my written letters, I thought I would try to type. Having been blessed with a secretary for the last twenty years, I had found no need to type.

I am not a touch typist anyway. In college we called my method the Columbus method: "Land on one key and then search for another." Much to my surprise, the thoughts appeared much more completely in the typewritten material. In addition to having less mistakes, it was easier for me to see any omissions. This track of adaptation led us on to a user-friendly computer with a word processing program. Now I am able to write letters and feel that I am not totally isolated from the world of intelligent people.

Sleep

Sleeplessness has accompanied my journey into Alzheimer's disease. I feel as though I have forgotten how to fall asleep. I lay awake hour after hour every night. Sometimes I get only two or three hours of sleep. The less sleep I have, the more disturbed and confused I become. Depression, confusion, and paranoia accompany the sleep deprivation.

Before the surgery last spring, my mind held accurate photographs of all the places that I have traveled around the world. I could recall with vivid imagery the pleasant experiences I had in my life. I would turn my mind to this and to thoughts of prayer and thoughts of praise and slip off to sleep with great joy. Now with this diseased condition, when I let loose of my concentration my thoughts go into blackness. In this blackness, like the Bloom County cartoon strip, the terrible monsters from Milo's anxiety closet come out to haunt me. One night I spent hours facing down a tiger with bared fangs. Though my intellect knew this was only a figment of my mental pictures, my body reacted with all the adrenaline rush, perspiration, rapid breathing, and heart pounding of a real situation. And perhaps the worst part was that I could not move my body. I felt if only I could get up and start walking, reality would return. My body refused to respond to my will but rather responded to the unreal situation presented by my shorted-out brain.

I had to find a way to move from waking into sleep without getting caught in this never-never land of terror. I tried the usual radio talk shows and found them extremely distressing, because they were usually controversial subjects that got my mind whirling with the arguments raised. Music did not lull me to sleep.

As much as I hate to admit it, even the Bible on tape did not help. It rather awakened me as my mind would go back and pick up some familiar passage, think about it, think of when I had taught about it or preached on it, how it had been used, and then with all this stimulation sleep was gone. A relaxation tape made by my psychologist, Dr. Jack Tapp, gave me the first relief from this dilemma. His soft, persuasive voice talked me through the blackness to sleep. In fact, I used the tape for two weeks before I ever heard the end of it. But gradually even this lost its effect. If only I could find something else which was not stimulating to the imagination but was interesting enough to hold the concentration level out of the "black hole."

God answers our prayers in many interesting ways. A young couple, Phil and Debbie Rich, knowing I had lost my ability to read and wanting to comfort me, put their ingenuity to work and found some cassette tapes of Louis L'Amour. As unspiritual as this may seem, Louis L'Amour books of the American west have been favorites of mine for years. His word pictures had piqued my interest in the western scenery. I had used these books for years to turn off the whirl of my mind after late night committee meetings or counseling sessions. Again, I found myself turning on the same side of the tape for several nights before I finally heard it to the end. At last a way to help me past the "anxiety closet of my mind" and into the welcomed relief of sleep.

When I had finally heard all the tapes to the end I went to the public library and learned that not only could I get regular commercial books on tape but that since Alzheimer's disease is an organic cause for being unable to read, the vast store of recorded books for the blind are available to me free of charge. They are available to anyone who cannot read for some physical reason, even to those who are physically impaired so that they cannot hold a book. Forms are needed from two doctors to verify the condition, and information on how to apply is available from most public libraries.

Since sleep comes to me so erratically now, I determined that during these times of wakefulness, which may come at two in the morning, I would not get up. I turn on the tape machine and listen to these books. I realize that if I allow myself to set a pattern of getting up to watch television or wander around the house I will disrupt the sleep patterns of everyone in the family. Therefore, I consider it a part of my self-discipline to keep my sleep confined to normal hours, and I lie quietly listening to a tape through an earplug or pillow speaker. I hope this will delay the time when I will create the "thirty-six-hour day" for my family with twenty-four-hour days of no beginning or end.

Responses from Others

I have been a public figure for twenty-nine years. When someone's profession thrusts him into the public eye whether as a preacher, a performer, or a professional athlete, it involves giving up certain freedoms of privacy.

We explained this to our children when they were growing up complaining about their goldfish bowl existence, telling them that "it goes with the territory." The easiest way to deal with the situation when people's lives are an open book is just to be sure there are no pages they would be ashamed for Jesus Christ to read. If our lives please him, there is no need to fear what anyone else may say about us.

Since my life has been open for public view, there was no way to hide what was happening to me. My ruling elders had been aware that I was trying to deal with an undiagnosed illness for more than a year. When I finally learned that there is no chance that I will ever be any better than I am now, I had no choice but to make it known and resign. For five months prior to my resignation, I had only been able to work in a very limited capacity. Being unable to carry out the duties of the minister of a large suburban church and being a limited human being are two vastly different roles. Not being able to handle the ministerial role did not mean that I immediately became a blithering idiot. Rather, it meant that I am now limited in my activities. I must choose my "battleground," so to speak. I need more rest and recuperative time after social contacts. I may not remember your name but if I have known you I still know you. The disease interferes with the access passageways especially to the names of things but I still know the thing. It is the vocabulary, not the concept, that is gone at this early stage.

As soon as my diagnosis was announced, some people became very uncomfortable around me. I realize that the shock and pain, especially to those who have a parent with this disease, are difficult to deal with at first. It was strange that in most cases I had to make the effort to seek out people who were avoiding me and look them in the eye and say, "I don't bite. I am still the same person. I just can't do my work anymore. I know that one of these days I will not be in here anymore, but for now, maybe for another year or two, I am still home in here and I need your friendship and acceptance."

Usually the response was one of great relief. Over and over the answer came, "I'm so glad you said that. I just didn't know what to say. I didn't know how to treat you. I didn't know if you could still laugh."

I am still human. I laugh at the ridiculous disease that steals the most obvious things from my thoughts and leaves me spouting some of the most obscure, irrelevant information when the right button is pushed. I want to participate in life to my utmost limit. The reduced capacity, however, leaves me barely able to take care of my basic living needs, and there is nothing left over for being a productive member of society. This leaves me in a terrible dilemma. When I go out into society I look whole. There is no wheelchair, no bandage, or missing part to remind people of my loss. It is difficult to meet the question, "What do you do?" When I answer, "I am a retired minister."

The next line hurts, "You look awfully young to be retired."

When you answer, "I have Alzheimer's disease," there is a strange look and uncomfortable silence. When Mayor Steve Clark and Commissioner Clare Oesterle, on behalf of the Board of Dade County Commissioners, presented me with a certificate of appreciation, this strange treatment was illustrated. Commission meetings are aired live on a cable channel and again in the evening for the benefit of those who are working during the day. That evening my family and I watched the presentation on television. During the shifting back to their seats, some of the commissioners, unaware that their microphones were open, were laughing and commenting, "He sure talks fine for someone with Alzheimer's."

For some reason some segments of society have a hard time dealing with a person who is just partly here. If you are unable to carry on all the responsibilities of your work, you should be bedfast or at least drooling on yourself.

One of the children at church illustrated this very well. After the final sermon and tearful farewell party and our very abbreviated trip, we returned to church to worship. This precious child of about eight years old, unhampered by the restrictions of manners, greeted me with his honest question, "Dr. Davis, why aren't you dead yet?" I gently explained, "The disease I have just kills your brain a little at a time, and I will probably be around for a while longer. I will worship here at the church even though I can't be the minister anymore."

As I have visited many nursing homes in my twenty-nine years of ministry, I have seen many people afflicted with one kind of dementia or another. When I relate to them, I do not do so with the assumption that they are silly, old, helpless people. I see the person they once were. If I did not know the person before the dementia, I tried to learn about them from a friend or relative. There is still a part of that vital person living inside that sometimes helpless-looking body, a person who deserves to be treated with dignity. Just because a person is incontinent or requires feeding does not give some eighteen-year-old twit the right to call them "dearie," or "sweetie."

Watching some of the Alzheimer's day care centers featured on television gives me the "willies." I could never bear to be talked to and treated like a child at summer camp. "All right boys and girls, let's all stretch our arms to the music; let's dance the hokey pokey."

I am repulsed by activity directors on cruise ships, much less some twenty-year-old trying to get me to play childish exercises to rock music. I'm sure I would try to get back to my room and if stopped in this attempt I would become churlish and belligerent. If the insensitive director continued to push or became condescending and began to pat my arm, I would probably explode with all the violence pent up in my six-foot-seven frame. If I were then restrained or tied in my chair, my fury would take me right out of my mind.

Why? Is this a result of Alzheimer's disease? No, this is how I would react now in my best state of mind. I cannot stand the beat of rock music or the bouncing around of even senior citizen aerobic exercise classes. Human dignity demands that I have the right of refusal for any activity or entertainment that I do not perceive as entertaining. I deserve the right to withdraw from any situation and to go to a place of quiet and calm that I have appreciated over the years.

As a caring professional minister, I have learned many things over the years. A person even in a comatose condition often hears what is said in the room.

Relatives have been surprised on many occasions to learn that the comments they made in the presence of a comatose individual have been repeated to them when the patient regains consciousness. A person in whatever state of dementia deserves to be treated with all dignity and respect. In my twenty-nine years in the ministry, I have always called people by their title or Mr. or Mrs. until our friendship put us on a first name basis. I have never appreciated nurses and aides who greet me with over-familiarity.

When I called on persons suffering from any kind of mental loss, I let them tell me whatever was on their mind, and tell it as many times as they felt necessary. Then I tried to gently guide their thoughts back to an earlier, happier time. As they relaxed with their comforting memories, I then guided the conversation to the goodness of God and encouraged them to pray with me.

In Alzheimer's disease there is the loss of the personality, a diminished sense of self-worth. A highly productive person has to wonder why he is still alive and what purpose the Lord has in keeping him on this earth. As I struggle with the indignities that accompany daily living, I am losing my sense of humanity and self-worth. Blessed is the person who can take the Alzheimer's patient back to that happier time when they were worthwhile and allow them to see the situation in which they were of some use. I have a basket of letters from these angels of mercy who have written to remind me of a time that I shared God's strength with them and helped them. These have been my sustenance during these dark months of loss.

How One Goes into Society

I am not yet ready to be a hermit, even though there are times when I must insulate myself and regroup my diminishing resources. When I go into a large group of people, I know my friends, but the stimulus comes too quickly for my brain to sort out names. I smile and say hello to everyone. If I see someone approaching me, I try to ask the first question. It will be a timely question but one that makes little difference what the answer is. It may be as general as, "What do you think of the Miami Dolphins this year?" or "Isn't this weather incredible?" Sometimes this will buy me enough time to bring to mind some personal information so that I can ask about their work or family. This puts the burden of the first answer on them, and it allows me to sort things out and get them in their proper perspective. Blessed is that person who comes up to me and tells me his name first and reminds me of some experience we have shared. Usually this kind of approach on their part suddenly triggers a flow of memories that is almost impossible for me to recall by just reaching into the blankness.

Much of my life has been spent in the midst of large crowds of people. Now I find the maximum size group of people for me is no more than eight or ten. In larger groups I go into such overload that I have to withdraw and leave the group early. I still need social contact, but it must be limited to just a few people at a time and with little stimulation. Extraneous noise, such as a loud television set, a barking dog, or children who constantly interrupt and vie for attention produce overload so that I can no longer participate in the conversation. I develop a headache and begin to cough uncontrollably. The only remedy for this is a quiet, dark room.

Letting Go Release

As a pastor, I have been through many heart-breaking situations with parents who had a dementia of one kind or another. The difficulty they brought on themselves and their children because they refused to recognize their diminished capacity for good decision-making was tragic. I have seen them give away fortunes and do many other foolish things. I do not want this to happen to me.

I have given my wife the ability to make all decisions for the family. An attorney set up a durable power of attorney for her so that when I become totally incapacitated she will not have to resort to the courts for the authority to use our resources. She has the authority to make any legal decision on my behalf. I cannot function with any external pressure weighing on me. Since I can no longer do mathematical calculations, it would be foolish for me to hang on to the financial decision-making.

It is humiliating to give up our areas of responsibility. There is a distinct feeling of the loss of self and all that we have been. Yet all is not gone. I have chosen to give up those areas where I will be met with failure or my wife would be filled with aggravation at having to live with the consequences of my foolish decisions. It is better to release willingly those areas and concentrate on the areas where I still have some ability. Just as my wife gave up her right to self-determination when she married me and vowed to love, honor, and obey, so now in my weakness I willingly relinquish to the woman who has modeled the wife in Proverbs:

A wife of noble character who can find? She is worth far more than rubies. Her husband has full confidence in her and lacks nothing of value. She brings him good, not harm, all the days of her life. (Prov. 21:10–12)

This act of relinquishing to her has relieved me of many of the things that would rob me of peace.

From In a Tangled Wood:
An Alzheimer's Journey

JOYCE DYER

CHAPTER THREE: PLAQUES AND TANGLES

This is madness, I think. "This is madness," I say out loud. But I know better.
This is Alzheimer's disease.

Marion Roach, *Another Name for Madness*

1

TANGLEWOOD is a tiny and simple world, but still a world far too complicated for most of the people living here. A thousand times a day, residents of
Tanglewood ask where their rooms are and where they sit for dinner. Names
printed in black marker and pasted to bright backgrounds appear on dining
room tables, on doors of rooms, above beds. The construction-paper backgrounds are color-coded. Each resident has become a Crayola crayon in a box
of twenty-four. My mother's color is consistently, always, purple.

A long table runs across one side of the living area. A heavy piece of glass
protects its surface, but also weighs down a photograph display of residents.
Their names are printed boldly on strips of paper taped above each picture.
A banner appears at the top: "Seniors at Tanglewood. Summer 1994."

Mr. Miller just arrived at Tanglewood and still knows his name, and where
he eats, and how to find his room. Mr. Miller always wears his baseball cap
tightly on his head to keep his brains from spilling out and says the same thing
a hundred times a day to anyone who will listen. "Have you seen Sandra Miller?
Tell her I'm looking for her."

But for residents who no longer can read, or have forgotten their names, the
signs become useless. Lost men and women sit at tables and with thick yellow
thumbnails pick and scratch the heavy tape that bolts their names to the furniture.

2

When I arrived for an early winter visit in 1994, I noticed that my mother seemed to have something tucked in her pants. Her slender waist and small stomach protruded in unnatural ridges. I pulled the elastic waistband toward me and heard the sound of fabric slapping plastic. My mother was wearing a diaper, a Depend brief for adults.

She was becoming occasionally incontinent. This had not been a good week for her; there had been many accidents. For some time now, an aide had been taking her to the bathroom every four hours. But even that wasn't working. Annabelle had forgotten what a toilet was, after using one for over eighty years.

She would sit on the cold seat, but would no longer understand the purpose for being there. She could not urinate on command. Her body processes were beyond her control. Sometimes she would refuse to cooperate altogether, scream "No!" and strike the arms and chests of attendants who were trying to pull her pants down or help her bend her knees and crouch.

When I visit my mother, I am keenly aware of urination. I check immediately to see if she is in a Depend or wearing her own underpants. We visit her toilet several times, and once in a while she understands what to do. If I use the toilet first in front of her, she seems to show more interest.

Once she guided me into a room not her own, and stood for ten minutes staring directly at the toilet bowl. Like a bird discovering a new birdbath in a somewhat familiar garden, she angled her head several times in confusion. Then, she clasped the safety rail on one side with her left hand and leaned over slightly to flick the water in the bowl with her right. Finally, she turned around, backed in, pulled down her pants, sat, and peed.

I saw her grin as she closed her eyes.

3

There are many varieties of dementia. Alzheimer's is just one. My mother also suffers from multi-infarct, known as mixed dementia. At least three times since being admitted to Tanglewood, she has had "transient ischemic attacks," or TIAs, temporary warning signs of possible stroke. On two such occasions, she just passed out at dinner, fell off her chair and onto the floor. I always race to the unit after receiving calls about these episodes, but when I arrive my mother is usually sitting quietly in her seat, unaware that anything unusual has happened.

Often she is smiling, perhaps secretly proud that nothing so minor will ever take her from this earth. Alzheimer's is the opponent she must fear, the opponent worthy of my mother—not some feeble villain of the vascular system.

I know a stroke will never kill her. I know it for a fact.

4

Famous people who have died from Alzheimer's disease: Norman Rockwell, Sugar Ray Robinson, Edmund O'Brien, Rita Hayworth, Otto Preminger, E. B. White, Ross McDonald, Joyce Chen. Famous people who have cared for someone with Alzheimer's: Mike Myers, Jay Rockefeller, Angie Dickinson, Keith Hernandez, Deborah Hoffmann, Shelley Fabares, Nancy Reagan. Lewis Thomas called it a "disease-of-the-century." He said, "It is the worst of all diseases, not just for what it does to the patient, but for its devastating effects on families and friends." Thomas singled it out in 1980 as the one disease that ought to be targeted by the government for special research funding. He urged private foundations that currently have a large stake in the "Health-Care Delivery System" to commit half their endowments to research on senile dementia, knowing the government cannot handle this disease alone.

No one can.

5

My mother was diagnosed with Alzheimer's when she was seventy-six years old. She visited the doctor, much against her will, and was given an MSQ (mental-status questionnaire examination) and a CAT scan. "DAT," her diagnosis read. Dementia of the Alzheimer Type. Profound brain atrophy.

Due to the late onset of her disease, I am not at extremely great risk.

But I am at higher risk than others, and I know it.

No physical symptom that mimics brain atrophy is casual to me. If I feel my head cloud from a headache or heat, I picture brain cells dying behind my eyes. When I misplace a folder or show the slightest hesitancy about finding my parked car—or a word, especially a word—I panic.

Sometimes I think I will kill myself if I find out this is my fate.

But maybe I will not.

I used to ask my father how he did all he did, how he, a very impatient man by nature, stood the tension and demands of my mother's illness with such humor and grace. "She's like an old dog," he would say. "I've gotten kind of used to her over the years."

My mother's illness has been both the greatest task she has ever asked of me, and the greatest gift she has ever given. It has broken me in half, and made me whole in a way I could never have been without it. It has destroyed me completely, but healed me for all eternity. How can I explain such remarkable contradictions?

Her illness made my father a great man. A truly great man whom I came to adore.

As brutal and incomprehensible as it might sound, even to me, perhaps most especially to me, I think I would let it happen, should it happen to me.

6

Since my mother entered Stage 3 of her disease, the final stage, the following drugs have been prescribed: Ativan, Thorazine, milk of magnesia, Darvocet, aspirin, estrogen, Senokot syrup, Sinequan, Provera, and Thera-M vitamins. She has been on doses of Thorazine as high as 75 mg, when severely agitated, and as low as 10 mg. She took her first dose of Thorazine in 1993, for "obsessiveness, compulsiveness, hitting, kicking, psychotic behaviors." I am always told when the dosage is upped or lowered. And I am never happier than when my mother is on only 10 mg. Or on none at all.

Other drugs that those with Alzheimer's have been given include Hydergine, Cognex, Haldol, Stelazine, Compazine, choline combined with lecithin, and neuropeptides. Eldepryl, originally prescribed for Parkinson's disease, seems to increase sociability in people with Alzheimer's, but results are inconclusive. Ibuprofen, the drug contained in such pain relievers as Advil, Motrin, and Nuprin, has been the promising focus of a fourteen-year Johns Hopkins University study. It seems to reduce the risk of developing Alzheimer's disease by as much as 30 to 60 percent. And tacrine, now approved for sale, as well as Exelon, a promising drug currently being tested, shows evidence of slowing or temporarily reversing the disease.

Lamps continue to flicker late into the night at research centers throughout the world, looking for magic.

7

The county where my mother resides reports 8,517 cases of Alzheimer's disease. In the region where she lives, 50,000 people are afflicted with Alzheimer's, enough to fill a football stadium. In the state that Annabelle Coyne has always called home, in the state where my mother will live out her life and be buried beside my father when she dies, 170,944 people are gradually losing their minds.

8

If you were to board a hovercraft and fly over two human brains, one normal and one diseased by Alzheimer's, you would notice some remarkable differences.

If you had a giant PET scanner with you, an imager built for the gods, the AD brain would exhibit huge oceans of purple in the center, not healthy green or turquoise islands. Purple shows fluid in the brain, fluid that increases as more and more brain cells die. When you return, you'll never like purple again. You will fold your priestly robes into a cedar chest and leave the order. You will avoid grape jelly the rest of your life.

The normal brain has folds in the cerebrum called *sulci*. They are narrow and shallow. But a brain diseased by Alzheimer's exhibits deeper valleys, and much wider. The valleys widen as the brain shrinks. Neurons lose their intricate branches and fill up with abnormal protein deposits, called tangles. Outside the nerve cells plaques form, graveyards for dead or dying neurons.

The disease has built a labyrinth from which no one can ever escape. It has gouged out the brain with a forklift. Even without your scanner you can see the valleys of death.

You could drop a huge silver ball into one of the wide crevices of an Alzheimer's brain from your craft and never find it again. It would roll forever in the pinball machine from hell.

You don't want to crash over the deadly surface of a brain like this. There's no way out.

9

Frances moves in perpetual motion. She sits in her wheelchair and shakes from the top of her right shoulder to the little toe of her right foot. She is in an uncontrollable flutter. She is a seventeen-year locust, incapable of producing sound except through the constant movement of her wings.

The parts of her brain that control her muscles are being destroyed, day by day, cell by cell. She has tangles from Alzheimer's, and tangles from progressive palsy. Frances's brain is all knotted up.

And so is Reggie's.

Reggie is constantly on parade, wearing a T-shirt that says "Over the Hill" and marching rigidly over the same ground every day. He seems practically paralyzed—and is. He can move his lower body, but his arms are as inflexible and rigid as a mannequin's. His hands clump in fists and his fingers seem to have disappeared into his palms. His features are as fixed as those on the face of a coin. Nothing ever moves—not eyebrows, lips, not even skin. In the four years I have known him, his expression has never changed.

Reggie belongs on Mount Rushmore with Washington, Jefferson, Lincoln, and Theodore Roosevelt.

I sometimes wonder what Reggie was doing when his face decided to turn to stone.

10

A phone message is on my answering machine when I arrive home from a morning of errands. It's Esther's. "Now, don't worry," she begins. And then, the terrifying words I dread even spoken in Esther's calm tones, "But your mother..."

My mother had been standing behind a rocker, watching a small group dance to music during an activity period. She had lost consciousness and fallen to her knees, her hands still clinging firmly to the back of the chair. Nurses rushed to her side. She quickly snapped awake and allowed herself to be guided to a sofa. They observed her for half an hour. Then, as she lifted herself up, the nurses holding tightly to her arms, her entire right side, and her left arm, began to twitch. Her body jerked uncontrollably in a fit of seizure—an occasional twist to the disease that appears in late stages. She began a horrible dance, a Saint Vitus dance, a dance that can only be danced alone.

Esther sat my mother in a G/C, a geriatric chair that restricts movement, and began to administer oxygen. She pulled the chair beside her at the nurse's station. She had called my mother's doctor and been advised to monitor her carefully for one hour and summon an ambulance if my mother did not improve or respond.

For one hour, Annabelle stared into space, unable to follow a face or a finger trying to pull her back to Tanglewood. She twisted and jerked to music no one else heard. Completely gone, she permitted the oxygen mask to remain in place, for exactly one hour. Then, almost as if a timer had been set in her dead head, my mother tore the mask from her face, blinked her eyes, smiled slyly at the aides and nurses gathered lovingly around her, and skipped away down the hall.

Once more, she had evaded her executioner.

11

Victoria likes to sit by the TV. Not because she likes TV but because she likes to pull hard on the steel cart that supports it. Victoria's hands are like yard clippers, like Venus flytraps. They grab and pinch and pull and tear whatever they can reach.

She sits in a vinyl chair, rolling up her turquoise pants far above her knees. Victoria has beautiful legs, and perhaps she remembers this about herself. Her calves are muscular and have not discolored and bulged out with veins like those of the rest of the women in the unit.

She is busy today. She takes a Kleenex and stuffs it in the toe of her slipper, pushing the slipper almost out of reach—but not quite. Fetch the Slipper is her favorite game. She supports herself on the arms of the chair and tries to rise. But her beautiful legs no longer know what to do. Dim signals sent out by her brain are returned marked "Address Unknown." She raises her rear six inches off the vinyl and then drops back to her sitting position. Again and again, a hundred times an hour, she tries to rise but invariably falls back into her seat.

Her only other movement is to grab hold of blouses, shirts, TV carts, arms, anything that she might trap. She has torn sleeves off uniforms, ripped fabric belts from waists, scratched forearms, and upset juice carts. Victoria is strong and quick. If she has you in her vise, you must strain to free yourself. And when you do, and run away, she howls and sobs like a little child.

The nurses gently scold her, but know there will be no remembering. There is no point to a reprimand. When they lift her from her seat into a wheelchair, they swiftly grab her under the arms and let her flail like a spider. She points her arms high into the air, turning thumbs and index fingers into pistols, laughs wildly, and tongues a sound.

"Da-da-da-da-daaa!" she repeats over and over, shooting the demons that have done this to her.

12

In the late spring of 1994, I discovered that my mother had forgotten not only her bladder but also her bowels. We were sitting outside in the patio on a cool day when I realized how foreign her own body had become to her.

She suddenly grew extremely restless. She began pacing the walk. Then she went to each corner of the enclosure and pressed her right shoulder firmly against it. She proceeded to rub her body up and down the seams of the building, up and down the bricks and boards.

Finally she stopped her frenzied activity at the fourth corner, the corner where Tanglewood abuts the nursing wing. She pushed her back hard against the bricks and bent her legs slightly. Her face flushed. She looked at me in terror. I tried to pull her toward the Tanglewood entrance, but she stood stiff and immovable.

Slowly, she took her right hand and slid it inside the back of her sweatpants. She brought it out after a few moments, heaped with her own warm excrement. I had no idea what to do.

Shaking, I grabbed a tissue from my purse, but she would not release her grasp and let me remove the waste. Instead, she began throwing it against windows and walls and white doors. It was everywhere and she wouldn't stop until it was all gone. Her hand was colored brown and under her nails were pieces of feces. But at last she let me clasp her wrist and clean her.

It was then that I asked the nurses about her bowel habits. They said this had been going on for several weeks. They were not surprised and told me it was common in the late stages of the disease. I was not to be alarmed. It was normal.

In the unit itself, they would find pieces of my mother's excrement in the grooves of wooden handrails (her favorite hiding place), in corners, on light bulbs. Once they smelled it at night warmed by the glow of a lamp. Another time they found steaming coils on a wool welcome mat I had bought my mother for Christmas. It was woven with the words "Home Sweet Home."

On one occasion she had proudly placed a neatly formed ball of it on the counter of the nurse's station and stuck a pencil she had found unguarded smack in the center, like a birthday cake for a one-year-old.

CHAPTER FOUR: NURSES AND STAFF

If there is wisdom to be found, it must be in the knowledge that human beings are capable of the kind of love and loyalty that transcends not only the physical debasement but even the spiritual weariness of the years of sorrow.
Sherwin B. Nuland, "Alzheimer's Disease," from *How We Die*

1

Carolyn is huffing down the hall toward Tanglewood. I see her flowered blouse, her trademark, a mile away. She has a piece of paper in her hand loaded with signatures.

"Have you been reading about Walt Disney?" she asks me as we approach the unit together, her glasses slipping down her nose. "Disney is trying to build near Manassas. I have a petition already completed. They can't do that. This is sacred, hallowed ground!"

I agree, and hold the door for her as she enters Tanglewood in front of me.

2

Mrs. Goldman. Admitted in February of 1994. Mrs. Goldman is a small woman, the matriarch of the unit at ninety-nine years. "Ninety-nine," she says to anyone who will listen. "It's better to go earlier. Good Lord."

Mrs. Goldman sits on a chair upholstered in dark pink vinyl. A chair that gives her a view of nearly everything that's going on. She can see the television screen in the central area by leaning just inches to her left. Even without leaning she can hear the sound of Vivien Leigh pleading with Clark Gable on a video of *Gone With the Wind*, one of the unit's favorite films. "Oh, Rhett. I'm so cold and hungry."

She sits with her walker in front of her, dressed as she dressed thirty years, fifty years, seventy years ago. "My husband did this to me. He always was good to me. I don't understand. He thinks I can't take care of myself and do the shopping. You never know when you get old what will happen. I had a beautiful house."

An aide stops to listen. She strokes Mrs. Goldman's hair. "You're entitled to your opinion, Mrs. Goldman. Everyone is."

3

"Relax," says Esther. "Just relax, Stanley."

Stanley is in a wheelchair, shaking all over. He wears a fleece sweat suit, the typical attire of both men and women in Tanglewood. They look like dabs of primary color, Olympic athletes, gumdrops: purple, black, turquoise, red mounds of cotton and Spandex. Stanley is dressed in Reebok tennis shoes and bright gold sweats—the Golden Fleece of Tanglewood. A nervous aide is trying to push him as quickly as she can toward his room and his private bath. But Stanley drags his feet and nearly topples head first onto the floor.

He winces, moans, then screams. "Can't hold it!"

Esther quietly, powerfully, rises from her seat behind the nurse's station and places her hand on the arm of Stanley's chair. "Relax," she exhales. She rests her hand on his stomach, close to the groin. She lifts his feet that have been scuffling across the close-napped carpet and slides them onto the footrests she locks in place. "Relax, Stan," she smiles.

He stops shaking. The aide continues her brief journey down the hall to Stanley's room.

4

Esther is from West Virginia. She loves the mountains. She loves her religion. She loves the hymns sung by visiting church groups.

Esther works the day shift and has been at The Woods twenty-five years, five of those at Tanglewood. She is one of the founders who argued for a special wing for people like my mother. When Esther is on duty, the residents are spoiled. They know it and they love it.

Esther doesn't mind spills or messes. In the four years I've been coming to Tanglewood, I've never seen her irritated, annoyed, short-tempered. Once I saw an angry resident punch Esther in the stomach because Esther was trying to lift her from her chair so that her diaper could be changed. Esther caught her breath and then looked directly in her enemy's eye. "Dana," Esther said, in the tone of a strict but loving parent, "no more. That's enough. Come with me. It's over." The woman nodded her head and echoed Esther's last words, "Come with me. It's over." She walked with Esther, hand in hand, down the hall.

Esther always has a story to tell me about Annabelle when I arrive. She loves my mother. I hope my mother dies during her shift.

5

I stand near the nurse's station talking with Esther. I place my elbow on the counter and rest my chin in the palm of my right hand and listen to her voice. It nearly rocks me to sleep. She tells me about her vacation. She'll be going to a special Florida beach with her grandson, she says, where the sand is always cool, like baking powder from a red tin can, not like sand at all.

As she talks, three male residents drift to the counter like ghosts. They stand side by side, arms folded, staring at Esther—much as I am.

"They think this is a bar," she laughs. She pats, then squeezes, each of the six hands. The men turn, almost in step, and say something about cars and sons and keys in a half-human roar. They lower their heads like Minotaurs and waddle down a leg of their labyrinth looking for something they will never find because they have forgotten what it is.

6

My mother quickly grabs an unattended piece of paper from the counter top of the nurse's station. She folds it three times and then leads me toward the patio. It will be my task the rest of the afternoon to recover the sheet and return it to the nurse on duty when I leave.

We sit under the umbrella table and relax. My mother smiles and stares at me with blue clouded eyes, eyes so much like the sky today that it is remarkable. She looks at her right hand and is surprised to see the paper that she holds. She unfolds it and tries to read, but can only growl, "Gee, yee, gee." She shrugs her shoulders, refolds the paper, and places it tightly in my hand. She laughs and stares off somewhere else.

I open the paper and start to iron it back to its original condition with my hand. I look down at it as my fingers try to heal the spectacular folds my mother has created, and read:

All Nurses and Nurses' Aides
Please Plan to Come.

Inservice
June 28, 1994
HOSPICE
Comfort-Oriented Care for the Dying
7:00 A.M.
2:00 P.M.
3:00 P.M.

Although I know I cannot attend any of these sessions—my world is on the other side of the nurse's station—I also know that this announcement was somehow meant for me.

7

Carolyn comes in at 3:00 P.M. She seldom arrives without something for the unit. A small box of her discarded books, flowered blouses frayed at the sleeves or collar, records from the '50s, a huge blossom of one sort or another from her garden of perennials.

When Carolyn takes a break, you'll find her reading in the lounge, enjoying a cup of coffee. She reads the works of the good writers.

Carolyn loves the difficult evening hours right after supper best. She will gather people around her by the record player and the bookshelves. Sometimes she'll read to them from children's books. Or she'll tell them a story that she told her own children years before.

She knows exactly what popular songs residents loved when they were young, and she plays them on the turntable. "Remember that, Fannie?" she'll ask with excitement. Occasionally a word from a familiar refrain, always from the refrain, is recovered by a resident. One person listens to a collection of Gershwin songs and yells, "'S won-der-ful!" The person next to her surprises herself by chiming in "'S mar-ve-lous!" Carolyn cries "Good!" and sings the whole line: "'S won-der-ful! —'S mar-vel-ous!—You should care—for me!"

But the good cheer soon fades. The residents lose interest. They grow restless and begin to rub foreheads and become angry for no reason other than a missed beat in their brains, for no reason other than the sun is going down. Carolyn reads the cues quickly, glides to the nurse's closet, locates a small black case, and returns to her stage.

Some residents recognize the case and become still. They smile and hold each other's hands. A few who remember applaud. They look at the long case and the two shiny locks on its edge.

Carolyn snaps the locks open and removes the pieces of a silver flute. She assembles it, wets her lips, and trills.

8

Al works the evening shift. He arrives at Tanglewood around 3:00 P.M. and stays to 11:00 P.M. Al loves sports, especially baseball. He walks with a mild limp, and smiles easily. He takes care of the men in the unit, lifting them, carrying them to restrooms and beds and dinner tables. He sets the tables himself sometimes, helps change the linen on the beds and the towels in the bathrooms. He tightens Benny's bowling suspenders and zips up pants. He is a strong man.

"Are you OK, Mr. Miller?" you'll hear him say. And you'll see him sit among the men and talk or laugh, or be silent with them, as they choose.

He asks Stanley who will win the game on Saturday. He flips a rubber baseball in his right hand. His language is as simple as the language the residents speak.

Sometimes, before dinner, music is played to a circle of listeners, the way it was when my mother's seizure occurred. Al becomes a prince. He makes women forget they cannot walk. They throw their canes into a heap. He magically lifts ancient bodies formerly soldered to wheelchairs into his arms and ballroom dances to the music on the record player.

Color comes into the cheeks of the women for just a minute. Someone hits a balloon into the air. A toast is made with pineapple juice in pill cups.

The music winds to an end and the needle scratches its finale. The women move more slowly once again and begin their search through a pile of walkers and canes for something to hold them up.

9

On July 30, 1988, my parents visited me in Boone, North Carolina. I was there for a month-long seminar. We had difficulty locating a restaurant close by, so we traveled to Blowing Rock up the road and entered the Green Park Inn. It seemed like a mistake at first. The prices were high and the whole idea of the place different from what my family was used to. Clearly this was a spot for rich people from the Piedmont. The women were manicured and jeweled; the men, right out of Fitzgerald novels, were dressed in cool linen suits. They came to hold one another and to dance to the live big band music paid for by the restaurant's high prices.

But soon all of that moved to the background. Things shifted when I heard my father ask Annabelle to dance.

It was now the summer of their fifty-second wedding anniversary. She was not even sure where she was when my father extended his hand to her in the Green Park Inn. Before we had gone to dinner, she had proudly shown me around her motel room and talked about her "new house." We had examined gleaming tile, closets, Kleenex dispensers, velvet paintings in red and black, and bed quilts with wide bars of color. When she left the motel, she grew frightened, and absolutely still.

"Will you dance with me, Annabelle?" he asked, lifting her from her chair, his great buck teeth lighting the way through the dark, like headlights.

She looked alarmed, but trusted him, knowing she had no strength but his. They walked arm in arm to the dance floor. He stood erect, remembering other days. My mother softly placed her hand in his and rested her arm across the collar of his cheap white shirt.

He pumped his arms up and down as the music began, and exaggerated his steps like a mechanical monkey to help my mother follow. But it was too difficult for her. Once a graceful dancer, my mother no longer could keep her feet from becoming tangled and she started to pull away. Her body did not remember enough anymore. It remembered something, but not enough for the Green Park Inn.

Without pausing, my father leaned over and bent softly to the ground. He lifted my mother's right foot and placed it on top his left. Then as he stood, he raised her body gently until her left foot rested on his other shoe. They danced for over an hour like that. He carried her on his feet, carried her full weight, carried her like a swan carries a cygnet on its back.

They danced to "Alice Blue Gown." I could hear my father humming loudly off key whenever the sound of the band dimmed. I unconsciously began to mouth the words of the refrain, words as common in our house as "The Lord's Prayer" and "The Star-Spangled Banner." Words you saluted, or stood at attention for. "Till it wilt-ed I wore it, I'll al-ways a-dore it, My sweet lit-tle A-lice blue gown."

They danced as they had danced at Summit Beach Park and the East Market Center when they were young. They danced with eyes closed, my father helping his wife remember the fun of being young, the inevitable connection between a saxophone and your feet, the feel of warm bodies close together. Once I saw him whisper in one of her deaf ears. Across the room, I may have heard her laugh.

10

Esther brings some apple juice to the woman in green. She strokes Gloria's henna hair and buttons the cuffs of her blouse. Esther yawns leisurely and turns. "You're lovely," Gloria shouts in Esther's direction. "Keep it that *way*. I don't mean north and south. I mean the way you are."

11

Maggy works in the nursing wing but sometimes substitutes in Tanglewood. "I watch your mother in the patio out the window of my wing," she tells me as she coaxes Annabelle to take her medicines, buried in applesauce and frozen yogurt. "She picks in the soil, rips up weeds and things. Did she have a garden?"

"A small garden," I say. "She was wonderful, really."

"Still is," Maggy corrects me.

A young aide chimes in. "Annabelle was mad at me yesterday, weren't you, Annabelle?" The aide throws her lower lip into a pout and my mother laughs and pats the girl's face with her hand. "She took her supper outside and I made her come in. She was getting red as a beet and I worried she'd faint. She's my favorite person in the unit because she's so feisty." I suddenly remember the first day we admitted my mother. She pretended to know all the people who warmly greeted her. But after she realized that something was wrong, she ran to the patio and tried to throw herself over the fence, bloodying her arms and legs.

The aide seems to be dreaming, just as I am. "She's so spunky," she continues, talking more to herself than anyone else. "I can see myself being like her when I'm old. I'd *like* to be like her." I feel as if this young aide and I have secretly formed a pact, pricked our fingers together and become blood sisters for the remainder of our lives.

"She had me late in life," I tell Maggy, just making conversation after the young aide drifts dreamlike toward another resident. "Doctors told her that with one ovary there would be little chance of children. It was a myth, of course, but she believed it and it almost came true. At nearly forty, there I was."

"Then you're a miracle!"

"Yes," I reply. "I guess I'm a miracle."

12

Jackie pulls a chair beside us. "She's doing fine," she whispers. "I know it's not easy. But you calm her."

I feel the hot tears swell in my eyes and look away. I can't even thank her for saying this. Jackie sits with us, in the hurry of the middle of her afternoon. She sits and sits, as if she's invited us both to her home for lemonade in the summer when there's nothing else to do.

"Your mother has so much energy. What did she do when she was young?" Jackie asks.

And I tell her the story of my mother, who was different from other women, different without even knowing it, without my even knowing it then.

"I can see that in her even now," she says when I finish. "I can see it all. Deep down is a spirit that's still her. She's the same really, isn't she?"

Jackie leaves us, quietly moving to the cart to distribute medications. I feel my hands begin to shake.

I look at my mother. She's staring at the birds in the small cage across the room. Her rocker soothes her and her eyes close to slits. I take my thumb and trace her cheekbone. I rub the skin and watch it become young in my hands. The lines vanish, then reappear. Vanish, then reappear.

I remember being her young daughter, rubbing the rouge into her cheeks this way. She taught me how to find the bone and trace it. And then she placed the color on my finger and let me smooth it in. I could have stared at her forever. I still could.

My thumb moves softly from front to back, again and again. I watch the lines return and disappear. They will someday be the lines that already have begun to form across my own face.

I close my eyes. My mother's lines vanish altogether and all I feel is silk.

Two Poems

EUGENE HIRSCH

I HOLD YOUR HANDS:
RAVAGES OF ALZHEIMER'S DISEASE

I hold your hands in mine.
You wince and stretch back,
bewildered, into childhood.
In that instant,
from the middle of my eye,
I see you oh so quickly
growing more and more alone.
You pole the canals of Venice,
logged by their water
that creeps
through your mortar,
your lath, the trenchant
paths inside your eyes.
Do you remember my name?

The portrait of one
who loves you soars
above the rotunda,
fending off foreign
charms and spells that drop
through your brittle shell
to prey upon your mind.
And now, in a moment,
from the middle of yourself,
you no longer speak.

I hold your face in mine.
But you leap aghast,

your ins and outs
urging you to turn,
to make of me the beast
that haunts you
as the suns sets red
behind the silhouette
of the last chimney,
revealing the deep night
and its walkabout,
down the stairs and into
imaginary streets,
wet with the rain
of a million tears.

For you are king
of distant whims.
While I sleep
my dreaming
fusion flights,
the cherry-box
inside your breath
sings secrets
from the sweetness
of our forgotten past.

In Search

I find my way in search,
in darkened rooms

laced by windows, or
where the windows

ought to be, or
used to be, or

where canvas sea oats
simulate outdoors

in place of portals, or
where they ought to be, or

where a poem or a sonata
finds an abandoned street,

footsteps climbing, clamor
sounding the stairs,

to track me
where I ought to be, or
where my flagellant images

drive me, or
where I have driven my mind

into caves and blow holes,
hidden madness wandering

through relics, or
through the foggy bottom at dawn,

churning round to spin,
spiraling to win,

only to spin
where I have been before, or

ought to have been,
or wished to have been, or,

never having tasted of the being,
just touching myself tonight

among sounds of the salt-froth
sea, muffled in the distance.

A Wonderland Party

JEAN WOOD

I was the white rabbit,
And she was Alice, I'd say.

We took our two mad hatters
To a restaurant dinner,
Valentine's Day.

Fragments, phrases . . . her husband
Made no more sense than mine.
I listened to him—
A new nonsense,
In no way taxing.

And she listened to mine.
How curiously relaxing!
Let's have some wine!

We made up their minds and ordered.
My husband showed the waiter his tie
With tennis racket print three times.

We spread their bread,
And cut their meat,
And sugared their tea,
Then paused to eat.
Camaraderie!

She and I,
With one great thing in common,
Talked of everything else.

We learned about one another.

And each other's
Husbands . . . then, and when.

Needs diminished . . .
We nearly finished
A carafe!
How good to laugh!

We'll do it again!

Notes on Contributors

CONRAD AIKEN (1889–1973). Born in Savannah, Georgia and educated at Harvard University, Conrad Aiken became a poet and novelist. He is noted for his *Selected Poems* (1930), which won the Pulitzer Prize and his *Collected Poems*, which won the 1954 National Book Award. "Silent Snow, Secret Snow" is one of his most notable short stories.

PHILIP BOOTH (1925–) has won critical acclaim for his poetry's simplicity and power. Often anthologized, his poem "Panic" can be found in his book *First Available Light* (1976). His other books include *The Islanders* (1961), *Beyond Our Fears* (1967), and *Margins* (1970). He currently teaches at Syracuse University and often uses the Northeast seacoast as a setting for his poetry.

JOHN G. BRADLEY, M.D. practices medicine in Decatur, Illinois, and is on the faculty at Southern Illinois University School of Medicine.

HALE CHATFIELD (1936–). Educated at Wesleyan and Rutgers Universities, Hale Chatfield resides in Huntsburg, Ohio, and teaches English and Writing at Hiram College. He is the founder and editor of the *Hiram Poetry Review*, and his books include *The Young Country and Other Poems* (1959), *At Home* (1971), and *Water Colors* (1977).

PHILLIP V. DAVIS teaches in the Department of Medical Humanities at Southern Illinois University School of Medicine.

ROBERT DAVIS was a Christian pastor in Miami, Florida, until Alzheimer's Disease interrupted his ministry. He chronicled the course of his disease with the help of his wife, Betty. This is one of the few first-person accounts of the experience of an Alzheimer's patient.

EMILY DICKINSON (1830–1886). A quiet author whose life of seclusion led to more than a thousand poems, Emily Dickinson has become a nearly mythical figure to millions. Her poetry is known for its idiosyncratic punctuation and its resemblance to church hymns. Dickinson died from Bright's disease in the same house in which she was born; she published only seven poems in her entire lifetime.

JOYCE DYER (1947–). The Director of Writing and an Associate Professor at Hiram College, Joyce Dyer attended Wittenberg University and attained her Ph.D. at Kent State University. Her publications include *The Awakening: A Novel of Beginnings* (1993) and *In a Tangled Wood* (1996).

RALPH ELLISON (1914–1994). Born in Oklahoma City, Ralph Ellison is noted for not only his short stories and essays, but his scriptwriting as well. A trumpeter, Ellison studied music in Harlem, where he met Langston Hughes and Richard Wright, who encouraged him to write fiction. His other writings include the short story "Battle Royal" (1947) and scripts for television shows including the *Alfred Hitchcock Hour* and *Star Trek*.

LAURA ESQUIVEL (1957–). Mexican novelist and screenwriter Laura Esquivel makes her home in Mexico City. She is most noted for her 1989 screenplay and novel *Like Water for Chocolate*. She has worked as a teacher and a writer/director for a children's theater. Her other screenplays include *Chido One* (1985) and *Little Ocean Star* (1994).

SETH FARBER, who often appears on radio and TV, is a practicing counselor in New York City. Dr. Farber is active in the Network Against Coercive Psychiatry.

WILLIAM FAULKNER (1897–1962) received the Nobel Prize for Literature in 1950. Though he served in the Royal Canadian Air Force in WWI, he never saw overseas service. He wrote nearly one hundred short stories, one of which is his famous "A Rose for Emily." His many novels include: *As I Lay Dying* (1930), *Light in August* (1932), and *The Hamlet* (1940).

JANET FRAME (1924–), a New Zealand author, is known for her complex and disturbing novels. She won the 1989 New Zealand Book Award for her novel *The Carpathians*. Some of her other works are *Owls Do Cry* (1957), *Living in Maniototo* (1979), and *Envoy from Mirror City* (1985). She also published a book of poetry entitled *The Pocket Mirror* (1967).

CHARLOTTE PERKINS GILMAN (1860–1935). A lecturer and author of books on women's rights and socialism, Charlotte Perkins Gilman was noted for her book *Women and Economics* (1899). However, she became most famous for her often-anthologized short story, "The Yellow Wallpaper," which was inspired by her own nervous breakdown and subsequent treatment by the famous Dr. S. Weir Mitchell.

STEPHEN JAY GOULD (1941–) is a geology professor, paleontologist, and philosopher of science. He attained his Ph.D. at Columbia and has taught at Harvard since 1967. As an author, he has contributed more than one hundred articles to scientific journals. Among his other writings are *The Mismeasure of Man* (1981) and *Eight Little Piggies: Reflections in Natural History* (1993).

GRAHAM GREENE (1904–1991). A noted English novelist and essayist, Graham Greene's writings often dealt with major spiritual issues. The son of a headmaster, he was educated at the University of Oxford and worked for the London Times. His many novels include *The Man Within* (1929), *Rumour at Nightfall* (1931), and *The Ministry of Fear* (1943).

IAN HACKING (1936–). Originally from Vancouver, Canada, Ian Hacking teaches at many different universities. His many interests include the philosophy of science, the philosophy of language, the philosophy of mathematics, and philosophical questions about pathology. His many books include *The Logic of Statistical Inference* (1965) and a *Concise Introduction to Logic* (1971).

JOY HARJO (1951–), a Creek Indian, was born in Tulsa, Oklahoma. Her poetry mirrors the rhythm of her native language and often relates her struggle to avoid assimilation into the dominant culture. She now teaches at the University of Colorado, Boulder. Her many books include *She Had Some Horses* (1997) and *In Mad Love and War* (1990).

SEAMUS HEANEY (1939–) was awarded the 1995 Nobel Prize for poetry. Originally from Northern Ireland, he now resides in both Dublin and in America. He teaches at Harvard University, and his many books include *Station Island* (1985), *The Haw Lantern* (1987), and *The Spirit Level* (1996).

LINDA HOGAN (1947–), poet, novelist, playwright, and screenwriter, teaches English at the University of Colorado, Boulder. She is a member of the Chickasaw tribe and writes about the global community and Native American culture. She has authored several collections of poetry, including *Calling Myself Home* (1979), *Savings* (1988), and *Book of Medicines* (1993).

KIM HOPPER is a medical anthropologist who works as a research scientist at the Nathan S. Kline Institute for Psychiatric Research. He has conducted ethnographic and historical research on homelessness in New York City and is the cofounder of the National Coalition for the Homeless. In addition, he is a contributor to *Homeless in America*.

SUSANNA KAYSEN, whose memoir about her mental illness and two-year experience in a psychiatric hospital is excerpted here, is the author of three novels. She lives in Cambridge, Massachusetts.

MAXINE HONG KINGSTON (1940–). The daughter of Chinese immigrants, Kingston combines autobiography and fiction to portray memories of Chinese American life and fantasies of Chinese history and culture. She now teaches at the University of California, Berkeley. Her books include *Woman Warrior* (1976) and *Tripmaster Monkey: His Fake Book* (1989).

TOMASSO LANDOLFI (1908–) was born in Pico, Italy, where he still lives. He has published novels, translations, and a collection of short stories.

CAROL LEVINE has been editor of the *Hastings Center Report,* executive director of the Citizens Commission on AIDS, and editor of *Taking Sides: Clashing Views on Controversial Bioethical Issues,* which has gone through several editions.

TONI MORRISON (1931–). A Pulitzer (1988) and Nobel Prize (1993) winner, Toni Morrison has been praised for her lyrical language and her inventive and original plots. Her novels—among them, *The Bluest Eye* (1970), *Sula* (1973), and *Beloved* (1987)—often include fantastic and mystical events.

PETER NICHOLS (1927–), author of such award-winning plays as *Joe Egg* (1967) and *The National Health* (1969), also writes movie scripts ("Georgie Girl") and plays for television.

FLANNERY O' CONNOR (1925–1964) spent most of her life in her hometown of Milledgeville, Georgia. Like her father, she was stricken with lupus erythematosus, from which she eventually died. Her two novels are *Wise Blood* (1952) and *The Violent Bear it Away* (1960). However, she was probably best known for her short stories, in which she utilized both the grotesque and her Roman Catholic background.

WILFRED OWEN (1893–1918) was a native of Shropshire, England, and attended London University. During WWI he became a company commander in the British army. He was hospitalized for shell-shock after the Battle of Somme and was killed in action after returning to the front. Owen's antiwar poems made him a voice of pacifism.

TIM O' BRIEN (1946–) served in the Vietnam War and has written about it frequently. His third book, *Going After Cacciato* (1978), won the National Book Award in 1979.

EDGAR ALLEN POE (1809–1849) was an orphan of traveling actors and was raised by well-off foster parents. He published his first book of poems at age eighteen. As a poet and writer of stories, he is remembered for his macabre and haunting writings such as "Murders in the Rue Morgue," "The Purloined Letter," and "The Raven."

RAINER MARIA RILKE (1875–1926) was an Austro-German poet and novelist. Influenced by the French symbolists, Rilke tried to eliminate vague lyricism from his poetry. His writings include *Life and Song* (1894), *Stories of God* (1900), and *The Book of Pictures* (1902).

ANNE SEXTON (1928–1974) suffered her first mental breakdown just before the death of her first child. After her second breakdown, her psychiatrist encouraged her to write poetry. In this poetry, she wrote not only of her breakdowns, but the problems she faced as a woman.

PETER SHAFFER (1926–), English playwright of such award-winning plays as *Amadeus* and *Royal Hunt of the Sun,* also won the Tony Award for Best Play for *Equus.* He lives and works in London.

LESLIE MARMON SILKO (1948–) was born on a Laguna Pueblo Indian Reservation. She studied at the University of Mexico, and her writing explores the conflict between Native American values and the values of the dominant culture. *Storyteller* (1981), *Almanac of the Dead* (1991), and *Yellow Woman* (1993) are among her many novels.

JOHN STEINBECK (1902–1968) was born in Salinas, California. He worked as a reporter in New York and also filed dispatches from battle fronts in Italy and Africa during WWII. He is famous for classics such as *The Grapes of Wrath* (1939), *The Winter of Our Discontent* (1961), and *East of Eden* (1952). He was known for his sympathy towards the downtrodden, and he won the Nobel Prize for Literature in 1962.

ANNE TYLER (1941–), American novelist educated in the south, has several award-winning novels to her credit, including *Dinner at the Homesick Restaurant* (1982), *The Accidental Tourist* (1985), and *Breathing Lessons* (1988).

EUDORA WELTY (1909–) is known for her engaging female characters and her sympathy for the distorted and deformed. Her numerous short stories—such as "Why I Live at the P. O." (1941), "A Worn Path" (1941), and "The Bride of Innisfallen" (1955)—have captured generations of readers. She was born and raised in Jackson, Mississippi, and its impact can be seen in the Southern influence in her writing.

JEAN WOOD lives and writes in Sanibel, Florida.

VIRGINIA WOOLF (1882–1941) was a major influence on English literature. A powerful writer, she succeeded as an essayist, novelist and critic. Though plagued by nervous breakdowns, she wrote some of the most thought-provoking pieces of her time. These writings include: *To the Lighthouse* (1927), *A Room of One's Own* (1929), and *The Waves* (1931).

IRVIN D. YALOM is the author of the novel *When Nietzsche Wept*. He also wrote *Lying on the Couch* (1996) and several basic textbooks including *Theory and Practice of Group Psychotherapy* and *Existential Psychotherapy*. Currently he is Professor Emeritus of Psychiatry at the Stanford University School of Medicine and the general editor of *Treating the Elderly*.

Permissions Acknowledgments

Index

What's Normal?

was designed by Will Underwood;

composed in 10½-point Adobe Minion on an Apple

Quadra system using QuarkXPress by The Book Bage, Inc.;

printed by sheet-fed offset lithography on 50-pound

Turin Book Natural Vellum stock (an acid-free,

totally chlorine-free paper), notch bound

in signatures with paper covers printed in

two colors coated with polypropylene matte

film lamination by Thomson-Shore,

Inc.; and published by

The Kent State University Press

KENT, OHIO 44242